A [illegible]
PUB[illegible]C HEALTH

A Short Book of
PUBLIC HEALTH

Second Edition

VK Muthu

MBBS DPH MSc (Applied Nutrition)

Formerly

Faculty of Rural Health and Sanitation

Gandhigram Rural Institute, Gandhigram

Dindigul District-624302

Tamil Nadu, India

JAYPEE

JAYPEE BROTHERS MEDICAL PUBLISHERS (P) LTD

New Delhi • London • Philadelphia • Panama

Jaypee Brothers Medical Publishers (P) Ltd

Headquarters

Jaypee Brothers Medical Publishers (P) Ltd
4838/24, Ansari Road, Daryaganj
New Delhi 110 002, India
Phone: +91-11-43574357
Fax: +91-11-43574314
Email: jaypee@jaypeebrothers.com

Overseas Offices

J.P. Medical Ltd
83 Victoria Street, London
SW1H 0HW (UK)
Phone: +44-2031708910
Fax: +02-03-0086180
Email: info@jpmedpub.com

Jaypee-Highlights Medical Publishers Inc
City of Knowledge, Bld. 237, Clayton
Panama City, Panama
Phone: +1 507-301-0496
Fax: +1 507-301-0499
Email: cservice@jphmedical.com

Jaypee Medical Inc
The Bourse
111 South Independence Mall East
Suite 835, Philadelphia, PA 19106, USA
Phone: +1 267-519-9789
Email: joe.rusko@jaypeebrothers.com

Jaypee Brothers Medical Publishers (P) Ltd
17/1-B Babar Road, Block-B, Shaymali
Mohammadpur, Dhaka-1207
Bangladesh
Mobile: +08801912003485
Email: jaypeedhaka@gmail.com

Jaypee Brothers Medical Publishers (P) Ltd
Bhotahity, Kathmandu, Nepal
Phone: +977-9741283608
Email: kathmandu@jaypeebrothers.com

Website: www.jaypeebrothers.com
Website: www.jaypeedigital.com

Inquiries for bulk sales may be solicited at: jaypee@jaypeebrothers.com

A Short Book of Public Health

First Edition: 2005
Reprint: 2006, 2008
Second Edition: ***2014***

ISBN 978-93-5152-228-7
Printed at

Dedicated to

The memory of my beloved parents

Preface to the Second Edition

I am happy that the second edition of the title *'A Short Book of Public Health'* is being brought out by the publisher. The book has been revised completely incorporating up-to-date information on public health to cater the needs of students of public health as well as health professionals. The contents of the book have been organized into 10 sections, which in turn have been divided into 33 chapters. Chapter 1 contains new topics such as 'Disease elimination and eradication strategies' and 'Drug resistance'. In Chapter 2, 'Immunity and Immunizing agents' are described. Many communicable diseases, which did not find place in the first edition, have now been incorporated in this edition. A new section 'Environment and Health' has been added. The section 'Healthcare System in India' has been completely revised. National Health Policy 2002 and National Rural Health Mission (2005-2012) are newly incorporated topics.

VK Muthu

Preface to the First Edition

This book is an attempt to bring out a smaller volume on public health specially to cater the needs of students and public health personnel like sanitary inspectors, nurses and doctors. It may be useful to others, as well as a guide to refer to. My 19 years of teaching of public health has made me quite aware of the need for such a book.

I have used the usual format adopted by textbooks of Social and Preventive Medicine. The language used will be easy to understand and enhance the clarity of the principles and concepts. Only the minimum needed to understand the subject has been incorporated in this book.

The contents have been organized into 9 chapters. Chapter 1 discusses strategies for providing health care, concepts in preventing diseases, etc. Chapter 2 deals with epidemiology of communicable diseases. Chapter 3 deals with non-communicable diseases. Demography, family planning, and maternal and child health are discussed in Chapter 4. Chapter 5 deals with nutrition and Chapter 6 describes school health service and principles of health education. Chapter 7 deals with occupational health. Health systems and healthcare programs in India are dealt with in Chapter 8. Chapter 9 covers topics like basic statistics in health care, disinfection procedures, vector control methods, immunization schedule, etc.

VK Muthu

Acknowledgments

The book has been compiled from various sources. I wish to express my sincere thanks for all those sources. I also wish to express my gratitude to M Sankarapandian for his help in the compilation of the topic 'Basic Statistics in Health Care'.

I also thank Shri Jitendar P Vij (Group Chairman), Mr Ankit Vij (Managing Director) and Mr Tarun Duneja (Director-Publishing) of M/s Jaypee Brothers Medical Publishers (P) Ltd, New Delhi and Bengaluru Branch.

Contents

Section 1: Introduction

Section 2: Epidemiology of Communicable Diseases

Part A: Principles of Control and Prevention

Part B: Specific Infections

Section 3: Non-communicable Diseases

Section 4: Demography and Family Welfare

Section 5: Nutrition

Section 6: Health Education and School Health Service

Section 7: Environment and Health

Section 8: Healthcare System in India

Section 9: Health Care in India: Vision and Mission

Section 10: Epidemiology and Biostatistics

SECTION

1

Introduction

CHAPTER

1

Concepts in Health Care

❑ EVOLUTION OF MEDICINE AND PUBLIC HEALTH

Medicine has developed from primitive method of treating ailments to the present scientific form. During the industrial revolution, there arose the necessity to think in terms of public health. The idea of public health was mooted to protect the public from illnesses brought about by the pollution caused by industries and the insanitation caused by overcrowding in industrial slums. Public health, as defined by World Health Organization (WHO) expert committee, is the science and art of preventing disease, prolonging life and promoting health and efficiency through organized community, efforts for the sanitation of environment, the control of communicable infections, the education of the individual in personal hygiene, the organization of medical and nursing services for early diagnosis and preventive treatment of diseases and the development of social machinery to ensure for every individual a standard of living adequate for the maintenance of health. So organizing these benefits as to enable every citizen to realize his birth right of health and longevity. This definition is based on the definition of CEA Winslow, a former Professor of public health at Yale University. Public health is a universally recognized concept. But, while applying the principles of public health, societies and nations are found lacking in initiative.

Hygiene is defined as the science of health; the science dealing with the establishment and maintenance of health in the individual and the group. It embraces all factors, which contribute to healthful living. The word hygiene is derived from Hygeia, the

Goddess of Health in Greek mythology. Preventive medicine now means promotion of health and prevention of illness, and is used as a synonymous term with public health.

Community health has replaced the terms public health, preventive medicine and social medicine in some countries.

Social medicine, by derivation, is the study of man as a social being in his total environment. It is concerned with all the factors affecting the distribution of health and ill health in population including the use of health services. It is not a new branch of medicine, but rather an extension of public health idea. The term now is displaced by the term community medicine.

Community medicine is the new term now used to denote what were previously known as public health, preventive medicine, social medicine and community health.

Curative medicine, also known as clinical medicine, which is involved in the treatment of patients, is found to work as an independent and separate health activity instead of functioning as an important component of public health. The phenomenal growth of curative medicine into specialties and superspecialties has affected the very delivery of health care in a coherent and holistic way. Medicine has become too costly to be available to the most needy, since it is practiced in a commercial fashion. The corporate hospitals show more interest in specializations like heart or kidney transplant that fetch huge money rather than involving themselves in the provision of primary health care to the masses. Only government institutions cater to the poor that also badly falling short of the requirements. It is found that tertiary care consumes most of the healthcare budget, while primary health care and health promotion get only step-motherly treatment.

A civilized society should make medical and health care available to all based on need and not on paying capacity. But unfortunately, in the present world plagued by materialistic culture, medicine has been hijacked by the money-minded to function on commercial lines. The concept of socialized medicine, which makes free medical care available for all, is observed only in socialist and communist countries.

Public health, as a separate discipline, has vastly widened its scope. Now it has within its ambit, all aspects of human activity that affect health. The definition of WHO that 'health is a state of complete physical, mental and social well-being, and not merely the absence of disease or infirmity', amply illustrates this fact and gives a clear signal that public health needs the cooperation of all disciplines involved in human development and cannot be promoted by the health sector alone.

It has to be understood that the dearth of knowledge is not responsible for the ill health prevalent in most communities. It is the social problems that contribute to the high prevalence of morbidity by coming in the way of the practice of public health and the use of the available scientific knowledge to prevent diseases and promote health. This fact has been clearly spelt out in the Alma-Ata declaration, which delineates equitable distribution, appropriate technology, intersectoral coordination and community participation as cardinal principles to provide primary health care to all.

❑ HEALTH FOR ALL AND PRIMARY HEALTH CARE

In the modern world, providing health care to all has become the responsibility of the state. Civilized societies should be able to provide health care based on one's need and not on his/her paying capacity. World societies are continuously trying to improve the health of the constituent members. But it can be easily said that the world is nowhere near the ideal system of providing health care to all. The WHO, as a global agency for health promotion, is also formulating healthcare strategies to be implemented in member countries. Taking note of the inequitable distribution of health services between the urban and the rural, and between the rich and the poor, UNICEF and WHO jointly came out with a health policy to provide basic health services to all. In 1977, WHO health assembly resolved to launch a movement called Health for All by 2000 AD and fixed ambitious targets for promotion of health to be achieved in stages. Providing right kind of food for all by 1985, essential drugs by 1986 and basic sanitation, safe water and immunization against six infectious diseases by 1990 were some of the targets fixed besides many others. The joint WHO-UNICEF conference held at Alma Ata in Russia in the year 1978 endorsed the WHO concept of Health for All by 2000 AD and suggested a new approach called primary health care to provide health for all.

Primary health care is defined as "essential health care made universally accessible to individuals and acceptable to them, through their full participation and at a cost the community and the country can afford." Primary healthcare concept was evolved based on four principles namely:

1. Equitable distribution (of healthcare facilities).
2. Community participation.
3. Multisectoral approach.
4. Appropriate technology.

Aims of primary health care are the following:

1. Promotion of food supplies and nutrition.
2. Providing health education about health problems and their control.
3. Provision of safe water supply and sanitation.
4. Promotion of maternal and child health, and family planning.
5. Providing immunization against infectious diseases.
6. Prevention and control of locally endemic diseases.
7. Treatment of common diseases and injuries.
8. Provision of essential drugs.

'Health for All by 2000 AD' movement was not as successful as anticipated and many of the targets fixed could not be achieved. The failure was primarily due to the kind of social conditions that existed in the nations, particularly the developing countries. Community participation, which is of paramount importance in the implementation of healthcare programs, was conspicuous by its absence. It is not surprising because community participation cannot be enlisted in any community, which is plagued by communalism, casteism, regionalism, political rivalry and the like. Unless social harmony is ensured through mass movements, community participation will only be a mirage.

Here it is pertinent to observe that simply changing strategies, with new and attractive names (first comprehensive health care; now primary health care) without attacking the basic social issues that come in the way of implementation of programs, cannot bring about tangible results commensurate with the amount and energy spent on such programs.

❑ CAUSATION OF DISEASES

Disease affects man when he is exposed to harmful influences in his environment. The interaction between man, his environment and agent factors decides the genesis of pathological process. These three aspects, viz. agent, host and environment form that is called the epidemiological triad (Fig. 1.1).

Occurrence of infectious diseases either as a single case or as an epidemic and their distribution in the community is decided by the agent-host-environment interaction. This agent-host-environment model of disease causation has helped in the understanding of many diseases, especially the communicable diseases. But in the case of chronic diseases (e.g. coronary heart disease, cancer, hypertension, diabetes, etc.) this model is not able to explain the pathogenesis adequately.

The agents known to cause diseases in man are:

1. Biological agents, e.g. bacteria, fungi, virus, protozoa, etc.
2. Nutritional factors, e.g. either deficiency or excess of nutrients like vitamins, minerals, fat, etc.
3. Physical agents, e.g. excessive heat and cold, humidity, atmospheric pressure, radiation, sound, etc.
4. Chemical agents, e.g. gases, heavy metals, insecticides, carcinogens, etc.
5. Mechanical factors, e.g. friction, crushing injuries, fractures, etc.
6. Endogenous factors, e.g. excess or deficiency of hormones, deficiency of immunoglobulins and chromosomal abnormality.

Lifestyle practices like dietary habits, smoking, alcoholism and some behavioral patterns are the host factors that are involved in causing diseases in man.

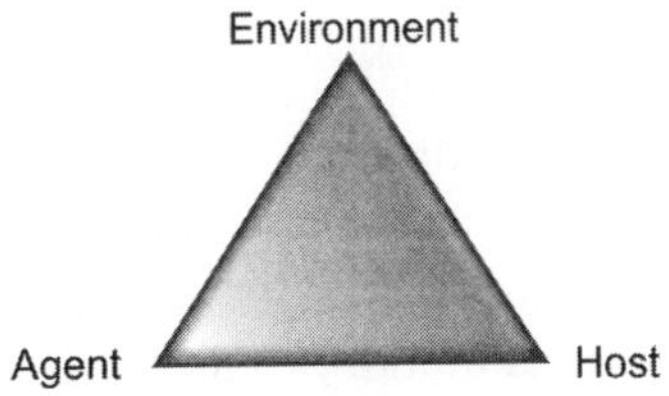

Figure 1.1: Epidemiological triad

The environment in which man lives is also an important

determinant of disease in man. All living and non-living things with which man is in constant interaction form his environment. Air, water, food, industrial and housing conditions are the main physical factors that affect man's health. Besides the physical environment, man is also exposed to biological environment composed of bacteria, viruses, plants, rodents, insects and animals, which may cause diseases. Psychosocial environment is another, which may make man vulnerable to diseases. Family and social climate, poverty, urbanization, migration to new environments, cultural and traditional habits, and customs all are capable of affecting man's health.

The fact, which is now well recognized in respect of diseases in man, is that diseases have multifactorial causes as single cause theory of diseases proposed earlier is unable to explain the pathogenesis of many diseases affecting man.

❑ CONCEPTS IN PREVENTION OF DISEASES

Public health is the science and art of preventing diseases, prolonging life and promoting health by community efforts. This can be accomplished by improving environmental sanitation, providing health education and curative services, and by improving the standard of life so as to enable every citizen to realize his/her birthright of health and longevity.

The term community medicine is now used almost as a synonym for what was previously known as public health, preventive medicine, social medicine and community health.

From the definition, it is clear that prevention of diseases is one of the important goals of public health. Three levels of preventive strategies are described and they are primary, secondary and tertiary prevention. Primary prevention aims to prevent the diseases from occurring at the first instance, while the aim of secondary and tertiary preventions is to limit the severity and/or the spread of diseases by proper treatment and rehabilitation.

In primary prevention, factors known to cause diseases are removed so that diseases will not occur. Health promotion (good food, sanitation, clean environment, healthy lifestyles, etc.) and specific protection (immunization, supplementation with specific nutrients, etc.) constitute primary prevention.

Early diagnosis and treatment is the aim of secondary prevention given with a view to prevent the diseases from becoming serious and to prevent the development of secondary cases in the community. This comes under the purview of clinical medicine. Tuberculosis and leprosy are the two communicable diseases for which early diagnosis and treatment are imperative to prevent their spread to susceptible contacts.

The aim of tertiary prevention is prevention of potential consequences of diseases. Disability limitation and rehabilitation constitute tertiary prevention. Instituting appropriate treatment early will prevent further complications. For example, in leprosy, proper treatment will prevent complications like clawing of hand, and loss of fingers and toes. The objectives of rehabilitation are:

1. To restore function (e.g. correction surgery in leprosy) by medical and surgical procedures (medical rehabilitation).
2. To train vocationally so that the individual can earn his/her livelihood (vocational rehabilitation).
3. To integrate socially with the family and the society (social rehabilitation).
4. To instill self-confidence (psychological rehabilitation).

❑ DETERMINANTS OF HEALTH

World Health Organization defines health as a state of complete physical, mental and social well-being, and not merely the absence of disease or infirmity. The definition clearly indicates that health is multidimensional. Therefore, many factors are involved in determining health. They are:

1. Genetic factors, environment (physical, biological and psychological).
2. Lifestyles (smoking, drug abuse, personal hygiene, food habits, etc.).
3. Poverty as well as affluence.
4. Healthcare facilities available.

It therefore implies that prevention of diseases and promotion of health, require a multipronged attack and health sector alone cannot do that.

Among the various determinants of health, the most amenable for modification is the physical environment. Providing a conducive physical environment (protected water, sanitary conveniences, clean environment, good food, etc.) involves a lot of spending and therefore, it is often said that 'public health is purchasable'. Many underdeveloped countries are unable to spare enough funds for improving environmental sanitation. At the same time it has to be understood that creating facilities like water supply and sanitation by spending huge amount alone cannot improve health. Awareness on the importance of healthy lifestyles must be created among people simultaneously. Only then healthcare programs will become successful leading to perceptible change in the level of health.

❑ DIMENSIONS OF HEALTH

'Health is a state of complete physical, mental and social well-being and not merely the absence of disease or infirmity' is the definition of health by WHO. From the definition, it is evident that health has three dimensions namely physical, mental and social. It is important to realize here that social well-being is not only just one of the dimensions of health but also a quintessential one. Social well-being has been defined as the quantity and quality of an individual's interpersonal ties and the extent of involvement with the community. A good social environment should make every individual feel that he/she has contributed or can contribute to the welfare of the society. In the same way the society also should make every individual's life happy and enjoyable. Mere absence of ill health does not make an individual's health complete. A balanced mind is needed to lead a socially and economically productive life. Though an individual's capabilities are determined by heredity, it is the social environment that decides what the individual actually does. Therefore, a conducive social environment is vital for conditioning the individual's behavior. The relationship between the society and an individual can be compared to that between a phonograph and a music disk. The music in the disk can be brought out faithfully only when the phonograph is of high quality.

Social Well-being (Prerequisite for Health)

Physical health has been studied extensively and many sophisticated systems have been developed to improve it. Advancement in tertiary care is phenomenal and now a dying man can be kept alive indefinitely albeit without much use. Mental health has also been studied sufficiently though mental health programs are not that adequate. But it is distressing to note that the societies have not bothered to study properly the importance of social conditions in providing health. Poverty and illiteracy are the two important factors that come in the way of creating a healthy society. About 45% of world population (2.8 billion) lives on just 2 US dollars a day or less. The richest 20% enjoy 86% of the collective gross world product (GWP), while the poorest 20% have access only to 1% of the total GWP. The poor suffer worse health and die younger, have higher than average child and maternal mortality, high levels of disease and more limited access to health care and social protection. For the poor, health is an important economic asset. When ill or injured, the entire households become trapped in a downward spiral of lost income and higher health costs. It is essential to understand that poverty is the result of injustice. A just society will not allow poverty to exist. Nobel laureate Amartya Sen has portrayed poverty as denial of opportunity. About 26% of world's population (1 billion) is non-literates of which two thirds are women and 98% of them are in developing countries. Illiteracy is a social problem, not an individual problem. When children are humiliated or discriminated against on the basis of class, race or caste, learning is made harder. So it can be easily inferred that rampant illiteracy is due to denial of opportunity to the vast majority. Illiteracy can lead to marginalization and mistreatment.

Therefore, to improve public health a just society free from social tensions is necessary. Creation of an egalitarian society in which wealth is distributed to all based on requirement, health care is made available to all based on the need and not on paying capacity, food, water, and sanitation is available to all based on physiological requirement, is an important step to provide health for all and this cannot be achieved by technological development alone. Unfortunately, societies try to provide the basic physical needs of the populations by spending vast sums of money on technologies. The phenomenal growth of computer sciences is a pointer to this. Adequate attention is not being given to the social causes that prevent creating just societies in the world. As already pointed out health of the masses is not satisfactory not because of dearth of technological development and expertise, but because of the inequitable distribution of the existing wealth and healthcare facilities due to social problems discussed already.

❑ MEASUREMENT OF HEALTH

As health is influenced by many factors, its measurement also involves approaches from different dimensions. Therefore, many indicators have been used to assess health. Health indicators are needed to identify how healthy people are in a given population and to take remedial steps. It is also useful in comparing health conditions between different population groups.

Indicators of morbidity and mortality, disability rates, nutritional status indicators, healthcare delivery indicators, utilization rates, indicators of social and mental health, socioeconomic indicators and health policy indicators are now being used to assess health status of populations. An index called physical quality of life index (PQLI) is also used in this connection.

Physical health is measured by morbidity and mortality rates, life expectancy, etc. Incidence and prevalence rates and disability rates will indicate the quantum of sickness (morbidity) and hence the status of health in the community. Mortality indicators like crude death rates, disease-specific and age-specific death rates indirectly throw light on health situation. Anthropometric measurements like weight for age, weight for height, height for age, mid-arm circumference and skin-fold thickness, which reflect the nutritional status of children, are also used as indicators of health of the community. Doctor-population ratio, population per health center/sub-center, etc. reveal the level of accessibility to health care.

Incidences of crime, suicide, homicide, violence, juvenile delinquency, alcohol and drug abuse, and the like indicate mental health condition.

Socioeconomic conditions like per capita gross national product (GNP), literacy level, per capita calorie availability, housing conditions, etc. are also used as indicators of health. Similarly, health policy indicators like proportion of GNP spent for health-related activity highlight the priority accorded for health.

❑ GLOBAL DISEASE ELIMINATION AND ERADICATION AS PUBLIC HEALTH STRATEGIES

Global disease elimination and eradication as public health strategies are given below. It is adapted from WHO bulletin, OMS volume 76, supplement number 2, December 1998.

Infectious Diseases

Bacterial Diseases

Congenital syphilis, trachoma and *Haemophilus influenzae* type b (Hib) infection in some countries are candidates for elimination, but no bacterial disease was judged to be a current candidate for eradication.

Parasitic Diseases

Dracunculiasis (guinea worm disease) eradication is in progress. Although no additional parasitic disease was considered to be a current candidate for eradication, the increasing availability of potent, long-acting drugs brings extraordinary opportunities for overcoming onchocerciasis (river blindness) and lymphatic filariasis. The effectiveness of the strategy for controlling the triatomid vectors provides similar opportunities for the control of American trypanosomiasis (Chagas' disease). The workgroup concluded that onchocerciasis and lymphatic filariasis (caused by all wuchereria and most brugia infections) could be eliminated and possibly eradicated in the future. For the 5% of cases of lymphatic filariasis caused by *Brugia malayi*, which has an animal reservoir also (in Southeast Asia), elimination of disease is feasible, but not infection. Similarly, for Chagas' disease where animal reservoirs exist, elimination of disease is feasible, but not infection.

Viral Diseases

Poliomyelitis eradication is in progress. Measles and rubella were concluded to be possible candidates for eradication within the next 10–15 years. Developing countries should proceed cautiously to more costly measles elimination programs so that the poliomyelitis eradication effort is not undermined. Experience gained from regional and country interventions should be used to refine the strategies for eventual eradication.

The eradication of rubella as an add-on to measles eradication was felt to be biologically plausible. Rabies, yellow fever and Japanese encephalitis were considered not suitable candidates for eradication because of the existence of animal reservoirs. Hepatitis A virus eradication was concluded to be biologically feasible. Though hepatitis B virus was not considered to be a current candidate for eradication, the workgroup recommended immunization in all countries to maximize the likelihood of eliminating transmission of hepatitis B virus.

Principal Indicators of Eradicability

In theory, if the right tools were available, all infectious diseases would be eradicable. In reality there are distinct biological features of the organisms and technical factors of dealing with them that make their potential eradicability more or less likely. Today's categorization of a disease as not eradicable can change completely tomorrow either because, research efforts are successful in developing new and effective intervention tools or because, those presumed obstructions to eradicability that seemed important in theory prove capable of being overcome in practice. Three indicators were considered to be of primary importance:

1. An effective intervention is available to interrupt transmission of the agent.
2. Practical diagnostic tools with sufficient sensitivity and specificity are available to detect levels of infection that can lead to transmission.
3. Humans are essential for the lifecycle of the agent, which has no other vertebrate reservoir and it does not amplify in the environment.

❑ CANDIDATE DISEASES FOR ELIMINATION OR ERADICATION

Candidate diseases for elimination or eradication are given below. It is adapted from WHO bulletin, OMS volume 76, supplement number 2, December 1998.

Bacterial Diseases

Congenital Syphilis

Syphilis elimination is biologically feasible because no naturally occurring non-human host exists for the disease, serological tests for diagnosis are relatively accurate (> 95% sensitive and specific) and curative treatment is available. Early syphilis can be treated with a single injection of penicillin. The biological feasibility of syphilis elimination including the elimination of congenital syphilis has been demonstrated in most of the developed world.

Diphtheria

Eradication is not currently feasible because preliminary evidence suggests that circulation of toxigenic *Corynebacterium diphtheriae* might persist even in populations with fairly high childhood immunization coverage and might be difficult to detect and sustainable reservoirs for the toxin gene might exist in non-human mammals.

Factors favoring eradication: These are as follows:

1. Humans are the only known sustained reservoir.
2. An inexpensive and safe toxoid vaccine exists.
3. High coverage with this vaccine appears to reduce circulation of toxigenic strains of *C. diphtheriae* in the human population and to prevent disease.
4. Seasonality exists for both respiratory and cutaneous diphtheria, making transmission of toxigenic strains more vulnerable to interruption.

Factors hindering eradication: Are given below:

1. The phage carrying the toxin gene can occasionally be found in non-diphtheria *Corynebacterium* species infecting animals

(this may represent an ineradicable reservoir for reintroduction of toxin gene into non-toxigenic *C. diphtheriae* strains).

2. Infection with a toxigenic strain can either be direct or in situ by a phage carrying the toxin gene, infecting a commensal non-toxigenic *C. diphtheriae* strain.
3. An asymptomatic carrier state exists, even among immune persons and circulation appears to be able to continue under some settings even in populations with fairly high childhood immunization rates.
4. Immunity to diphtheria is not lifelong. A minimum of three doses is required for effective primary immunization and periodic booster doses are required throughout adult life to maintain protective titers. In addition, immune persons are not distinguishable from susceptible persons except by serological or Schick testing.
5. In countries with low incidence, both the clinician and laboratory can easily miss the diagnosis of diphtheria and empirical antibiotic treatment can prevent recovery of the organism.
6. Limited epidemiological, clinical and laboratory expertise is available on diphtheria.
7. Political will may be lacking because the disease burden is low in developed countries and is perceived to be relatively low in developing countries.

Haemophilus influenzae Type B Infection

Several aspects of Hib disease and Hib vaccines make elimination possible. Hib is a uniquely human pathogen with no known reservoir in the environment. Hib polysaccharide protein conjugate vaccines are highly effective (efficacy of 90%–100%) in preventing disease and should provide long-lasting protection. Hib conjugate vaccines also can interrupt transmission by preventing asymptomatic carriage and are thereby able to protect unvaccinated persons through herd immunity.

Leprosy

Elimination of leprosy may be feasible. Although other animals (e.g. armadillos) carry *Mycobacterium leprae,* humans are believed to be the organism's major reservoir and multidrug therapy (MDT) is curative. However, prolonged incubation period of leprosy makes recognition of a disease-free area difficult. Asymptomatic carriers of *M. leprae* may infect other people and the frequently chronic and mild symptoms may be difficult to detect without systematic screening of populations.

Neonatal Tetanus

Because tetanus spores are ubiquitous in the environment, eradication is not biologically feasible. Elimination (achieving rates < 1/1000 live births) is feasible only if high levels of coverage with appropriate strategies are achieved.

Strategies: Key strategies to accomplish the objective are as follows:

1. Achieving and maintaining high vaccination coverage levels for at least two doses of potent tetanus toxoid (TT) among reproductive-aged women in high-risk areas.
2. Promoting clean delivery, cord care practices and other surgical procedures performed on neonates (including the following practices shown to reduce risk.
3. Handwashing by the delivery attendant, delivery on a clean surface, use of a sterile or clean cutting tool and application of a topical antimicrobial to the umbilical stump wound).
4. Targeting women with a history of nuchal translucency (NT) in previous infants.

In June 1998, the Scientific Advisory Group of experts for WHO recommended that TT be replaced with tetanus-diphtheria (Td) vaccine.

Pertussis

Factors hindering eradication: Whole-cell and acellular pertussis vaccines are most effective only in preventing severe disease and may have little impact on acquisition of infection, preventing mild disease and decreasing transmission to other individuals. Pertussis vaccines require multiple doses for protection, hence they require a highly organized vaccine delivery system; immunity following vaccination wanes and in the absence of booster vaccinations in older children and adults, susceptible adolescents and adults will exist. Adequate herd immunity to block pertussis transmission in a sustained fashion (> 90% level of population immunity may be needed) may not be attainable even with 100% coverage. The efficacy of currently available acellular and whole-cell vaccines is, at best, 90%. Side effects associated with whole-cell pertussis vaccines are a major concern among healthcare providers and parents. Although new acellular pertussis vaccines cause fewer adverse reactions, they are significantly more expensive, especially when resources are limited in many countries.

Factors favoring eradication: Humans are the only reservoir for *Bordetella pertussis.* Whole-cell and acellular pertussis vaccines are highly effective in preventing severe disease. Seasonality exists for pertussis epidemics, making transmission more vulnerable to interruption and long-term carrier state is not thought to occur.

Trachoma

Elimination of blinding trachoma is possible, but eradication of *Chlamydia trachomatis* seems impossible. Trachoma has disappeared from North America and Europe because of improved socioeconomic conditions and hygiene.

Tuberculosis

Control measures are the same for developed and developing countries. However, the quality of these measures and the degree of their application differ greatly.

Elimination of tuberculosis (TB) is feasible for the reasons outlined below:

1. Infectious TB is relatively easy to identify by sputum test for acid-fast bacilli (AFB). Tuberculosis is treatable and curable with cure rates approaching 100% when modern short-course chemotherapy is used. Highly effective regimens are available. Early diagnosis and effective treatment significantly reduce transmission. Directly observed treatment short course (DOTS) strategy with direct supervision to ensure cure is available now.

2. Infected persons at increased risk of developing infectious TB can be identified through tuberculin screening of high-risk populations. Tuberculosis is preventable by the administration of isoniazid-preventive therapy (chemoprophylaxis) to those at risk of developing the disease. More recent studies in developing countries have also found isoniazid preventive therapy to be effective in HIV-infected persons also.
3. Humans are the primary reservoir of TB. Except for dairy cattle infected by *Mycobacterium bovis,* no other important animal or environmental reservoir of infection exists.
4. In developed countries TB has retreated into focal pockets that can be targeted for intensified control efforts. However, eliminating TB in these countries depends in part on global elimination because of imported cases. Although improved screening and prevention programs targeting immigrants from countries with high TB rates will reduce the number of imported cases, tuberculosis in foreign-born persons will continue to occur until TB is eliminated globally.
5. The World Bank has shown that short-course therapy (DOTS) is one of the most cost-effective health interventions available.

Parasitic Diseases

Chagas' Disease or American Trypanosomiasis

World Health Organization (WHO) has targeted elimination of domestic transmission of Chagas' disease. Because it exists as a zoonosis, complete eradication is not feasible; however, control of human transmission is considered achievable by eliminating domestic insect vector populations.

Lymphatic Filariasis

The International Task Force for Disease Eradication considers lymphatic filariasis to be one of only six eradicable or potentially eradicable diseases. Factors favoring eradication include inefficient transmission (several 100 infective mosquito bites are required to produce a fertile adult worm pair) and at least for *Wuchereria bancrofti,* the absence of a non-human reservoir. Because new drugs and drug combinations are now available that profoundly suppress microfilariae levels in the blood for 12 months after a single dose, elimination is possible with annual single-dose mass treatment.

Onchocerciasis

In 1993, the International Task Force for Disease Elimination did not list onchocerciasis as one of the six diseases suitable for eradication. However, blindness caused by onchocerciasis could be eliminated. The difficulties in eradication include:

1. The long life span of the adult worms.
2. The occurrence of reinfections.
3. Lack of vaccines and acceptable drugs to kill the adult worms.

If transmission can be interrupted with a free and easily deliverable medicine, the disease could potentially be eradicable. Repeated ivermectin treatment might affect the fecundity of adult female worms or longevity of adult male worms, thus reducing the duration of mass treatment programs to less than the life span of the adult parasites (8–15 year). The problem is, unlike lymphatic filariasis, restricted to rural Africa and Latin America. Thus, onchocerciasis may now be eligible to be included in the list of diseases for potential eradication.

Schistosomiasis

Comprehensive control programs, including mass treatment with antischistosomal drugs, health education, application of molluscicides and other measures have reduced the prevalence dramatically in many areas. Though control programs have not usually led to elimination or eradication of transmission, they have led to elimination of transmission. Schistosomiasis has been eradicated from Japan and Montserrat. Control interventions probably will stop transmission in Indonesia, Islamic Republic of Iran, Morocco and Saudi Arabia during the next few years.

Viral Diseases

Hepatitis B Virus Infection

Humans are the only known host for hepatitis B virus (HBV). The initial vaccination series confers protection against chronic infection for at least 15 years and HBV transmission has been eliminated in populations 10 years after introduction of routine infant vaccination. Potential infectivity of chronically infected persons decreases because of the decline in HBV titer (HBsAg positive). The combined effects of immunization and declining infectivity make elimination of HBV infection feasible. The increased use of effective antiviral agents to treat chronic HBV infection could hasten its elimination.

Measles

Humans are believed to be the only reservoir capable of sustaining transmission of the virus. Acquired immunity after illness is permanent. Live attenuated measles virus, when administered at the recommended ages, produces > 85% immunity after one dose and > 90% immunity after two doses and vaccine-induced immunity is long lasting. Widespread vaccination (mass campaigns and routine vaccination) has resulted in interruption of measles virus transmission in a number of settings. However, sustaining elimination in large populations or regions is difficult because of importations of measles virus from endemic areas, which is facilitated by the frequency of air travel. This experience suggests eradication of measles is technically feasible with existing vaccines, but will require a coordinated global effort over a relatively short period of time.

Rubella and Congenital Rubella Syndrome

According to the International Task force for Disease Eradication indicates that rubella and congenital rubella syndrome (CRS) can be eradicated. The following factors favor elimination/eradication of rubella/CRS:

1. Humans are the only reservoir for rubella.
2. Rubella vaccine is highly effective in preventing rubella and CRS.

3. A combination vaccine with measles exists and because of this combination vaccine, rubella elimination/eradication can be combined with the already existing measles elimination/eradication efforts.

Yellow Fever

Although yellow fever can never be eradicated because the virus is maintained in natural animal reservoirs, human disease can be effectively eliminated by vaccination with the proven 17D vaccine or in urban areas, by mosquito control.

❑ EMERGING INFECTIOUS DISEASES

Emerging pathogens are those that have appeared in a human population for the first time or have occurred previously, but are increasing in incidence or expanding into areas where they have not previously been reported, usually over the last 20 years (WHO, 1997). Re-emerging pathogens are those, whose incidence is increasing as a result of long-term changes in their underlying epidemiology (Woolhouse, 2002). By these criteria, 175 species of infectious agents from 96 different genera are classified as emerging pathogens. Of this group, 75% are zoonotic species. Improved methods of surveillance, epidemiological studies and the continuous development of more advanced methods of diagnosis have allowed us to detect new pathogenic species of microorganism or to associate a known microorganism with a new or atypical set of disease symptoms. Furthermore, the agents of several diseases that were thought to have been controlled are re-emerging as a result of adaptive changes in the pathogen and changes to the immunological status of the people.

Man has been able to control many communicable diseases, which were once a threat to health and very survival by using scientific methods and technologies. But this conquest is far from complete as new emerging infectious diseases and re-emergence of old infectious diseases are seen to confront him in recent times.

Toxic shock syndrome in intrauterine device (IUD) users caused by *Staphylococcus aureus* infection of the genital tract, Lyme disease caused by *Borrelia burgdorferi* in USA due to reforestation and increase in deer population, increase in the transmission of diseases such as shigellosis, giardiasis and hepatitis A to children and staff of child care centers, opportunistic infections by *Pneumocystis carinii*, *Cryptosporidium* and Cytomegalovirus due to immune suppression caused by chemotherapy, organ transplant and HIV, diarrheas caused by enterohemorrhagic strain (0157:H7) of *Escherichia coli* and gastrointestinal diseases caused by *Cryptosporidium* species due to changes in diet, food processing, globalization of food supply and contamination of municipal water supplies, hantavirus pulmonary syndrome caused by infected rodents, development of a new strain of *Vibrio cholerae* 0139 due to evolution and the severe acute respiratory syndrome (SARS), bird flu and chikungunya are the emerging infectious diseases in recent times. The latest in the list since 26th April 2009 is the swine flu pandemic. As of 31 of July 2009, 168 countries and overseas territories/communities have reported laboratory confirmed cases of pandemic (H1N1)/09. All continents are affected by the pandemic.

Drug resistance is an important factor in the re-emergence of infectious diseases and this phenomenon is due to widespread use of antibiotics. Tubercle bacilli, gonococci, pneumococci, hospital-acquired enterococci and staphylococci all have developed resistance to drugs already employed. Influenza virus has developed resistance to amantadine, *Candida* species to azole, *Trichomonas vaginalis* to metronidazole, malarial parasite to chloroquine, HIV to antiviral drugs and *Salmonella typhi* to commonly used drugs causing serious problems in their management. As a result, now prolonged hospitalization, higher death rates and higher health-care costs are caused.

Other factors responsible for the re-emergence of infectious diseases are:

1. Migration to previously uninhabited new areas.
2. Overcrowding.
3. Civil disturbances and war causing breakdown in sanitary and other public health measures.
4. Deforestation, reforestation and urbanization.
5. Erratic human behaviors such as drug abuse, improper sexuality due to breakdown in moral values caused by money-oriented media like cinema and television.

6. Increase in international travel and commerce.
7. Changes in food processing and handling, international trade in food.
8. Evolution of pathogenic infectious agents, development of resistance in infectious agents such as tubercle bacilli, malarial parasite and gonococci.
9. Resistance of insect vectors like mosquitoes to insecticides.
10. Immunosuppression of individuals caused by medical treatments or by new infectious agent like AIDS virus.
11. Deterioration of surveillance system for infectious diseases.
12. Social evils such as communalism, corruption, poverty and illiteracy, which are responsible for failure of programs.

The WHO suggests following measures to tackle this problem:

1. Strengthening of global surveillance.
2. Establishing national and international infrastructure to recognize, report and respond to new disease threats.
3. Developing applied research on diagnosis and epidemiological control of emerging infectious diseases.
4. Strengthening the international capacity for infectious disease control and prevention.

Tackling of social evils and issues that come in the way of implementation of health programs and proper use of scientific knowledge must form an integral part of the strategy in this regard.

Drug Resistance

The first case of resistant *Staphylococcus* was seen half a century ago. Now antimicrobial resistance has become a serious public health concern. Multidrug-resistant tuberculosis (MDR-TB) is no longer confined to any one country. Extensively drug-resistant tuberculosis (XDR-TB) also has arisen. Resistant malaria is on the rise. In the developed world, as much as 60% of hospital-acquired infections are caused by drug-resistant microbes. Many resistant infections generated in hospital settings may have migrated to the community at large is a worrisome feature.

Although antimicrobial resistance affects industrialized and developing countries alike, its impact is far greater in developing countries causing a dramatic escalation in the price of treatment.

In addition, MDR forms of diseases can become untreatable in any country, at any price, once the options have been exhausted. Pharmaceutical manufacturers have found it difficult to develop new antibiotics and other drugs fast enough to replace those that have become ineffective.

Factors Favoring Resistance

Natural selection of microbes: When a microbial population is exposed to an antibiotic, more susceptible organisms will succumb, while those resistant to the antimicrobial action will survive. These organisms can then either pass on their resistance genes to their subsequent generations by replication or to other related bacteria through conjugation whereby plasmids carrying the genes jump from one organism to another. This natural phenomenon is exacerbated by the abuse, overuse and misuse of antimicrobials in the treatment of human illness, and in animal husbandry and agriculture.

Complacency: Many drug manufacturers have turned away from intensive antibacterial research because of complacency that infectious diseases have been conquered and therefore, concentrated on seeking drugs for heart diseases and other chronic diseases. Further research into new drugs to combat bacterial infections was not pursued seriously.

Drug accessibilities: Poverty and inadequate access to drugs in poor countries continue to be the major problem in the development of resistance. Being unable to buy costly drugs, most patients are forced to resort to poor quality products or incomplete treatment. The prescribed treatment may not be followed. Once the symptoms disappear, people often stop taking the antibiotics thereby increasing the risk of developing drug-resistant forms of disease. In developing countries antibiotics can be bought over-the-counter without a prescription and self-medication is commonplace.

Misdiagnosis: Overworked healthcare workers, not equipped to deal with the large number of patients, inevitably go for 'defensive' and unnecessary prescribing. The absence of diagnostic facilities or their high cost in poorer countries forces the healthcare workers to engage in symptomatic treatment that often leads to misdiagnosis and/or prescribing the wrong medication. Quackery is also common in developing countries.

Spurious drugs: These are also a problem that directly contributes to antimicrobial resistance. These drugs may not contain the active ingredient, may contain the wrong ingredient or lesser than recommended concentrations of active medication, thus favoring resistance.

Preference for broad-spectrum antibiotics: Many healthcare workers avoid narrow-spectrum drugs in favor of broader-spectrum antibiotics that have wider applications. Unethical pharmaceutical companies pay a commission for recommending more expensive broader-spectrum medications in some countries. Such use of 'shotgun therapy' accelerates the natural process of resistance.

Drug advertising: Sometimes patients also demand for antimicrobials from medical personnel as a consequence of the information learnt from advertising media.

Lack of education about drug resistance: In developed nations, the issue of antimicrobial resistance is not addressed adequately in medical schools or is confined only to specialist training.

Inappropriate hospital prescriptions: In an analysis of 10 studies undertaken at teaching hospitals worldwide, researchers determined that between 40% and 91% of antibiotics prescribed in the hospitals were inappropriate. In Canada and the United States, approximately half of all outpatient prescriptions for antibiotics were found to be unnecessary.

In a study in Vietnam, over 70% of patients were given inadequate dosages.

Food and antimicrobial resistance: Antimicrobials are used to treat sick animals, as growth promoters in livestock and to rid cultivated foodstuffs of various destructive organisms. This low-level dosing for growth and prophylaxis inevitably results in the development of resistance in bacteria in or near livestock. It is well known that vancomycin-resistant *Enterococcus faecium* (VRE) has appeared in animals that may have 'jumped' into the human population. The emergence of VRE in food can be traced to the widespread use of avoparcin, the animal equivalent of the human antibiotic vancomycin, in livestock. Besides, when livestock production increases in developing countries, reliance on antimicrobials is likewise expanding, often without guidelines.

Globalization and resistance: As a result of international travel and trade, a microbe originating in one country can arrive in another country within a very short time, say 24 hours. For example, majority of multidrug-resistant typhoid cases originated in the six developing countries are now seen in the United States according to published reports.

Diseases once thought to be under control have become increasingly resistant to the currently available drugs. The specter of incurable infectious diseases looms large. The fight against TB, malaria, pneumonia, cholera, diarrheal diseases and HIV is severely affected.

Acute respiratory illness (ARI) and pneumonia: About 70% of chest infections are resistant to one of the first-line antimicrobials. This alarming situation is due, in part, to widespread confusion over the difference between viral and bacterial respiratory infections. Both forms present the same clinical symptoms that can often only be distinguished by expensive laboratory tests that are not available in many parts of the world. Treating viral illness with antibiotics is not only ineffective, but contributes to the development of resistance. This is particularly true when it comes to treating children.

Vaccines developed to prevent some of the bacterial pneumonias, e.g. Hib and Pneumovax vaccines offer some hope in combating resistance by reducing the number of infected individuals and thereby minimizing transmission, infection and the need for treatment.

Diarrheal diseases: Multidrug resistance is also occurring in microbes that cause diarrheal diseases. *Shigella dysenteriae* is resistant to almost every available drug. Today, nearly all *Shigella* are non-responsive to co-trimoxazole, while resistance to ciprofloxacin appears to be just around the corner. Cholera and typhoid organisms also acquire resistance easily. *Salmonella* typhi have developed resistance to first-line, second-line and now third-line drugs. In India two-thirds of reported cases in 1992 were chloramphenicol resistant.

Acquired immunodeficiency syndrome (AIDS): A small, but growing number of patients are showing primary resistance to antiretroviral drug zidovudine (AZT). When human immunodeficiency virus (HIV) develops resistance to one protease inhibitor it quickly becomes insensitive to the entire family of drugs, thus outwitting antiretrovirals. The resistance in HIV assumes greater significance because of the fact that those infected become reservoirs for resistant TB, leishmaniasis, pneumonia and other opportunistic infections.

Tuberculosis: It is staging a major comeback. It is becoming increasingly resistant to routine anti-TB drugs. About 5% of TB cases are found to be multidrug-resistant. There are estimated 40,000 new extremely drug-resistant, XDR-TB cases annually. The length of TB treatment also adds to the resistance crisis as many do not take the treatment completely. The DOTS strategy, if followed, minimizes the development of resistance by preventing treatment failure. With the arrival of MDR-TB and XDR-TB, the cost of treatment may rise to more than 100 times.

Malaria: It is reappearing in areas of the world formerly considered free. Resistance to chloroquine is now seen in 80% of the 92 countries where malaria continues to be a major killer. Resistance to newer second- and third-line drugs continues to grow. Mefloquine resistance emerged in Southeast Asia almost as soon as the drug was introduced. Artemisinin resistance has also been reported. Development of newer and more effective medicines becomes imperative in the containment of drug-resistant malaria.

Leishmaniasis: It is showing resistance to the antimonials at rates of 64% in some developing nations. Like MDR-TB, drug-resistant leishmaniasis results when treatment courses are too short, interrupted or when the courses consist of poor-quality or spurious drugs. In developed Mediterranean nations, drug-resistant leishmaniasis continues to spread as the number of patients coinfected with HIV increases.

Gonorrhea: Antimicrobial resistance in gonorrhea is one of the major healthcare disasters of the 20th century. In most of South-east Asia, resistance to penicillin has been reported in nearly all strains at an overall rate of 98%. Even newer and more expensive drugs like ciprofloxacin are showing an increasing failure rate.

Common worms: Another area where drug resistance poses a threat is in the treatment of food-borne and soil-transmitted helminths. Resistance of helminths to drugs is already a problem among livestock. In humans, though resistance has not yet emerged, it remains a real threat.

Hospital-acquired infections: Hospital wards are breeding grounds of resistant microbes, viz. Staphylococci, *Salmonella, Pseudomonas* and *Klebsiella.* For example, methicillin-resistant *Staphyloccocus aureus* and vancomycin-resistant *Enterococcus* are wreaking havoc in hospital wards around the world. So far, the only drug available to treat methicillin resistant *S. aureus* is vancomycin. Vancomycin itself falters in the face of a renewed attack by vancomycin-intermediate *S. aureus,* which is already seen in hospitals and nursing homes holding large numbers of immunocompromised patients. So far, the current preventive methods emphasizing aggressive infection control measures have only slowed the spread of resistant bacteria. That many resistant infections generated in hospital settings may migrate to the community at large is a worrisome feature.

Remedial Action for Reducing the Impact of Antimicrobial Resistance

The impact of antimicrobial resistance could be greatly reduced by integrated management of childhood illnesses, better prescribing practices, training for health workers, educating the public, using user-friendly packaging of drugs to encourage adherence and developing of simple-to-use tests that permit accurate diagnosis. Establishing national surveillance systems, which can detect and respond to antimicrobial resistance at an early stage, are very important in this regard.

❑ VACCINATION FOR INTERNATIONAL TRAVEL

General Considerations

Vaccination offers, for the traveler, the possibility of protecting from dangerous infections that may be encountered in a foreign soil. Vaccines do not fully protect 100% of the recipients. Therefore, all additional precautions against infection should be followed carefully regardless of any vaccines or other medication that have been administered. These same precautions are to be taken to reduce the risk of acquiring diseases for which no vaccines exist (WHO vaccine-preventable diseases, vaccines and vaccination, Chapter 6).

Planning Before Travel

Travelers are advised to consult a travel medicine clinic or personal physician 4–6 weeks before departure if the travel destination is endemic for any vaccine-preventable disease. Travelers should be provided with a written record of all vaccines administered preferably using the international vaccination certificate (which is required in the case of yellow fever vaccination).

The vaccines and the possible adverse reactions of the vaccines are explained in Tables 1.1 to 1.3.

TABLE 1.1: Vaccines for travelers

Category	Vaccine/Disease
Routine use	Diphtheria, pertussis, tetanus (DPT); hepatitis B virus (HBV); *Haemophilus influenzae* type b (Hib); measles, mumps, rubella (MMR); poliomyelitis (OPV* or IPV†)
Selective use for travelers	Cholera, influenza, hepatitis A virus (HAV) Japanese encephalitis, Lyme disease, meningococcal disease, pneumococcal disease, rabies, tick-borne encephalitis, tuberculosis (BCG‡), typhoid fever and yellow fever (for individual protection)
Mandatory vaccination	Yellow fever (for protection of vulnerable countries) Meningococcal disease (required by Saudi Arabia for pilgrims visiting Mecca for the Hajj (annual pilgrimage) or for the Umrah

*OPV, oral polio vaccine; †IPV, inactivated polio vaccine; ‡BCG, bacillus Calmette-Guerin.

TABLE 1.2: Common minor vaccine reactions

Vaccine/Disease	Possible minor adverse reaction	Expected frequency
BCG	Local reaction (pain, swelling, redness)	Common
Cholera	Oral presentation—none	–
Diphtheria, pertussis, tetanus (DPT)	Local reaction (pain, swelling, redness)	Up to 50%[a]
	Fever	Up to 50%
Hepatitis A	Local reaction (pain, swelling, redness)	Up to 50%

Contd...

Contd...

Vaccine/Disease	Possible minor adverse reaction	Expected frequency
Hepatitis B	Local reaction (pain, swelling, redness)	Adults up to 30%
		Children up to 5%
	Fever	1%–6%
Haemophilus influenzae type b (Hib)	Local reaction (pain, swelling, redness)	5%–15%
	Fever	2%–10%
Japanese encephalitis	Local reaction, low-grade fever, myalgia, gastrointestinal upset	Up to 20%
Lyme disease	Local reaction, myalgia, influenza-like illness	Up to 20%
Measles, mumps, rubella (MMR)	Local reaction (pain, swelling, redness)	Up to 10%
	Irritability, malaise and non-specific symptoms, fever	Up to 5%
Pneumococcal	Local reaction (pain, swelling, redness)	30%–50%
Poliomyelitis (OPV)	None	
Poliomyelitis (IPV)	None	
Rabies	Local and/or general reaction depending on type of vaccine (see product information)	15%–25%
Meningococcal disease	Mild local reactions	Up to 71%
Tetanus-diphtheria (Td)	Local reaction (pain, swelling, redness)[b]	Up to 10%
	Malaise and non-specific symptoms	Up to 25%
Tick-borne encephalitis	Local reaction (pain, swelling, redness)	Up to 10%
Typhoid fever	Depends on type of vaccine use (see product information)	–
Yellow fever	Headache	10%
	Influenza-like symptoms	22%
	Local reaction (pain, swelling, redness)	5%

[a]With whole-cell pertussis vaccine. Rates for acellular pertussis vaccine are lower.
[b]Rate of local reactions likely to increase with booster doses, up to 50%–85%.

TABLE 1.3: Uncommon severe adverse reactions

Vaccine/Disease	Possible adverse reaction	Expected rate per million doses[a]
Bacillus Calmette-Guerin (BCG)	Suppurative lymphadenitis	100–1,000 (mostly in immunodeficient individuals)
	BCG-osteitis	1–700 (rarely with current vaccines)
	Disseminated BCG infection	0.19–1.56
Cholera	NR*	–
Diphtheria, pertussis, tetanus (DPT)	Persistent crying	1,000–60,000
	Seizures	570
	Hypotonic–hyporesponsive episode	570
	Anaphylaxis	20
Hepatitis A	NR	–
Hepatitis B[b]	Anaphylaxis	1–2
	Guillain–Barré syndrome (plasma-derived)	5
Haemophilus influenzae type b (Hib)	NR	–
Japanese encephalitis	Mouse-brain only—neurological event	Rare
	Hypersensitivity	100–6,400
Lyme disease	NR	–
Measles, mumps, rubella (MMR)	Febrile seizure	333
	Thrombocytopenic purpura	33–45
	Anaphylaxis	1–50
	Encephalitis	1
Meningococcal disease	Anaphylaxis	1
Mumps	Depends on strain—aseptic meningitis	0–500

Contd...

Contd...

Vaccine/Disease	Possible adverse reaction	Expected rate per million doses[a]
Pneumococcal	Anaphylaxis	Very rare
Poliomyelitis (OPV†)	Vaccine-associated paralytic poliomyelitis	1.4–3.4
Poliomyelitis (IPV‡)	NR	–
Rabies	Animal brain tissue only—neuroparalysis	17–44
	Cell derived-allergic reactions	rare
Rubella	Arthralgia/arthritis/arthropathy	None or very rare
Tetanus	Brachial neuritis	5–10
	Anaphylaxis	1–6
Tick-borne encephalitis	NR	–
Typhoid fever	Parenteral vaccine—various	Very rare
	Oral vaccine—NR	–
Yellow fever	Encephalitis(< 6 month)	500–4,000
	Allergy/anaphylaxis	5–20
	Hepatic failure	Rare

*NR, none reported; †OPV, oral polio vaccine; ‡IPV, inactivated polio vaccine.
[a]Precise rate may vary with survey method.
[b]Although there have been anecdotal reports of demyelinating disease following hepatitis B vaccine, there is no scientific evidence for a causal relationship.

❑ INTERNATIONAL CERTIFICATE OF VACCINATION

The certificate must be printed and completed in English and French. An additional language may be added. The international certificate of vaccination is an individual certificate. It should not be used collectively. Separate certificates should be issued for children. The information should not be incorporated in the mother's certificate. An international certificate is valid only if the yellow fever vaccine used has been approved by WHO and if the vaccinating center has been designated by the national health administration for the area in which the center is situated. The date should be recorded in the following sequence – day, month, year, with the month written in letters, e.g. 8 January 2001. A certificate issued to a child who is unable to write should be signed by a parent or guardian. For illiterates, the signature should be indicated by their mark certified by another person. Although a nurse may carry out the vaccination under the direct supervision of a qualified medical practitioner, the certificate must be signed by the person authorized by the national health administration. The official stamp of the center is not an accepted substitute for a personal signature.

SECTION

2

Epidemiology of Communicable Diseases

PART A

Principles of Control and Prevention

CHAPTER

2

Common Terms and Concepts

❑ COMMON TERMS

Infection

Infection is defined as the entry and development or multiplication of a microorganism in man or animals. It may be contained by the defenses of the body or may progress into a disease if immunity is lowered.

Gradient of Infection

Gradient of infection refers to different types of host responses to an infection. At one extreme, infection may result in death (fatality), at the other extreme it may just be an inapparent infection and in between it may be illness, mild to severe followed by recovery.

Inapparent Infection

Inapparent infection is the presence of an infection in a level below the threshold of clinical symptoms. Another synonymous expression for this is subclinical case. The importance of this phenomenon lies in the fact that people with inapparent infection (subclinical cases) will be much more in number than clinical cases during an epidemic. These cases may be equally and sometimes more infectious than overt cases. They also play an important role in determining the size of the susceptible to many infections in a population since this type of infection can induce protective antibodies.

Latent Infection

Latent infection is one in which the organism remains dormant and is not being shed from the host, but may get reactivated after some period (may be years). Herpes simplex virus and chickenpox virus are known to occur as latent infections.

Nosocomial Infection

When a patient contracts an infection during his/her stay in hospital, it is called nosocomial or hospital-acquired infection. A hospital-acquired infection is an infection that first appears between 48 hours and 4 days after a patient is admitted to a hospital or other healthcare facility. Hospital-acquired infections can be caused by bacteria, viruses, fungi or parasites. These microorganisms may already be present in the patient's body or may come from the environment, contaminated hospital equipment, healthcare workers or other patients. Hospital-acquired infections may develop from the performance of surgical procedures; from the insertion of catheters (tubes) into the urinary tract, nose, mouth or blood vessels. The most common types of hospital-acquired infections are urinary tract infections (UTIs), ventilator-associated pneumonia and surgical wound infections. Pneumonia is the second most common type of hospital-acquired infection. Inadequately sterilized syringes may transmit hepatitis B and acquired immunodeficiency syndrome (AIDS). Pseudomonas (surgical) wound infection is common in postoperative patients in hospitals. Improper ventilation in hospitals can favor transmission of respiratory diseases such as swine flu, tuberculosis, etc.

Cross Infection

Infection contracted from fellow patients or from hospital environment is called cross infection. Respiratory and alimentary canal infections may be contracted in this way when there is lack of cross ventilation and hygiene. Centralized air conditioning without proper maintenance of indoor air quality (IAQ) is a health hazard to patients as well as to patient attendees.

Iatrogenic Disease

Diseases or complications caused to patients as a result of treatment or investigation procedures in the hospital are called iatrogenic disease or physician-induced disease. Allergic and adverse reactions to drugs come under this category.

Infectious Disease

It is a disease resulting from an infection, e.g. tuberculosis, leprosy, malaria, etc.

Infestation

Infestation is the lodgment, development and reproduction of arthropods on the surface of the body or in the clothing, e.g. itch mite, lice. This term is also applied to the presence of parasite worms in the gut, e.g. ascariasis, ancylostomiasis. Presence of rodents in the rooms is also described as infestation.

Contamination

Contamination is the presence of an infectious agent on the body surface and also on or in clothes, beddings, toys, surgical instruments or dressings and in articles like water, milk and food.

Pollution

Pollution is the presence of offensive, but not necessarily infectious agents in the environment, e.g. water pollution, soil pollution.

Contagious Disease

Contagious disease is one that is transmitted through physical contact, e.g. scabies, sexually transmitted diseases (STDs), leprosy.

Communicable Disease

Communicable disease is one caused by a specific microorganism, which is transmissible from one person to another or from one animal to another or from environment to man or animal either directly or indirectly, e.g. cholera, typhoid, AIDS, etc.

Host

Host is defined as a person or animal that harbors an infectious agent under natural conditions.

Obligate Host

Obligate host is the only host for a specific organism. For example, man is the only host for typhoid bacilli.

Definitive or Primary Host

Definitive or primary host is the one in which a parasite attains maturity (e.g. man in teniasis) or passes its sexual stage (e.g. mosquito in malaria).

Intermediate Host

Intermediate host is the one in which larval or asexual stage of a parasite is spent during its life cycle (e.g. man in malaria).

Epidemic

Epidemic is the unusual occurrence of a disease or health-related event clearly in excess of usual occurrence in a community or region. Even one case of smallpox, if it occurs now anywhere will constitute an epidemic. The term `slow epidemics' is applied to describe the occurrence in excess of non-communicable diseases like diabetes mellitus, heart attacks, etc.

Endemic

Endemic refers to the constant occurrence of a disease in a region or population group in a particular frequency.

Hyperendemic

Hyperendemic refers to the presence of a disease at high incidence and or prevalence rate.

Holoendemic

Holoendemic is the situation in which there is high level of infection among child population beginning early in life and adults show fewer incidences (e.g. malaria).

Sporadic

Sporadic refers to the occurrence of a disease infrequently, irregularly and haphazardly, cases being separated widely in time and space with no connection between one incidence and another, e.g. polio, tetanus.

Pandemic

Pandemic is the epidemic affecting large number of people, major part of a nation, entire nation, a continent or the world (e.g. AIDs, influenza).

Exotic Diseases

Exotic diseases are the one that is imported into an area, where these diseases do not occur (e.g. rabies in UK, Australia, yellow fever in India).

Zoonotic Diseases

Zoonotic diseases are communicable diseases that are transmissible from vertebrate animals to man under natural conditions (e.g. rabies, plague, anthrax, salmonellosis, hydatid cyst, bovine tuberculosis, Kyasanur forest disease (KFD), monkeypox).

Zooanthroponosis

The infection is transmitted from man to vertebrate animals (e.g. human TB in animals).

Anthropozoonosis

Anthropozoonosis is transmitted from vertebrate animals to man (e.g. rabies).

Amphixenosis

The transmission is possible in either direction, i.e. man to animals or vice versa (e.g. *Trypanosoma cruzi* and *Schistosoma japonicum*).

Epizootic

Epizootic is the occurrence of epidemic in animals (e.g. anthrax, brucellosis, rabies, Q fever, Japanese encephalitis, equine encephalitis).

Enzootic

Enzootic is the constant presence of an infectious disease among animals at particular frequency (e.g. anthrax, rabies, brucellosis, endemic typhus).

Control

The reduction of disease incidence, prevalence, morbidity or mortality to a locally acceptable level as a result of deliberate efforts. Continued intervention measures are required to maintain the reduction, e.g. diarrheal diseases.

Elimination

Elimination of a Disease

It is achieved when there is zero incidence of the specified disease in a defined geographical area as a result of deliberate efforts. Continued intervention measures are required to achieve elimination. For example, neonatal tetanus can be eliminated by vaccination of all antenatal mothers and by safe delivery practices.

Elimination of Infection

It is reduction to zero of the incidence of infection caused by a specific agent in a defined geographical area as a result of deliberate efforts. Continued measures to prevent re-establishment of transmission are required. For example, measles and poliomyelitis infections can be eliminated by a continuous ongoing vaccination program.

Eradication

There is permanent worldwide zero incidence of an infection caused by a specific agent as a result of deliberate efforts. Once eradicated, intervention measures are no longer needed. For example, the one infection that has been eradicated globally is smallpox.

Extinction

The specific infectious agent no longer exists in nature or in the laboratory, e.g. none.

❑ MODES OF SPREAD OF COMMUNICABLE DISEASES

Communicable diseases spread from a reservoir to a susceptible host in many ways. A reservoir is the person or animal, arthropod, plant, soil or substance in which an infectious agent is able to thrive and from where it can be transmitted to another host. For many diseases, man himself is the reservoir. Human reservoir may be in the form of an overt clinical case, a subclinical case or a carrier.

Carrier state is a condition in which a man or animal harbors and excretes an infectious agent without overt clinical signs and symptoms. Temporary carrier state may be seen during the incubation period (incubatory carriers), in inapparent infections and during convalescence (convalescent carriers). Chronic carrier state is reported in diseases like typhoid. But lifelong carrier state is most infrequent. Carrier state is also described with reference to the route of exit of the infectious agent. Thus, there will be urinary carriers, fecal carriers and throat carriers. Epidemiologically carriers are more important than overt clinical cases. Identification of carrier state may not be easy and may require sophisticated investigations, but it is very important to control the transmission of communicable diseases.

Source is the material containing an infectious agent through which the actual transfer of the agent from the reservoir to a susceptible host takes place. For example, in pulmonary tuberculosis, man is the reservoir and sputum is the source through which the organism *Mycobacterium tuberculosis* is transmitted to another person.

A primary case is the one which is first introduced into a community. An index case is one which is first detected by an investigator. Secondary cases arise as a result of contact with a primary case. Secondary attack rate (SAR) may be high in certain diseases such as chickenpox, measles and whooping cough.

There are many animal reservoirs from which man can get infected, e.g. rabies from dogs and Japanese encephalitis from birds and pigs.

Soil and other inanimate objects may act as reservoir for some disease causing organisms (e.g. soil for *Clostridium tetani, Bacillus anthracis)*.

❑ ROUTES OF TRANSMISSION OF INFECTIOUS DISEASES

Transmission of infectious diseases from reservoir to susceptible hosts occurs either directly or indirectly.

Direct Transmission

Transmission of an infectious agent directly from the reservoir/ source to a susceptible host is called direct transmission. Close contact with the reservoir/source is therefore essential for this type of transmission. Direct transmission occurs through:

1. Direct contact.
2. Droplet infection.
3. Contact with soil.
4. Bite of an animal.
5. Placenta.

Direct Contact

Transmission occurs without an intervening agency from a reservoir or source to a susceptible host, e.g. transmission of STDs, AIDS through sexual intercourse and scabies through skin to skin contact.

Droplet Infection

Droplet infection is direct projection of droplet spray of saliva or nasopharyngeal secretions up to a distance of 30-60 cm into host's nose or mouth by acts like coughing, sneezing or talking. Examples for this type of transmission are common cold, diphtheria, tuberculosis, meningococcal meningitis, etc. Overcrowding and lack of ventilation facilitate this type of transmission.

Contact with Soil

Disease like tetanus and mycosis are transmitted directly from the soil to a susceptible host.

Bite of an Animal

Rabies is transmitted by the bite of a rabid animal (dog, jackal or fox).

Through Placenta

Transplacental transmission (vertical transmission) from the pregnant mother to the fetus occurs in diseases like syphilis, AIDS, German measles and hepatitis B. Drugs also may pass through placenta and affect the growing fetus.

Indirect Transmission

Indirect transmission requires a third agency between the source/ reservoir and the host and so the infectious agent should be able to survive till it reaches the susceptible host. Indirect transmission occurs through:

1. Vehicle.
2. Vector.
    a. Biological.
    b. Mechanical.
3. Air.
    a. Droplet nuclei.
    b. Dust.
4. Fomites.
5. Hands and fingers.

Through Vehicle

Here, the transmission takes place through vehicles like water, food, milk, milk products, ice, blood, serum, plasma or other biological products. Of these, water and food are the most frequently involved vehicles causing diseases chiefly in alimentary tract (e.g. diarrhea, typhoid fever, hepatitis A, food poisoning, intestinal parasites, etc.).

Through Vector

Vector is an arthropod or any living carrier that transmits an infectious agent to a susceptible host. Transmission through a vector may be mechanical or biological. Housefly is a mechanical vector, which simply carries pathogens on its body parts like mouth parts, legs and abdomen and deposits them on food articles. Diseases like infective hepatitis, typhoid, cholera and diarrhea are transmitted by housefly mechanically. Mosquito is a biological vector in which the disease causing organisms obtained through a bloody meal undergo development and/or multiplication before being transmitted to a susceptible host. Malaria and filariasis are transmitted by mosquitoes.

Biological transmission may be:

1. Propagative: The causative organism undergoes only multiplication in number in the vector, but there is no change in form of the organism, e.g. plague bacilli in rat fleas.
2. Cyclopropagative: The causative organism undergoes changes in both the number and the form, e.g. malarial parasite in mosquitoes.
3. Cyclodevelopmental: The causative organism undergoes only development, but no change in number, e.g. microfilaria in mosquitoes.

Transovarian transmission is the transmission of the agent from the infected female to its progeny. Transstadial transmission is the transmission of the agent from one stage of life cycle of a vector to another stage, e.g. From nymph to adult stage as in the case of *Rickettsia conorii* in ticks.

Vector transmission is principally of three types. They are:

1. Man: Arthropod man (e.g. malaria).
2. Mammal or bird: Arthropod-man (e.g. plague, Japanese encephalitis).
3. Man: Two intermediate hosts man (e.g. fish tapeworm).

Through Air

1. Droplet nuclei: These are tiny particles of 1–10 microns in size formed by evaporation of coughed or sneezed out droplets of saliva or nasopharyngeal secretions. Droplet nuclei may also be formed in microbiological laboratories, in abattoirs or in autopsy rooms. These tiny particles may remain suspended in the air for long periods and may be carried to distant places by air current. Examples for such transmission are tuberculosis, influenza, chickenpox, measles, Q fever and many other respiratory infections.
2. Dust: Larger droplets formed during coughing, sneezing and talking may settle down on the floor, carpets, furniture or toys and the organisms may remain viable for quite some time. During cleansing operations like sweeping, dusting or bed making, these large droplets containing the organisms emanate in the form of dust and may be inhaled by susceptible hosts. Infected dusts may also settle on food and milk directly. Hospital-acquired (nosocomial) infections occur in this way. Examples for transmission through infected dusts are tuberculosis, streptococcal infections, etc.

Through Fomites

Fomites are inanimate substances, other than food, water or milk, through which transmission of pathogenic organisms can occur. Soiled clothes, towels, handkerchiefs, cups, spoons, toys, pencils, door handles, lavatory chains, syringes, surgical dressings are some of the fomites involved in the transmission of communicable diseases. Diseases transmitted through fomites include diphtheria, typhoid, bacillary dysentery and eye and skin infections.

Through Unclean Hands and Fingers

Lack of personal hygiene is the cause for transmission of pathogens through unclean hands and fingers. Pathogens from skin, nose or feces may be transmitted in this way. Typhoid, dysentery, infective hepatitis, intestinal worms, staphylococcal and streptococcal infections are transmitted by soiled hands and fingers.

Susceptible host

A susceptible host is a person who is vulnerable to get affected by a pathogenic microorganism. The susceptibility may be due to lack of immunity. A microorganism after gaining entry into a susceptible host must reach the appropriate site (site of election) for multiplication. For example, hepatitis A virus after its entry through the alimentary canal reaches liver, multiplies there and causes hepatitis.

Incubation period: When a pathogenic microorganism enters into human body it cannot immediately cause disease. It takes time to multiply sufficiently and cause pathology in the site of election. Then only the signs and symptoms of the disease develop. This time interval between the entry of microorganisms and the development of signs and symptoms is called the incubation period. This period may be short (2–3 days), intermediate (10 days to less 3 weeks) or long (several weeks to months or years) depending upon the type of organism and the host response. It is short in diseases like cholera and influenza, while it is long in leprosy, tuberculosis and rabies. In typhoid the incubation period is of median length, i.e. 10–14 days.

Knowledge of incubation period is useful:

1. To trace the source of infection and contacts.
2. To determine the period of surveillance or quarantine.
3. To prevent infectious diseases by using immunoglobulin and antisera.
4. To identify whether an epidemic is point source or propagated.
5. To assess the prognosis of an infectious disease.

Generation time refers to the interval between the receipt of infection and the maximal infectivity. The period of infectivity may terminate prior to clinical recovery or may continue for sometime after recovery. Even cases in which the agent can be recovered, may transmit the infection only for a short period. Portal of entry is the route through which the infectious agent enters a host. Portal of exit is the way in which the agent gets excreted from the host. In typhoid, the organism gains entry through mouth and gets excreted in feces. Site of predilection is the tissue or organ in which the organism thrives and causes pathology. For example, in the case of infective hepatitis, the causative hepatitis A virus settles in liver cells causing hepatitis and in Japanese encephalitis the virus affects brain.

❑ IMMUNITY

The defence mechanisms in animals and man play a crucial role in maintaining health. Immunity is the term used to describe the phenomenon by which it is possible to recognize, destroy and eliminate foreign substances (bacteria, viruses and other antigenic substances). Immunity is effected mainly by:

1. Antibodies (immunoglobulins secreted by B lymphocytes—humoral immunity).
2. Phagocytes (like macrophages or polymorphs activated by lymphokines secreted by stimulated T lymphocytes cell-mediated immunity).

Cell-mediated immunity is more vital for health and survival. A child born with defective humoral antibody production can survive for as long as 6 years, while severe defect in cellular immunity can result in death within 6 months afterbirth. Both types of immunity (humoral and cell mediated) operate in tandem in the defence of the body from infectious agents. Immunity is natural, but can also be acquired.

Natural Immunity

A species may be immune to a particular organism by virtue of its bodily constitution or its environment (e.g. frogs are immune to anthrax). Natural defence may be present in the form of enzymes (e.g. lysozymes) and protective covering outside. Immunity developed as a result of clinical or subclinical infection is called active immunity. Immunity derived by babies from the mother through the placenta is called passive immunity, which gives protection to newborn babies for a few months afterbirth.

Acquired Immunity

In contrast to natural immunity, acquired immunity is obtained by vaccination. Antigenic substances (e.g. tetanus toxoid) induce active immunity. Antisera and immunoglobulins [human or animal [e.g. antitetanus serum (ATS), hepatitis B immune globulin (HBIG)] confer passive immunity.

Active Immunity

Humans and animals develop active immunity when they are challenged with an antigenic substance like bacteria, virus or toxins through an overt or subclinical infection and by vaccination. Such immunity is long lasting and specific, but takes a longer time to develop.

Passive Immunity

Passive immunity is obtained by acquiring antibodies either through vaccination with antisera or from mother to fetus through placenta. Such immunity is rapidly induced, but it does not last long. Also there is danger of allergic reactions like serum sickness and anaphylactic shock to the animal sera. However, human sera (e.g. human tetanus immunoglobulin) show less reactogenic propensity.

Herd Immunity

Herd immunity is the term used to describe the level of immunity in a community. When most people are found to have protective antibodies to a specific organism, say typhoid bacilli, the community is said to have a high level of herd immunity against typhoid. The level of herd immunity can be raised by a continuous ongoing vaccination program. Herd structure, which includes not only host species (people), but also other alternate hosts, possible insect vectors, environmental and social factors that will facilitate or inhibit the spread of an infectious disease, plays an important role in the level of immunity in the herd (population). Subclinical and clinical infections also contribute to herd immunity.

When herd immunity level is high in a community, occurrence of an epidemic is highly unlikely as susceptible individuals are surrounded by immune persons. But whether high herd immunity alone is sufficient to eradicate an infectious disease, is doubtful. Other factors like source reduction and improvement of environmental sanitation may also be essential to eliminate infectious diseases. However, in the case of tetanus, herd immunity does not offer protection to susceptible individuals as it is not spread from a case to a susceptible host.

Cross Immunity

When immunity against an infectious agent confers protection against another closely-related organism, it is called cross immunity. Bacillus Calmette-Guérin (BCG) vaccination is known to give some protection against leprosy both the organisms being acid-fast bacilli. It is believed that yellow fever is absent in Asia because of the presence of another closely-related virus, dengue in the region.

❑ IMMUNIZING AGENTS

Immunizing agents are of two types; either they induce active immunity or provide passive protection.

1. Which induce active immunity (antigenic preparations)?
   a. Live vaccines.
   b. Inactivated or killed vaccines.
   c. Toxoids.
   d. Cellular fractions.
2. Which provide passive immunity (antibody preparations)?
   a. Normal immunoglobulins.
   b. Specific immunoglobulins.
   c. Antisera or antitoxin.

Antigenic Preparations

These vaccines contain immunogenic substances, which evoke antibody formation and other immune mechanisms in the recipient. They may be prepared from live attenuated organisms or killed or inactivated organisms, cellular fractions or inactivated toxins or combination of these. Subunit vaccines and recombinant vaccines are recent preparations, which have less adverse effects.

Live Vaccines

Live vaccines, being more potent than killed vaccines, produce a durable immunity. These should be stored at optimal temperature. Storage of vaccines at the specified low temperature (sub-zero) from the places of manufacture till they reach the beneficiaries is described as cold chain maintenance. Cold chain maintenance is essential to keep the potency of the vaccines intact. Ice-lined refrigerator, cold box, vaccine carrier and flasks are some of the appliances used for cold chain maintenance.

Live vaccines are contraindicated in individuals with immune suppression as in the case of diseases like leukemia, lymphoma or malignancy and in persons on treatment with corticosteroids or alkylating agents. German measles vaccine is contraindicated in pregnancy.

Inactivated or Killed Vaccines

Killed or inactivated organisms are used in these preparations. These vaccines are less efficacious than live vaccines, but are useful in immunodeficient individuals in whom live vaccines are contraindicated and they can be stored at 2°C–10°C.

Toxoids

Some organisms such as *Clostridium tetani* and *Corynebacterium diphtheriae* produce toxins, which are responsible for causing disease. Therefore, the toxins and not the organisms themselves are used to prepare vaccines. These toxins are inactivated to produce toxoids, which are used to induce immunity. Toxoids are highly efficacious and safe.

Cellular Fractions

Certain vaccines are prepared from cellular fractions and not from the whole organisms (e.g. meningococcal, pneumococcal polysaccharide vaccines and hepatitis B vaccine and HBsAg polypeptide vaccine).

For ease of administration, combined vaccines are also available. Examples are DPT (diphtheria + pertussis + tetanus), DT (diphtheria + tetanus) and MMR (measles + mumps + rubella). Polyvalent vaccines contain two or more strains of the same species. For example, polio vaccine contains all the three strains. There are Type 1, Type 2 and Type 3. Vaccines are prepared either as plain vaccines or with an adjuvant and also as freeze-dried preparations. Adjuvant vaccines are more efficacious than plain vaccines. Adjuvants added are aluminum phosphate, aluminum hydroxide and water in oil. Freeze-dried preparations are more stable than liquid vaccines.

Antigenic Vaccines

The different types of antigenic vaccines are given in Table 2.1.

Antibody Preparations

Antibody preparations are administered to give immediate protection for the needy, as they are readymade antibodies. They are administered either as intramuscular (IM) or as intravenous (IV) injections. Peak blood levels are reached after 2 days of injection. They should not be given immediately after active immunization against all diseases except tetanus and hepatitis B.

TABLE 2.1: Different types of antigenic vaccines

Vaccines	Examples
Live-attenuated vaccines	
Bacterial	Bacillus Calmette-Guérin (BCG), typhoid oral, plague
Viral	Oral polio, yellow fever, measles, rubella, mumps, influenza
Rickettsial	Epidemic typhus

Contd...

Contd...

Vaccines	Examples
Inactivated or killed vaccines	
Bacterial	Typhoid, cholera, pertussis, CS meningitis, plague
Viral	Rabies, salk (polio), influenza, hepatitis B, Japanese encephalitis, Kyasanur forest disease (KFD)
Toxoids	
Bacterial	Diphtheria, tetanus, botulism

Local adverse reactions like pain, sterile abscesses are common. Rapid systemic reactions like flushing, rigor, dyspnea, shock (anaphylactic type) during or within minutes of administration and late systemic reactions like urticaria, arthralgia, pyrexia or diarrhea within hours or days of injection can occur. Systemic reactions are less common and can be prevented by prior administration of hydrocortisone.

Normal Immunoglobulins

There are five major types of immunoglobulins and they are IgG, IgD, IgM, IgA and IgE. All antibodies are immunoglobulins. Normal immunoglobulins present in human blood are harvested and used as vaccines against some infections (Table 2.2).

Specific Immunoglobulins

While normal immunoglobulins are present in all, specific immunoglobulins are produced in response to vaccination with specific antigens or after suffering from specific infections. Specific immunoglobulins are used against some infections either for prevention or treatment or for both (Table 2.3).

TABLE 2.2: Normal immunoglobulin preparations and their use

Disease	Target	Dose	Use
Hepatitis A	Family contact, institutional outbreaks	Immune globulin (IG) 0.02 mL/kg body weight	Recommended for prevention
	Travelers exposed to unhygienic conditions in developing countries	IG 0.02–0.05 mL/ kg every 4 month	Recommended for prevention
Hepatitis non-A, non-B	Percutaneous or mucosal exposure	IG 0.05 mL/kg	Optional for prevention
Rubella	Women exposed during early pregnancy	IG 20 mL	Optional for prevention
Measles	Infants less than 1 year old or immunosuppressed contacts of acute cases within 6 days of exposure	IG 0.25 mL/kg; 0.5 mL/kg if immuno-suppressed	Recommended for prevention

TABLE 2.3: Specific human immunoglobulin preparations and their use

Disease	Target	Dose	Use
Hepatitis B	Percutaneous or mucosal exposure	Hepatitis B immune globulin (HBIG) 0.05-0.07 mL/kg, repeat in 1 month	Recommended for prevention
	Newborns of mothers with HBsAg	0.05 mL at birth, 3 and 6 month	Recommended for prevention
	Sexual contacts of acute hepatitis B patients	0.05 mL/kg, repeat after 1 month	Optional for prevention
Varicella Zoster	Immunosuppressed contacts of acute cases or newborn contacts	Varicella-zoster immune globulin (VZIG) 15–25 unit/kg (minimum 125 unit)	Recommended for prevention

Contd...

Contd...

Disease	Target	Dose	Use
Rabies	Those exposed to rabid animals	RIG 20 IU/kg	Recommended for prevention
Tetanus	Following significant exposure of unimmunized or partially immunized person or immediately on diagnosis of disease	250 unit for prophylaxis; 3,000–6,000 unit for therapy	Recommended for prevention or treatment

Antisera or Antitoxin

Antisera or antitoxin are prepared from the sera of animals like horses. For diseases like tetanus, diphtheria, botulism, gas gangrene and snakebite, we still depend on animal preparations as human immunoglobulin preparations are either not available or costly. Adverse reactions in the form of serum sickness or anaphylactic shock may occur (Table 2.4).

TABLE 2.4: Antisera/antitoxin preparations and their use

Disease	Dose
Diphtheria	500–1,000 international unit of diphtheria antitoxin (ADS), IM to contacts immediately after exposure. Protection not more than 2–3 week.
Tetanus	1,500 international unit of tetanus antitoxin (ATS*-horse), subcutaneous or IM soon after injury.
Gas gangrene	Polyvalent antitoxin—10,000 unit of *Clostridium perfringens,* 5,000 unit of *Clostridium septicum,* 10,000 unit of *Clostridium oedematiens*—IM or IV.
Rabies	40 international unit/kg of antirabies serum (ARS).
Botulism	10,000 unit of polyvalent antitoxin every 3–4 hour.

*ATS, antitetanus serum

Hazards of Immunization

Local reactions like pain, swelling, tenderness, sterile abscess and general reactions like fever, malaise and headache can occur.

Faulty techniques in the preparation of vaccine like inadequate inactivation or detoxification and faulty sterilization methods may result in adverse reactions. Improper sterilization of needles and syringes can lead to abscess formation and spread of hepatitis B and AIDS (Table 2.5).

TABLE 2.5: Contraindications to vaccines

Vaccine	Contraindications
All vaccines	A severe adverse event following a dose of vaccine (e.g. anaphylaxis,* encephalitis/encephalopathy or non-febrile convulsions) is a true contraindication to further immunization with the antigen concerned and a subsequent dose should not be given. Current serious illness.
Live vaccines (MMR,† BCG, yellow fever)	Pregnancy, radiation therapy (i.e. total body radiation).
Yellow fever	Egg allergy. Immunodeficiency (from medication, disease or symptomatic HIV infection‡).
BCG	Symptomatic HIV infection.
Influenza, yellow fever	History of anaphylactic reactions as a following egg ingestion. No vaccines prepared in hen's influenza vaccines should be given (vaccine viruses propagated in chicken fibroblast cells, e.g. measles or MMR vaccines, can usually be given however).
Pertussis-containing vaccines	A serious reaction to a dose of DTP. The pertussis component should be omitted for subsequent doses and diphtheria and tetanus immunization completed with DT vaccine. Evolving neurological disease (e.g. uncontrolled epilepsy or progressive encephalopathy). Vaccines containing the whole-cell pertussis component should not be given to children with this problem. Acellular vaccine is less reactogenic and is used in many industrialized countries instead of whole-cell pertussis vaccine.

*Generalized urticaria, difficulty in breathing, swelling of the mouth and throat, hypotension or shock; †MMR, measles, mumps and rubella; ‡In many industrialized countries, yellow fever vaccine is administered to individuals with symptomatic HIV infection or who are suffering from other immunodeficiency diseases provided that their CD4 count is at least 400 cells/mm^3 and if they plan to visit areas, where epidemic or endemic yellow fever actually occurs. *(Adapted from* Vaccine-preventable diseases, vaccines and vaccination (WHO) chapter 6, 2005).

Hypersensitivity reactions can occasionally occur. Antisera (e.g. ATS) can give rise to serum sickness or anaphylactic shock. Neurological complications may also be seen occasionally. Post-vaccinal encephalitis and encephalopathy after antirabies vaccine (ARV) and smallpox vaccines respectively are examples.

Provocative reaction like provocative poliomyelitis after the administration of alum precipitated toxoid (APT) against diphtheria may be produced.

Precautions to be Taken

Testing for sensitivity must be done prior to administration of any antitoxin or antiserum. A drop of the preparation instilled into eye will produce pricking sensation, if the person is hypersensitive to the preparation or 0.2 mL of preparation diluted with (1:10) saline may be injected intradermally in the skin over anterior aspect of forearm. Sensitized persons will develop a wheel and flare within 10 minutes. But, one should bear in mind that reactions can occur even after a negative sensitivity test. Adrenaline and hydrocortisone with an extra sterile syringe should always be kept ready while giving antiserum. Adults should be injected 0.5 mL of adrenaline IM immediately after a reaction followed by 0.5 mL every 20 minutes if systolic blood pressure is below 100 mm of Hg. Antihistamine like chlorpheniramine maleate in 10–20 mg dose may also be given. All people who have received serum injections should be asked to wait for at least half an hour for observation before sending back home. National immunization schedule and new vaccines are detailed in Tables 2.6 and 2.7 respectively.

TABLE 2.6: National immunization schedule for infants, children and pregnant women

Vaccine	When to give	Dose	Route	Site
For infants				
BCG	At birth or as early as possible till 1 year of age	0.1 mL (0.05 mL until 1 month age)	Intradermal	Left upper arm
Hepatitis B*	At birth or as early as possible within 24 hour	0.5 mL	Intramuscular	Anterolateral side of mid thigh

Contd...

Contd...

Vaccine	When to give	Dose	Route	Site
Oral polio vaccine (OPV)-0	At birth or as early as possible within the first 15 day	2 drops	Oral	Oral
OPV 1,2 and 3	At 6 week, 10 week and 14 week	2 drops	Oral	Oral
Diptheria, tetanus and pertussis (DPT) 1,2 and 3	At 6 week, 10 week and 14 week	0.5 mL	Intramuscular	Anterolateral side of mid thigh
Hepatitis B 1,2 and 3	At 6 week, 10 week and 14 week	0.5 mL	Intramuscular	Anterolateral side of mid thigh
Measles	9–12 month (give up to 5 year if not received at 9–12 month age)	0.5 mL	Subcutaneous	Right upper arm
Vitamin A 1st dose	At 9 month with measles vaccine	1 mL (1 lakh IU)	Oral	Oral
For children				
DPT booster	16–24 month	0.5 mL	Intramuscular	Anterolateral side of mid thigh
OPV booster	16–24 month	2 drops	Oral	Oral
Japanese encephalitis†	16–24 month with DPT/OPV booster	0.5 mL	Subcutaneous	Left upper arm
Vitamin A‡ (2nd–9th dose)	16 month with DPT/OPV booster, then one dose every 6 month up to the age of 5 year	2 mL (2 lakh IU)	Oral	Oral
DPT booster	5–6 year	0.5 mL	Intramuscular	Upper arm

Contd...

Contd...

Vaccine	When to give	Dose	Route	Site
Tetanus toxoid (TT)	10 year and 16 year	0.5 mL	Intramuscular	Upper arm
For pregnant women				
TT-1	Early in pregnancy	0.5 mL	Intramuscular	Upper arm
TT-2	4 week after TT-1§	0.5 mL	Intramuscular	Upper arm
TT-Booster	If received 2 TT doses in a pregnancy within the last 3 year*	0.5 mL	Intramuscular	Upper arm

*In select states, districts and cities; †SA 14-12-2 vaccine, in select endemic districts after the campaign; ‡The 2nd to 9th doses of vitamin A can be administered to children 1–5 year old during biannual rounds, in collaboration with ICDS; §Give TT-2 or booster doses before 36 weeks of pregnancy. However, give these even if more than 36 weeks have passed. Give TT to a woman in labor, if she has not previously received TT. (*Adapted from* Immunization Handbook for Medical Officers (revised edition, 2009) Department of Health and Family Welfare. Ministry of Health and Family Welfare, GOI, 2009).

❑ PREVENTION AND CONTROL OF COMMUNICABLE DISEASES

Main aim of public health measures is to prevent diseases. At times because the preventive measures are not undertaken properly, we do get epidemic form of communicable diseases.

In such situations, we have to resort to control of the epidemic. Prevention and control of communicable diseases are achieved by:

1. Control of the reservoir of infection (treatment of cases, subclinical cases and carriers).
2. Breaking the chain of transmission (control of vectors, vehicle, etc.).
3. Equipping the susceptible people to resist the diseases by activating their defence mechanisms by immunization.

Continuous surveillance mechanisms should operate to assess the situation with regard to the number of cases at a specific time, the environmental factors that help or inhibit the transmission, the behavior and mobility of population, their immune status,

TABLE 2.7: New vaccines

Disease and vaccine	Age	Dose	Schedule	Route and site	Booster	Main contraindications (refer to manufacturer)
Measles, mumps, rubella (MMR)	12–15 month	0.5 mL	1 dose	SC Upper arm	No	Advanced immunodeficiency or immunosuppression, pregnancy, severe allergic reaction to vaccine component or following a prior dose
Measles, rubella (MR)	16–24 month	0.5 mL	1 dose	SC Upper arm	No	Advanced immunodeficiency or immunosuppression, pregnancy, severe allergic reaction to vaccine component or following a prior dose
Typhoid Whole cell typhoid vaccine Vi polysaccharide vaccine	 6–9 month onwards At or after 2 year	 0.25 mL/0.5 mL 0.5 mL	 2 doses 4 week apart 1 dose	SC Upper arm IM	 3–5 year 3 year	Severe allergic reaction to vaccine component or following a prior dose

Contd...

Contd...

Disease and vaccine	Age	Dose	Schedule	Route and site	Booster	Main contraindications (refer to manufacturer)
Typhoid oral Ty 21 a	5 year and above		3 capsules on alternate day	Oral Mouth	3–7 year	
Streptococcus pneumoniae	Below 6 months	0.5 mL	3 doses given at ages 2,4,6 month (minimum interval 4 week)	IM	12–15 month (minimum interval 8 week)	Severe allergic reaction to vaccine component or following a prior dose
Pneumococcal PCV7	7–11 month		2 doses 4 week apart	Upper arm	No	Moderate or severe acute illness
	12–23 month		1 dose			
	24–59 month		1 dose			
Pneumococcal PPV23	> 2 year (high risk)	25 μg in 0.5 mL	1 dose	IM or SC Upper arm	No	

Contd...

Contd...

Disease and vaccine	Age	Dose	Schedule	Route and site	Booster	Main contraindications (refer to manufacturer)
Hemophilus influenzae type B HibPRP-T, PRP-OMP and PRP-CRM 197 conjugate vaccine	Initiate at 6 week	0.5 mL	6, 10, 14 week	IM	No	Severe allergic reaction to vaccine component or following a prior dose
				Upper arm		Moderate or severe acute illness
Rota virus diarrhea Rotarix™	Initiate before 12 week		6 week, 10 week (no later than 24 week)	Oral		Severe allergic reaction to vaccine component or following a prior dose of vaccine; infants with H/O intussusceptions/ intestinal malformations
				Mouth		
RotaTeq™			2,4,6 month(to be completed by 32 week)			

Adapted from Immunization Handbook for Medical Officers (revised edition 2009). Department of Health and Family Welfare. Ministry of Health and Family Welfare, GOI, 2009.

the vectors if any, etc. in order to bring the disease under control. Only when the surveillance mechanisms are not functioning properly, disease incidence and prevalence rise. Removal of the weakest link in the chain of transmission may be all that is necessary to control a communicable disease. However, attention to all the three aspects namely the reservoir, host and the mode of transmission of the disease, though costly, may become necessary in some situations.

Control of Reservoir

Controlling the reservoir is essential to stop the spread immediately. The cases, subclinical cases and carriers, animal reservoirs and vectors constitute the reservoir pool.

Early diagnosis is important to treat all the cases, to start epidemiological investigations and to start control measures. However, subclinical cases and incubatory carriers may pose problem in the control.

Notification of an infectious disease to local health authority helps to initiate control measures quickly. Diseases, which are considered a serious threat to the health of the public, are to be notified statutorily. However, notifiable diseases vary from country to country and also from one state to another within a country.

Notification is done by the attending physician, head of the family, teachers, religious and political leaders or anyone including lay people and it can be done even on suspicion. Certain diseases are to be notified to World Health Organization (WHO) by the National Health Authority (NHA) under the International Health Regulations (IHR). The infectious diseases reportable under the IHR (2005) include unusual diseases such as smallpox, wild poliovirus infection, human influenza (new subtype), severe acute respiratory syndrome (SARS); epidemic-prone diseases such as cholera, pneumonic plague, yellow fever, viral hemorrhagic fevers, West Nile fever and diseases of special regional concern such as dengue fever.

Epidemiological investigations, with regard to geographical situation and climatic condition, character of the disease causing agent, reservoir, vector and vehicle, social, cultural and behavioral patterns of people and the susceptible host population, will help in the effective control of infectious diseases.

Ring immunization is a method in which the susceptible population is encircled by a ring of immune persons. This method was adopted to eradicate smallpox in 1960s and 1970s and now being used in the eradication of polio and measles.

Isolation of the sick from the rest during the period of communicability is useful in the control of diseases like cholera, diphtheria, pneumonic plague, etc. But, in diseases in which inapparent or subclinical cases, outnumber clinical cases (iceberg phenomenon), isolation may not be of much use, e.g. mumps, influenza. Physical isolation is now replaced by chemical isolation in the control of diseases like leprosy and tuberculosis in order to prevent the concealment of the symptoms by the sufferers for fear of ostracization by the community. The infected persons are treated vigorously with chemotherapeutic agents and are made non-infective quickly; and thereby prevent the transmission of the infectious agent from the cases to susceptible hosts.

Quarantine is a method in which apparently healthy individuals are kept under observation for the maximum known incubation period of the communicable disease. Quarantine is practiced for specific infectious diseases at airports and seaports, where people from foreign endemic countries arrive. It also may be applied to train, bus or other carrier passengers. Quarantine as a method of disease control has become outdated now.

Treatment of cases and carriers plays an important role in the control of spread of an infectious disease. In diseases like leprosy and tuberculosis, early treatment is of utmost importance to reduce the severity of the diseases as well as to interrupt transmission. When a disease is endemic mass treatment may be resorted to wherein all people in the area irrespective of whether they have the disease or not are treated, e.g. trachoma, filariasis.

Blocking the Transmission

This part of the control measure comes mainly under the purview of public health personnel. Diseases like cholera, diarrhea, dysentery, typhoid, infective hepatitis, gastroenteritis, etc. are transmitted from one person to another through vehicles like contaminated water, food or milk. So, purification of water, food hygiene and pasteurization of milk will prevent the transfer of pathogens. Personal hygiene measures like hand washing before and after food, avoiding open defecation, control of fly breeding all will prevent the spread of waterborne and foodborne infectious diseases. Control of vectors like housefly and mosquitoes; and keeping the environment clean so that the breeding of these vectors is prevented, can arrest the transmission of vector borne diseases like malaria, filariasis. Transmission of respiratory diseases like tuberculosis, diphtheria, whooping cough, etc. can be controlled by having proper ventilation and avoiding overcrowding. Health education to people against indiscriminate spitting and to cover their nose and mouth, while sneezing and coughing is also important in this regard.

Improving the Resistance of the Host

The susceptible host or people at risk can be protected to some extent by immunizing them either actively or passively. Diseases like diphtheria, polio, tetanus and measles have been controlled by active immunization. There are vaccines for many diseases, while at the same time we have not been able to produce vaccines for many other diseases like malaria, leprosy, AIDS, etc. Temporary protection by means of either human immunoglobulins or animal antitoxin or antisera also can be given to susceptible individuals. The important problem in vaccination programs in developing countries is the difficulty in cold chain maintenance. Peoples' participation is also not good. But, it should be borne in mind that vaccination programs are only supplements and the main endeavor should be to improve the nutrition, environmental sanitation and the standard of life of people through long-term programs for socioeconomic development.

Chemoprophylaxis

Prevention of communicable diseases by administering appropriate drugs to susceptible people is called chemoprophylaxis. Infectious diseases like malaria, plague, rheumatic fever, STDs, etc. can be prevented by this method. Healthcare personnel in infectious disease control, tourists entering endemic regions and family contacts of infectious cases can be protected by this strategy.

Other Measures

Measures like enactment of public health laws in parliament have contributed for the control of many diseases. But, at the same time, it should be realized that the behavioral change of people and their active participation in health programs alone can bring about a radical change in the health and disease scenario of any nation.

❑ SURVEILLANCE

Surveillance is described as the scrutiny of all aspects of occurrence and spread of diseases undertaken with the aim of bringing about an effective control. Surveillance has three basic component activities—data collection, analysis and dissemination.

It is not just mere reporting of cases, but includes laboratory investigation to confirm the diagnosis, detection of source of infection and routes of transmission, identification of all cases and the susceptible contacts, collection of morbidity and mortality data and their consolidation and rapid dissemination of the knowledge to those who are responsible for the control measures.

Surveillance is called active surveillance when it is done by specially employed people in vertical or special programs. Sentinel surveillance is the collection and analysis of data by designated institutions selected for their geographic location, medical specialty and ability to accurately diagnose and report high quality data. Interested and competent physicians or institutions can be the active sentinel centers. This system may be less costly than developing and maintaining ongoing notification system. Generally, sentinel surveillance is useful for answering specific epidemiologic questions, but because sentinel sites may not represent the general population or the general incidence of disease, they may have limited usefulness in analyzing national disease patterns and trends. If already existing facilities and staff (PHCs and hospitals) are involved in the process of surveillance it is called passive surveillance. WHO is maintaining surveillance system to monitor diseases like influenza, malaria, paralytic polio, louse-borne typhus, etc.

Both passive and active surveillance systems have advantages and disadvantages, which must be weighed when planning.

Passive systems can suffer from under reporting or compromised accuracy of reporting and show selection bias depending on the source of reports or laboratory specimens. Registries can be rather slow and expensive. However, passive systems can often be effective in an acceptable period. Active surveillance can produce early, timely and complete information, but methodology must be carefully developed and data interpreted. Active sentinel systems can also be expensive to maintain. No single surveillance tool is perfect and usually combinations of approaches will provide the best results.

Investigation of an Epidemic

Epidemics cause emergency calling for prompt control measures. The epidemiologist will have to travel to and work on locations in the field and the investigation is likely to be limited because of the need to take timely action. Epidemiologists, in field investigations, perform two things. First they collect particulars that describe the place of outbreak, i.e. the time of occurrence of the epidemic from where the epidemic was acquired and secondly what the characteristics of the illness are. These are the descriptive aspects of the investigation. Mostly these particulars will suffice to determine the source and the mode of transmission of the agent and to identify those at risk of developing the disease. However, in certain circumstances it will be difficult to determine the above facts from descriptive studies alone. Therefore, as a next step, analytical studies will have to be conducted in order to get the answers for the above questions. In analytical part of investigation, epidemiologists compare ill and well people; exposed and not exposed both believed to be at risk of contracting the disease in question to determine what exposure ill people had, which well people did not, using appropriate statistical techniques. If the differences between ill and well are greater than what one would expect by chance, inferences regarding the transmission and exposure to the disease can be drawn.

Steps

The following steps are usually involved in an epidemic field investigation:

1. Existence of an epidemic may be obvious in most situations like common source epidemics of cholera, jaundice etc. But, when there is some doubt, this can be ascertained by comparing the disease frequencies during the same period of previous years. To determine the existence of an epidemic one may need to collect information from schools or factories for absentee records, outpatient clinics, hospitals, laboratory records or death certificates. Simple survey of practicing physicians will strongly support the existence of an epidemic. Rapid household surveys in the community will throw light on the situation. To establish an epidemic, specific diagnosis is not important. Signs and symptoms will do. Usually two standard errors from the endemic occurrence are taken as epidemic threshold for common diseases such as influenza.
2. Verification of diagnosis on the spot by examining sample cases is all that is necessary to arrive at a diagnosis. Laboratory tests such as serology and/or isolation of the causative agent may be needed to confirm the diagnosis. If 15%–20% cases are laboratory confirmed that would do. However, several representative cases should be examined and confirmed by a physician.
3. Data collected is oriented with reference to time, place and person. This exercise should begin without waiting for the epidemic to end:
   a. By constructing an epidemic curve time clustering of cases can be observed, which may suggest whether it is a common source or a propagated (person-to-person) epidemic or both.
   b. Water supplies, milk distribution routes, sewage disposal outflows, prevailing wind currents, airflow patterns in buildings and ecological habitats of animals may play important roles in the dissemination of pathogens and in determining who is at risk of contracting the disease. If cases are plotted geographically a pattern of distribution may emerge. Such spot maps of cases (place distribution) will throw light on the vehicle or the mode of transmission. John snow was able to demonstrate that contaminated water in Thames was responsible for the classic cholera outbreak in London by using spot map.

c. Next the characteristics of the patient themselves (person distribution) in respect of age, sex, occupation and other factors that may be useful in portraying the uniqueness of the case population are examined.

Studying the time, place or person distribution or agent-host-environment relationship, possible source, causative agent, mode of spread and environmental factors related to the epidemic can be delineated.

4. Determine who is at risk of becoming ill. After the descriptive studies with reference to time, place and person distribution, a firm conclusion as to why and how the epidemic started can be arrived at. But still it is essential that some analytical studies are carried out to know that some other people in some other area are not at risk of developing the disease. This is done by looking for similar illnesses in other groups and comparing the illness rates in both the groups. Census of the entire population or subgroups depending upon the need must be taken by house to house visits. Size of the population is needed to compute the attack rates in various groups and subgroups.
5. Simultaneously rapid search for cases should be undertaken. For this purpose an accepted usual presentation of the disease with or without laboratory confirmation is taken as the guideline for case definition. A simple easily applicable definition should be used recognizing that some cases may be missed and some non-cases may be included. But, the case definition criteria once formed should be applied equally and without bias to all persons under investigation. Number of cases alone may not be sufficient. Particulars regarding name, age, sex, occupation, social class, travel, history of previous exposure, time of onset of disease, signs and symptoms of the illness, personal contacts at home, work, school and other places, special events like the parties attended, foods eaten and exposure to common vehicles such as water, food and milk, visits out of the community, history of receiving injections or blood products, attendance at large gatherings, etc. should be collected in the case sheet not only from cases but also from persons exposed, but unaffected.

Information collected should be relevant to the disease under study. If the disease under investigation is a waterborne or foodborne infection exposure to various water and food sources should be elicited. In diseases of person to person contact, frequency, duration and nature of personal contacts will have to be obtained. If the nature of the disease is unknown, questions relating to all possible aspects of transmission and risk should be raised. A case review form will ensure completeness and consistency of the data collected.

6. Search for new cases (secondary cases) should be carried out every day till the area is declared free of epidemic since the occurrence of the last case, for twice the incubation period of the disease.
7. Develop a hypothesis that explains the specific exposure that caused the disease and test the hypothesis by appropriate statistical methods.

   By the earlier exercises, the most likely source and the mode of transmission must have been ascertained. But still the most likely exposure that caused the disease must be found out by analytical studies. If the epidemic is a foodborne infection, the particular food among the various food items consumed by the affected persons that caused the disease must be identified by finding out the eating rates and attack rates with reference to all the items of food individually. By comparing these attack rates or exposure rates between the different food items the actual food that caused the epidemic can be found out.

   This phase of investigation is the most challenging one. The findings should be reviewed carefully; the clinical, laboratory and epidemiological features weighed and the possible exposures that could plausibly cause the disease hypothesized. If the exposure histories for ill and well are not significantly different, a new hypothesis should be developed, which may require resurveying of those at risk to obtain more pertinent information.
8. Compare the hypothesis with the established facts.

   Next it is essential to see that the hypothesis arrived at fits well with the known facts of the disease. For example, if it is an epidemic of food poisoning caused by staphylococci, the incriminated food should be one that can favor staphylococcal growth. If it is not the whole exercise should be reviewed and a new hypothesis tested. In a field investigation when the disease is undiagnosed, it is difficult to fit a hypothesis to the natural history of the disease in question.

9. Plan a more systematic study.

   More detailed and carefully executed studies are to be conducted to improve the specificity and sensitivity of the case definition and to establish the true number of persons at risk that is to improve the quality of numerator and the denominator. For example, serosurveys coupled with a more complete clinical history can often increase the accuracy of the case count and define more clearly those truly at risk of developing the disease. Repeat interviews of patients with confirmed disease may be useful to quantify the degree of exposure or dose response.
10. Hypotheses generated should be weighed and tested by comparing the attack rates between those exposed and those not exposed to each suspected factor.
11. Epidemic investigation also involves evaluation of ecological factors like sanitary status of hotels, water and milk supply, breakdown in water supply system, population mobility, atmospheric changes such as temperature, humidity and air pollution, bionomics of insects and animal reservoirs. This can give a lead to the source(s), reservoirs and mode of transmission.
12. Preparation of written report.

    The report of investigation should contain the findings and the recommendations.

Administrative/Operational Purposes

A document for action: The investigation report will form the basis for control and preventive action. Even if the investigation is not complete, still a reasonable assumption and recommendation can usually be made.

A record of performance: The report is also a record of accomplishment of the investigative team. Magnitude of health problems, changes in disease trends and the results of control and preventive efforts are brought out in the report.

A document for potential medical/legal issues: Reports prepared objectively, honestly and fairly may prove absolutely invaluable to consumers, practicing physicians or local and provincial health department officials in any legal action regarding health responsibilities and jurisdiction. Honest documentation of events and findings made available for interpretation and comment will serve the public better.

Scientific/Epidemiological Purposes

Enhancement of the quality of the investigation: The process of writing and viewing data in written form often generates new and different thought processes and associations in the minds of the epidemiologist. Committing to the paper the various findings of the investigation will lead to better understanding of the natural unfolding of the events. Previously unrecognized associations will sometimes emerge from a careful and step-by-step written analysis that may be critical in the final interpretation and recommendation. Written reports may stimulate further enquiry and fact finding in order to verify the earlier assumption.

An instrument for teaching epidemiology: The exercise of writing the results of an investigation constitutes an essential building block in learning epidemiology.

PART B

Specific Infections

CHAPTER

3

Respiratory Infections

Air has direct access to respiratory passage right up to the alveoli. Air is often the vehicle for the transmission of microorganisms from man to man or from environment to man. As the control of air quality is a difficult proposition respiratory infections are common.

Some important respiratory infections discussed here are the following:

- Smallpox
- Chickenpox
- Measles
- German measles
- Mumps
- Influenza
- Common cold
- Diphtheria
- Whooping cough
- Tuberculosis
- Meningococcal meningitis
- Severe acute respiratory syndrome (SARS)
- Avian influenza (bird flu) in humans
- Swine influenza in humans
- Acute respiratory infections (ARI).

❑ SMALLPOX

Smallpox Eradication—A Success Story

Smallpox was once a killer disease occurring throughout the world having an annual incidence of 10 million cases. An orthopox virus, the variola virus (variola major and variola minor) is the causative agent. WHO started the program of global eradication of smallpox in 1967. India's last case was reported in May 1975 and after a period of 2 years it was declared smallpox free in April 1977 by International Commission for Assessment of Smallpox Eradication. The last case reported in the world was in October 1977 in Somalia except for a laboratory accident in 1978 in Birmingham (UK). Since then the world is free from smallpox. WHO declared the global eradication of smallpox in May 1980 (Fig. 3.1).

The epidemiological features that favored the eradication of smallpox are:

1. The variola virus, the causative agent of smallpox, causes disease only in human beings and no extra human reservoir is known.
2. No carrier state is seen and subclinical cases played no significant role in the transmission.
3. The evolution of an outbreak is slow and therefore control is easy.
4. Secondary attack rate is low.
5. Availability of a potent vaccine, which conferred prolonged protection.
6. Lifelong immunity after recovery from the disease.
7. The disease is easily recognizable even by non-medical personnel and international cooperation.

Since the disease has been eradicated, it is no longer necessary to vaccinate anyone except those who handle vaccine virus for research and vaccine production and those who investigate human monkeypox cases directly.

Currently, variola virus is known to be stored in two facilities—the CDC in Atlanta and the Russian State Center for Research on Virology and Biotechnology, Koltsovo, Novosibirsk region, Russian federation. In the early 1980s, WHO recommended that all existing stocks of variola virus held in other countries be either destroyed or shipped to one of the two WHO-approved collaborating centers. All countries reported compliance.

The poxvirus infection in humans in future can come from two sources namely the laboratories, which preserve the virus and the animal poxviruses.

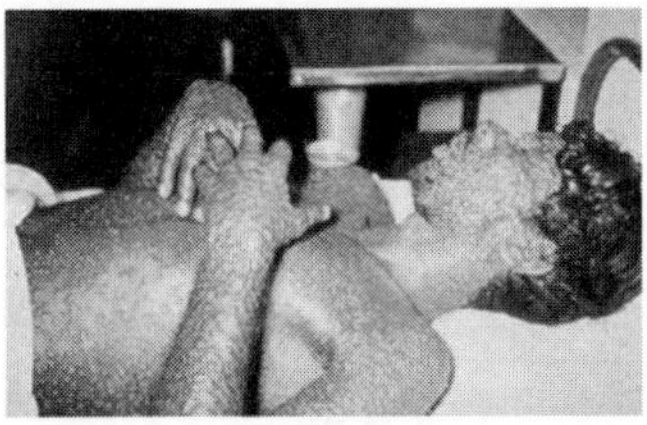

Figure 3.1: Smallpox in an adult [*Courtesy:* Barbra Rice, Centers for Disease Control and Prevention (CDC), Public Health Images Library, May 2001].

The other poxviruses that resemble smallpox virus are monkeypox, cowpox, camelpox, tanapox and tateropox. The monkeypox virus and the tanapox virus have caused diseases in man in Africa. Both are zoonotic diseases that affect man accidentally.

Antibodies against monkeypox virus were identified in several squirrel and monkey species as well as in other wild-caught animals in the endemic areas indicating that monkeypox virus may have a broad reservoir range. Immunity from smallpox vaccination protects against monkeypox with > 85% efficacy. However, currently available smallpox vaccines should not be used in monkeypox-endemic areas until the epidemiologic picture of monkeypox and the risks from vaccination are clarified.

Smallpox vaccine stock enough for 200 million people is maintained by WHO in Geneva, Toronto and New Delhi to meet the needs in the event of an accidental outbreak.

❑ CHICKENPOX

Chickenpox is a childhood disease affecting children below 10 years. It is a highly infectious disease with secondary attack rate (SAR) approaching 90%. It occurs in all parts of the world. Annual incidence is 80–90 million cases.

In India, it shows a seasonal trend occurring in summer months. Though it is mainly a childhood disease, current epidemiological data shows an increasing incidence of first infections in older age groups. The reason for this is not known, but this has important consequences as the infection is more serious in adults and pregnant women.

Causative organism is varicella-zoster (VZ) virus, the human (alpha) herpes virus 3. It is a double-stranded DNA virus belonging to the herpes virus family. Only one serotype is known.

Reservoir and Source

Man is the only reservoir. Cases, inapparent cases and herpes zoster cases constitute the reservoir pool. Nasopharyngeal secretion and vesicular fluid are the source of infective material. Scabs are not infectious. A hospital outbreak of chickenpox in which the source of infection was a cadaver has been reported in India.

Mode of Transmission

Chickenpox is transmitted through droplet infection and droplet nuclei. This virus can cross the placenta and infect the fetus.

Chickenpox can be contracted from herpes zoster (shingles) cases also. Herpes zoster is caused by the same VZ virus and it occurs in individuals who have already had chickenpox. The latent virus gets reactivated when immunity is lowered.

Factors Facilitating Transmission

Overcrowding, ignorance and viral shedding even before the appearance of rashes are some factors, which favor transmission.

Period of communicability commences 1–2 days before the appearance of rash and continues for 4–5 days after the appearance.

Incubation Period

Usually 2 weeks, but may vary between 7 and 23 days.

Clinical Manifestation

Clinical spectrum varies from a mild to severe illness with widespread rash. About 80% of all reported cases occur in children below 10 years of age.

Pre-eruptive stage characterized by sudden onset of fever, shivering, malaise and back pain is followed by eruptive stage after 24–48 hours. The rashes will be distributed more on the trunk (centripetal distribution) unlike in smallpox in which the rashes are present more on the face and extremities (centrifugal distribution). All forms of rashes (macule, papule, vesicle and pustule) can be observed at any point of time (pleomorphism) in chickenpox (Fig. 3.2), whereas in smallpox only one type of rash will be present at a given moment. The evolution of the rashes is completed by the 5th day after which scabbing begins. Scabs may remain intact for 1–3 weeks.

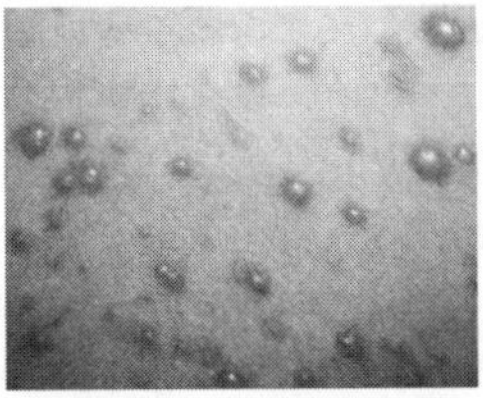

Figure 3.2: Chickenpox vesicles (pleomorphism) *(Courtesy:* Joe Miller-CDC)

Complications like secondary bacterial infection of the skin lesions and pneumonia in adults may occur. Very rarely encephalitis may be a complication. Usually an attack confers lifelong immunity. Herpes zoster manifests as rashes along the course of a peripheral nerve.

Prevention and Control

Japan was among the first countries to vaccinate against chickenpox. Field trials with the Japanese live attenuated vaccine have shown that it is safe and effective. Early childhood immunization is given (single dose) at 12–24 months of age. In adolescents and adults two subcutaneous doses, 4–8 weeks apart are advised.

A routine varicella vaccination program for healthy children would prevent 94% of all potential cases of chickenpox provided the vaccination coverage rate is 97% at school entry. But in India, chickenpox vaccine does not form part of the National Immunization Schedule. Since the vaccine is costly, not everyone can afford it. Thus chickenpox virus still exists in the community.

Contraindications are pregnancy, reaction to previous dose (including reaction to a component such as gelatin), any advanced immune disorder or cellular immune deficiency, symptomatic

HIV infection and severe illness. Adverse reactions include mild local reaction and mild illness with rash.

Control can be achieved by isolation of patients and separation of high risk individuals from cases. Cyclovir is an approved drug for the acute management of varicella in children and adults. When Cyclovir is given within the first 24 hours of the onset of rash in children, constitutional symptoms and pruritus are diminished. Number of lesions and the time for crusting are also reduced. In immunocompromised patients intravenous Cyclovir is indicated.

Children with varicella should not be given Aspirin because of the increased risk of Reye's syndrome, which is a serious condition that may affect all major systems or organs.

Immunosuppressed persons may be protected by giving varicella-zoster immunoglobulin (VZIG) within 72 hours of exposure.

❑ MEASLES (RUBEOLA)

Measles is an acute highly infectious childhood disease, which occurs both in endemic and epidemic form. Epidemics occur once in 2–3 years because of waning immunity among the people (Fig. 3.3).

There were an estimated 30–40 million cases of measles in 2000 causing some 777,000 deaths worldwide. Number of reported cases globally in 2011 has come down to 344,276. Number of measles deaths also has dropped from 777,000 in 2000 to 139,300 in 2010 globally.

Mostly children were the victims. The biggest decline (90%) occurred in the Eastern Mediterranean region.

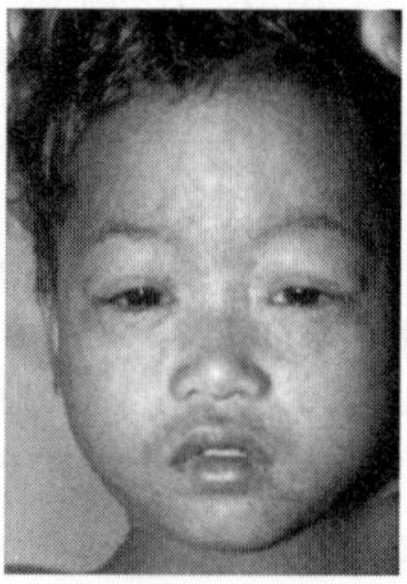

Figure 3.3: Measles *(Courtesy:* Centers for Disease Control and Prevention)

India is still haunted by measles despite the availability of an effective vaccine for over 40 years. The disease burden is high. 29,339 cases were reported in 2011, which is a little less than in 2010. Factors such as malnutrition, overcrowding and low socioeconomic status add to the mortality and morbidity.

Causative organism is an RNA paramyxovirus.

The virus has a single serotype although 23 genotypes have been identified. Infection by any genotype can induce lifelong immunity against all genotypes. All major epidemics in European region were associated with genotypes D4, D6 and B3. In India, genotypes D4 and D8 have been identified (WHO, Feb 2012).

Incubation period is 11–12 days usually, but may vary from 8 to 16 days. The patient is infectious from the prodromal period up to the first few days of the rash.

Reservoir and Source

Measles cases form the reservoir. No extra human reservoir is known. Inapparent infection and long carrier state is not seen. Respiratory secretion is the source of infective material.

Mode of Transmission

Measles is a highly infectious disease with secondary attack rate of over 80%. Transmission occurs by means of droplet infection and droplet nuclei and the virus enters through the respiratory tract. Unlike poliomyelitis, recipients of measles vaccine are not infectious to others.

Factors Facilitating Transmission

Overcrowding, population mobility, ignorance and superstitious beliefs favor transmission.

Clinical Manifestation

Measles is a disease of children. Infants below 6 months may not be affected if they have maternal antibodies. This disease runs a very severe course in malnourished children and the mortality is 400 times higher in the malnourished than in well-nourished children.

Two stages of the disease are described. During the initial pre-eruptive prodromal stage, the child will have fever, cough, sneezing, running nose and congestion of eyes, which may last 3–4 days. Two days prior to the appearance of rash, red spots with a pale surrounding called 'Koplik's spots' may be seen over the buccal mucosa opposite to the upper second molar tooth and it is a pathognomonic feature of measles. The eruptive stage is heralded by the appearance of maculopapular rashes first on the face and then over the trunk and extremities. The fever comes down 3–5 days after the appearance of rashes. The rashes begin to fade after 5–6 days and may leave a brownish discoloration on the skin.

Although usually a mild illness in children, measles can have serious complications and be fatal to children who are immunosuppressed. Among those who survive measles, up to 10% may suffer disabilities such as blindness, deafness and irreversible brain damage. Commonest complications are otitis media and pneumonia. Postmeasles diarrhea is another common complication, which often precipitates protein energy malnutrition (PEM) in infants. Serious complications like encephalitis may occur in 1 in 1,000 cases. Subacute sclerosing panencephalitis (SSPE) and multiple sclerosis (MS) may follow measles. Measles during pregnancy may result in prematurity, fetal wastage and congenital defects.

Prevention and Control

Immunizing agents both active and passive are available against measles. Immunoglobulin (human dose 0.25 mL/kg body weight with a maximum 15 mL) given within 3 days of exposure can protect those with deficient immunity.

Immunity can be induced actively by measles vaccine, a live attenuated vaccine. Freeze-dried measles vaccine has to be stored at recommended temperature. Now heat-stable vaccines are also available. One dose gives 95% protection for at least 15 years. Measles vaccine is advised for infants above 9 months of age, but not below that age because maternal antibodies may interfere with the antibody production. Susceptible contacts can be protected by measles vaccine, if the vaccine is given within 3 days of exposure. Very rarely serious complication like SSPE may be produced by the vaccine, the incidence of which is much less than that in natural infection.

Between 1985 and 1988, it was found that the children who received only 1 dose were not always protected from the disease. This led to the recommendation of a 2nd dose for children between the ages of 5 and 19 years to ensure protection. According to UNICEF, India is the only country in the world giving only 1 dose of measles vaccine. But according to experts 1 dose of measles vaccine is not sufficient to give protection to the whole population against measles.

It has also been found that the premature infants respond as well as the full-term infants to MMR vaccination and chickenpox vaccination. Therefore giving MMR and chickenpox vaccines on time to premature babies is the best way to protect these children from these diseases.

Measles vaccine is better avoided during pregnancy. It is contraindicated in immunocompromized children, those on steroid therapy and those with history of convulsions, allergy or eczema, acute illness and active tuberculosis.

Control is achieved by isolation, concurrent disinfection and immunization of contacts and by surveillance. Quarantine is impractical.

Eradication

Measles meets the technical criteria for eradication. Humans constitute the only natural reservoir for the causative virus and there are no healthy carriers of the virus (as in hepatitis B). An effective vaccine has been available for over 3 decades and today costs only US$ 0.26 for a single dose including safe injection equipment. Natural immunity to the virus is lifelong.

However, measles eradication is still a long way off. One reason is the priority given to polio eradication, scheduled for 2005. But in the meantime, efforts are being continued to reduce measles deaths throughout the world through immunization and vitamin A supplementation. Because measles is a highly contagious disease, the new plan calls for immunization of at least 90% of children worldwide. The current global vaccine coverage rate is only 85% (in 2010).

As the 1st dose of vaccine is only about 85% effective in developing countries, the plan recommends a 2nd dose of vaccine for all children, through either routine vaccination or mass immunization campaigns.

Measles Initiative

The measles initiative is a partnership led by the American Red Cross, the United Nations Foundation, UNICEF, the US Centers for Disease Control and Prevention and WHO, committed to reducing measles deaths worldwide. The measles initiative has been in operation since 2001 for reducing measles mortality in Africa. The measles initiative expanded its support to countries affected by measles in the Eastern Mediterranean, South-East Asia and Western Pacific regions of WHO. Since 2007, the measles initiative supports vaccination campaigns in all regions of the world, made possible by new funding from the International Finance Facility for Immunization.

WHO Measles Elimination Strategy

The WHO advocates a three phase strategy for measles elimination.

1. Catch up: This is a nationwide campaign to vaccinate all children between the ages of 9 months and 14 years regardless of measles history or vaccination status.
2. Keep up: This is the routine vaccination schedule in which the aim is to vaccinate at least 95% of children in each successive birth cohort.
3. Follow-up: It is conducted every 2–4 years after the catch-up phase. All children born after the catch-up phase are vaccinated.

Many countries around the world have adopted the three phase WHO strategy for eliminating measles and for decreasing mortality and morbidity. Not enough susceptibles will accumulate to cause an epidemic. Each importation will only lead to a few secondary cases (unlikely to be more than 100).

❑ GERMAN MEASLES (RUBELLA)

German measles, first described in Germany. It is a common exanthematous disease having worldwide occurrence. It occurs as an epidemic mostly in children, but also can occur in adults. It is known for its propensity to cause congenital defects in the newborn if infection occurs during pregnancy.

Rubella has worldwide distribution. Before the introduction of large scale rubella vaccination programs, the usual age range of infection was between 6 and 12 years in high-income countries and between 2 and 8 years in urban areas of low-income countries.

The incidence of rubella, including maternal infection, has decreased in countries implementing routine immunization against rubella with high coverage.

In 2011, 112,531 rubella cases and 214 cases of congenital rubella syndrome (CRS) were reported to WHO.

In India, comprehensive evidence about the true burden of CRS is not available. It is only now that the subject is sought to be revived on the country's health agenda. However, studies indicate that around 15%–30% of women in the childbearing age are susceptible to rubella in India. CRS accounts for 10%–15% of pediatric cataract. It is also the main cause of deafness in India.

Causative organism is an RNA virus of togavirus group. There is only a single serotype. It is a major cause of birth defects among the toxoplasmosis, rubella, cytomegalovirus and herpes (TORCH) simplex group of organisms causing congenital anomalies. Natural infection confers lifelong protection.

Incubation period is usually 18 days; but may vary from 14 to 21 days.

Reservoir and Source

No extra human reservoir is known. Cases of rubella form the reservoir. Subclinical cases also contribute for the transmission. Nasopharyngeal secretion is the source of infective material.

Mode of Transmission

Transmission is by means of droplet infection and droplet nuclei. It is the only togavirus known to be transmitted via the respiratory route. This virus can cross the placental barrier and infect the fetus in the womb. Period of communicability is several days before and several days after the appearance of rash.

Factors Facilitating Transmission

Overcrowding, ignorance, occurrence of subclinical cases and inadequate immunization coverage all favor transmission.

Clinical Manifestation

Rubella is usually a mild, self-limiting infection. Mild fever and malaise is followed by the appearance of maculopapular rash, the 'blueberry muffin' skin lesions, which spread rapidly from the face down the trunk. Lymphadenopathy is common and arthralgia may be present in 50% of adult cases. Testicular pain has also been reported. Serious complications are rare. Asymptomatic infection is common. Compared to measles, rubella is usually a milder illness with a shorter duration.

Complications include thrombocytopenia in about 1 in 3,000 cases and encephalitis in about 1 in 6,000 cases. Arthritis and arthralgia may affect up to 70% of adult females who become infected.

The importance of this disease lies in the fact that it can cause congenital defects in the newborn if the mother is infected during pregnancy—CRS. It was ophthalmologist Norman McAlister Gregg who first linked epidemic congenital cataracts (Fig. 3.4) in Australia to intrauterine rubella in 1941. Miscarriage, preterm birth and stillbirth are common when rubella is contracted in early pregnancy. The risk of defects drops as the pregnancy progresses. After 20

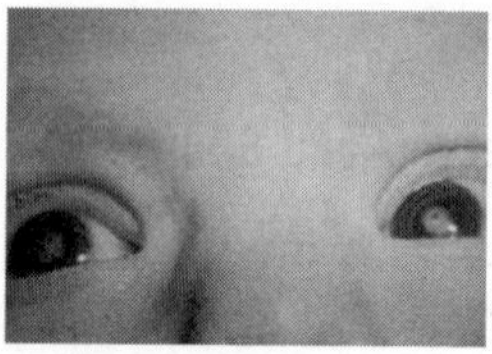

Figure 3.4: Congenital cataract in a newborn *(Courtesy*: Centers for Disease Control and Prevention)

weeks there is very little risk of defects. An attack confers lasting immunity as there is only one antigenic type of the virus.

Congenital rubella syndrome (CRS) affects three core organs namely the optic lens, the cochlea and the heart. CRS also causes diseases in the brain, lungs, liver, spleen, kidney, bone marrow, bones and endocrine organs. Encephalitis, mental retardation, pneumonia, hepatitis, thrombocytopenia, metaphyseal defects, diabetes mellitus and thyroiditis can be caused by rubella infection. Although cataracts, cochlear atrophy and patent ductus arteriosus were prevalent in typical CRS, other manifestations such as glaucoma, central auditory imperception and peripheral pulmonic stenosis were found to occur frequently.

Prevention and Control

As rubella is usually a mild, self-limiting infection, the aim of immunization is only to prevent congenital defects in the newborn by preventing the disease occurring in pregnant women.

Vaccination strategy now adopted aims to protect women of child bearing age (15–34 or 39 years) first and then to interrupt transmission by vaccinating all children currently aged 1–14 years and subsequently all children at 1 year of age. Infants under 1 year should not be vaccinated due to possible interference from persisting maternal antibodies. Rubella vaccine is contraindicated in pregnancy and in immunocompromised individuals.

Live attenuated virus vaccine (RA 27/3) given in a single dose of 0.5 mL subcutaneously induces antibodies in 95% of recipients and the immunity is lifelong. Combined mumps, measles and rubella (MMR) vaccine are also available.

Eradication of rubella and CRS is currently not a major global public health priority because other diseases such as poliomyelitis and measles have historically resulted in more morbidity and mortality. However, eradication of rubella should be possible since infection is limited to humans; prolonged shedding is limited to children with CRS and vaccine efficacy is high. Rubella immunization has been shown to be cost-effective in both developed and developing countries, if measles vaccine is coadministered and the coverage rates are more than 80%.

❑ MUMPS

Mumps is endemic throughout the world. Outbreaks may occur in schools and army camps. Mumps predominantly affects children, with 32% of reported cases worldwide in children aged 0–4 years and 53% in children aged 5–14 years.

Since the introduction of the combined MMR vaccine, there has been a decrease in the incidence of the disease. Those cases that still occur are usually in an older age group who are unvaccinated. In 2011, 718,858 cases have been reported to WHO.

In India there is no official figure for the prevalence of mumps. There were 301 children admitted with mumps between 1999 and 2003 at the Institute of Maternal and Child Health, Medical College, Calicut. Annual incidence is around 1,515.

Causative Organism

Causative organism is myxovirus parotitis (Rubulavirus), an RNA virus belonging to myxovirus group.

Reservoir and Source

Mumps cases (clinical and subclinical) constitute the only reservoir. Respiratory secretion is the source of infective material.

Mode of Transmission

Mumps is transmitted mainly through droplet infection. Transplacental transmission has also been established, but congenital defects in the newborn have not been observed. Secondary attack rate is 80%.

Incubation Period

The incubation period is 10–21 days.

Factors Facilitating Transmission

Overcrowding, ignorance, inadequate immunization coverage, incidence of inapparent cases (30%–40%) all favor transmission.

Clinical Manifestation

Clinically it is a mild disease, most cases recovering without any sequelae. About one third of cases are without symptoms. The prodromal feature like malaise is followed by the appearance of swelling of one or both the parotids and also the other salivary glands. Viremia may affect other organs like testes, ovaries, pancreas, heart, breast and the thyroid gland.

Although the disease is usually mild, up to 10% of patients can develop aseptic meningitis; a less common, but more serious complication is encephalitis, which can result in death or disability. Permanent deafness, orchitis and pancreatitis are other untoward effects of mumps. Mumps is a leading cause of acquired sensorineural deafness among children affecting approximately 5/100,000 mumps patients. Mumps infection during the first 12 weeks of pregnancy is associated with a 25% incidence of spontaneous abortion. But congenital malformations following mumps virus infection during pregnancy have not been found.

Prevention and Control

Live attenuated vaccine, which is available in a single dose of 0.5 mL IM, induces protective antibodies in 95% of vaccines. Combined MMR vaccine is also available. As mumps is a mild and self-limiting disease, vaccination may not be given routinely in children, but may be indicated in susceptible adults in whom the disease tends to be severe. Mumps vaccine is contraindicated in pregnancy and in immunocompromised individuals. Passive prophylaxis for contacts can be given with specific immunoglobulin obtained from convalescent sera.

Countries with high vaccine coverage have shown a rapid decline in mumps morbidity and mumps-associated encephalitis and deafness has nearly vanished in these countries.

Mumps elimination strategies:

1. Achieving high (more than 90%) coverage with a 1st dose of vaccine at the age of 12–18 months.
2. Ensuring a 2nd dose of vaccine.
3. Conducting catch-up immunization of susceptible cohorts.

A 2nd dose is not required when the 1st dose coverage is sufficiently high (i.e. more than 90%). The 2nd dose can be given by administering a second routine dose or by conducting periodic catch-up campaigns. In the initial catch-up campaign, the target age group should be the one in which susceptibility to mumps is highest. In most unvaccinated populations a majority of children acquire mumps infections before reaching the age of 10 years.

Control of mumps is difficult because of its occurrence as inapparent infection. However, isolation of cases, concurrent disinfection of patient's articles and surveillance of contacts may be useful in controlling this disease.

❑ INFLUENZA

Influenza is an international disease. While all other classic epidemic diseases (plague, smallpox, yellow fever and typhus) have been controlled, influenza still remains uncontrolled because it is caused by a virus, which periodically changes its antigens.

Many pandemics of influenza have occurred in the past including the catastrophic one that occurred during 1918–1919, which affected some 500 million and killed 20 million people. Successive pandemics occurred in 1957 and in 1968. Another pandemic was expected in the latter half of 1970–80 by studying the changing characteristics of the influenza antigen, which changed roughly once in 10 years. But the outbreak which occurred in 1976 did not become a pandemic because the population had already experienced this virus infection as it resembled the 1946–57 strain. In between pandemics, many epidemics occur at lesser intervals.

The WHO Global Influenza Surveillance Network, established in 1952, serves as a global alert mechanism for the emergence of influenza viruses with pandemic potential. The network comprises four WHO collaborating centers and 122 National Influenza Centers (NICs) in 94 countries. These NICs collect specimens; perform primary virus isolation and preliminary antigenic characterization in their countries.

Causative Organism

Influenza viruses type A, B and C cause disease in man. They belong to orthomyxovirus group. Type A exhibits highest antigenic variability and type B shows less while type C has no antigenic variability. The two surface antigens namely hemagglutinin (H antigen) and neuraminidase (N antigen) of the virus A and B are type specific and they undergo independent antigenic variation. The variation may be minor called antigenic drift or major called antigenic shift. The antibodies to H antigen are protective.

Mode of Transmission

Influenza is transmitted by droplet infection. Fomites also may play some role in the transmission.

Incubation Period

The incubation period is 18–72 hours.

Reservoir and Source

Cases and subclinical cases constitute the reservoir of infection. It usually affects children and young people, who have little immunity, like school age children in the age group of 5–14 years, but it can affect others as well. Pigs and ducks have also been found to be reservoirs. The respiratory secretion is the source of infective material and the period of infectivity is usually 1–2 days before and 1–2 days after the onset of symptoms.

Evolution of Disease

After entering the respiratory tract, the virus affects mainly the ciliated cells. The neuraminidase antigen facilitates the adsorption of the virus to surface epithelium. The ciliated cells are destroyed and shed. Therefore secondary bacterial invasion sets in. Viral pneumonia is seen only in severe cases.

Clinical Manifestation

The disease may be very mild or severe. Most of the infections are subclinical, which are mainly responsible for the transmission. The disease is characterized by abrupt onset of fever with headache and myalgia. In children type B infection may produce abdominal pain and vomiting. Uncomplicated cases resolve in 2–7 days.

Complications include pneumonia due to secondary infection, congestive cardiac failure or myocarditis and encephalitis. Congenital defects in the newborn may occur, if infection occurs during early pregnancy.

Confirmation of diagnosis is by demonstration of the virus antigen on the surface of the nasopharyngeal cells by immunofluorescence and the isolation of the virus in egg or monkey kidney cell culture.

Prevention and Control

Active immunization of the susceptible (old persons) and the high-risk individuals (policemen, hospital employees, transport workers) with killed or live vaccine can be effective in preventing the occurrence and spread of the disease. Vaccination is especially important when there is threat of a pandemic by a new virus because the whole population may be susceptible. But infection by the new strain may spread to all before the vaccine becomes available. Live intranasal vaccines produce local immunity in the respiratory tract. Chemoprophylaxis with the drug amantadine hydrochloride has also been found to be useful.

Isolation and quarantine are not practical because of the short incubation period, occurrence of subclinical cases and simultaneous spread in many areas.

Health education to avoid large crowds or known sources of infection during an epidemic may be beneficial.

The policy now is to reduce mortality during outbreaks by protecting the debilitated and the high risk groups with vaccine. Amantadine or rimantadine started within first 2 days of the illness may be beneficial as a therapeutic agent.

Global Influenza Virological Surveillance

The WHO, in collaboration with its collaborating centers and national centers of different countries, is carrying out continuous surveillance of influenza in order to spread the information about the strain and the control measures to all parts of the world.

❑ COMMON COLD

The common cold is one of the most common illnesses leading to more doctor visits and absences from school and work than any other illness every year. Children suffer more colds each year than adults due to their immature immune systems and to the close physical contact with other children at school or daycare centers.

Causative Organisms

More than 200 different viruses are incriminated in causing colds. However, majority of colds are caused by the rhinoviruses and the coronaviruses. Research has shown that rhinoviruses may survive up to 3 hours outside of the nasal mucosa.

Mode of Transmission

Highly communicable, the common cold often spreads through droplet infection. People can also contract cold through hand-to-hand contact of infected individuals or hand-to-infected-surface contact. After such contacts when a person touches his/her face/nose, the virus is transmitted.

Incubation Period

The incubation period is 2–3 days after the virus enters the body.

Mechanism of Disease Causation

The virus inflames the membranes lining the nose and throat.

Factors Facilitating Transmission

Schools in session increase the risk for exposure to the virus. People staying more indoors are in closer proximity to each other. Low humidity causes dry nasal passages, which are more susceptible to cold viruses.

Contrary to popular belief, cold weather or getting chilled does not cause a cold. The incidence of more colds during the cold season is probably due to the increased risk of exposure to the virus in schools and the tendency to stay indoors in closer proximity to each other during the season.

Clinical Manifestation

Stuffy, runny nose, scratchy, tickly throat, sneezing, watering eyes, low-grade fever, sore throat, mild hacking cough, achy muscles and bones, headache, mild fatigue, chills, watery discharge from nose that thickens and turns yellow or green are the most common symptoms.

The common cold and the flu (influenza) are two different illnesses (Table 3.1). A cold is relatively harmless and usually clears up by itself after a period of time although sometimes it may lead to a secondary infection such as an ear infection. However, the flu can lead to complications such as pneumonia and even death. What may seem like a cold, could, in fact, be the flu.

TABLE 3.1: Differences between cold and flu

Cold	Flu
Low or no fever	High fever
Sometimes a headache	Always a headache
Stuffy, runny nose	Clear nose
Sneezing	Sometimes sneezing
Mild, hacking cough	Cough, often becoming severe
Slight aches and pains	Often severe aches and pains
Mild fatigue	Several weeks of fatigue
Sore throat	Sometimes a sore throat
Normal energy level	Extreme exhaustion

Prevention and Control

The best way to avoid catching common cold is to wash one's hands frequently and avoid close contact with the infected people. When in the company of people with colds, nose or eyes should not be touched because hands may be contaminated with the virus.

People with colds should cover their face with hand kerchiefs while coughing and sneezing and then wash their hands immediately. As rhinoviruses may survive up to 3 hours outside of the nasal mucosa, cleaning surfaces with disinfectants that kill viruses can help to halt the transmission.

Currently, there is no medication available to cure or shorten the duration of the common cold. As use of Aspirin for treating viral illnesses in children has been associated with Reye's syndrome, it should not be used to treat colds, flu and chickenpox in children.

Colds can lead to secondary infections including bacterial middle ear and sinus infections that may require treatment with antibiotics. When a cold is accompanied by high fever, sinus pain, significantly swollen glands or a mucus-producing cough, a complication may be present that requires additional treatment.

❑ AVIAN INFLUENZA (BIRD FLU) IN HUMANS

Avian influenza, primarily an infectious disease of birds is now emerging as a disease of humans of late. As of 10 August 2012, since 2003, a total of 608 human cases of avian influenza with 359 deaths, were reported to WHO from 15 countries (Azerbaijan, Bangladesh, Cambodia, China, Djibouti, Egypt, Indonesia, Iraq, Laos, Myanmar, Nigeria, Pakistan, Thailand, Turkey and Viet Nam). Since January 2012, 30 human cases of influenza A (H1N5) have been reported to WHO. Egypt and Indonesia have encountered more cases and deaths. In India, there were outbreaks of this disease in poultry. But so far, no cases of human avian influenza have been reported from India.

Causative Organism

The H5 and H7 subtype of type A strains of the influenza viruses cause avian influenza in man.

Of the many strains of avian influenza A viruses, only four, namely H5N1, H7N3, H7N7 and H9N2 are known to have caused human infections. Since 1959 instances of human infection with an avian influenza virus have been documented on only 10 occasions.

Incubation Period

The incubation period is 7 days (WHO).

Reservoir and Source

Migratory waterfowl—most notably wild ducks are the natural reservoir of avian influenza viruses, which can be transmitted to domestic populations of birds and to commercial poultry. Some migratory waterfowl are known to carry the highly pathogenic H5N1 virus, sometimes over long distances and introduce the virus to poultry flocks along their migratory routes.

Soil contaminated with chicken feces (play area of children), swimming pools contaminated by dead or sick birds like ducks or other birds, live bird markets and the untreated bird feces used as fertilizer can be the source for transmission.

Mode of Transmission

Droplet Infection

The main mode of transmission from the reservoir/source to the susceptible humans is through droplet infection either directly from contaminated fingers, indirectly from items contaminated with bird feces or from small particle aerosol generated.

Human-to-human transmission has not been conclusively established. Avian influenza A viruses may be transmitted from animals to humans either directly from birds and avian virus-contaminated environments or through an intermediate host such as a pig.

When a pig is infected with both human influenza A virus and avian influenza A virus at the same time, the new replicating viruses could mix existing genetic information (reassortment) and produce a new virus that will have most of the genes from the human virus, but a hemagglutinin and/or neuraminidase from the avian virus. The resulting new virus might then be able to infect humans and spread from person to person.

Transmission among birds is through contact with contaminated nasal, respiratory or fecal material from infected birds. Fecal-to-oral transmission is the most common mode of spread between birds.

Factors Facilitating Transmission

Close contact with dead or sick birds is the principal source of human infection with the H5N1 virus. Outbreaks in backyard flocks are associated with a heightened risk of human exposure and infection.

Slaughtering, defeathering, butchering and preparation of infected birds for consumption, exposure of children to chicken feces when they play in an area frequented by free-ranging poultry and swimming in water bodies, where the carcasses of infected birds have been discarded or which may have been contaminated by feces from infected ducks or other birds can facilitate the transmission. Live bird markets can be another source for spreading avian influenza viruses.

Clinical Features in Man

Human infection with these viruses usually results in mild symptoms and very little severe illness. However, the highly pathogenic H5N1 virus can cause severe illness.

High fever and influenza-like symptoms are the initial features. Diarrhea, vomiting, abdominal pain, chest pain and bleeding from the nose and gums have also been reported as early symptoms in some patients.

Watery diarrhea without blood appears to be more common in H5N1 avian influenza than in normal seasonal influenza. Acute encephalitis may be the presenting feature in some cases.

Difficulty in breathing develops around 5 days following the first symptoms. Respiratory distress, a hoarse voice and a crackling sound during inspiration are commonly seen. Sputum production is variable and sometimes bloody. Almost all patients develop pneumonia. Another common feature is multiorgan dysfunction.

Leukopenia (mainly lymphopenia), mild-to-moderate thrombocytopenia, elevated aminotransferases and (in some instances) disseminated intravascular coagulation are the common laboratory findings.

Prevention and Control

The first line of defense for containing outbreaks is rapid culling of all infected or exposed birds, proper disposal of carcasses, the quarantining and rigorous disinfection of farms and the implementation of strict sanitary or 'biosecurity' measures. Restrictions on the movement of live poultry both within and between countries are another important control measure.

When culling fails or proves impracticable, vaccination of poultry in a high-risk area can be used as a supplementary emergency measure provided quality-assured vaccines are available and the recommendations of WHO are strictly followed. Poor quality vaccines may accelerate mutation of the virus and also pose a risk for human health as they may allow infected birds to shed virus, while still appearing to be disease free.

Isolation precautions identical to those recommended for patients with known SARS are to be observed.

Standard precautions include:

- Handwashing and antisepsis
- Use of personal protective equipment when handling blood, body substances, excretions and secretions
- Appropriate handling of patient care equipment and soiled linen
- Prevention of needle stick/sharp injuries
- Environmental cleaning and spills management
- Appropriate handling of waste.

Contact precautions include:

- Gloves and gown should be used for all patient contact
- Separate stethoscopes, disposable blood pressure cuffs, disposable thermometers, etc. should be used.

Eye Protection

Goggles or face shields should be used when within 3 feet of the patient.

Airborne Precautions

The patient should be placed in an airborne isolation room; such rooms should have monitored negative air pressure in relation to corridor with 6–12 air changes per hour and exhaust air directly outside or have recirculated air filtered by a high efficiency particulate air filter. If an airborne isolation room is unavailable, using portable high efficiency particulate air filters to augment the number of air changes per hour.

Fit-tested disposable respirator should be used when entering the room.

To date, epidemiological investigations have not linked any human cases to the consumption of poultry products. As a general rule, WHO recommends that all meats including that from poultry be thoroughly cooked so that all parts of the meat reach an internal temperature of 70°C. This temperature will kill an influenza virus and thus render safe any raw poultry meat contaminated with H5N1 virus. In countries affected by H5N1 outbreaks, eggs should also be thoroughly cooked as some studies have detected virus in raw eggs.

Travelers should avoid visits to live-bird markets in endemic areas. People who work with birds should use protective clothing and special breathing masks. Avoiding undercooked or uncooked meat reduces the risk of exposure to avian flu and other foodborne diseases.

Antiviral drugs notably oseltamivir (commercially known as Tamiflu) reduce the duration of viral replication and so can improve prospects of survival if administered within 48 hours of the onset of symptoms. The recommended dose in adults and adolescents 13 years and older is 150 mg/day (75 mg twice a day) for 5 days. Oseltamivir is not indicated in children less than 1 year of age.

Currently no vaccine is available to protect humans against the H5N1 virus that is seen in Asia. Vaccine development efforts are under way.

The US Food and Drug Administration (FDA), in 2007, has approved a vaccine for humans against the H5N1 influenza virus, which could be used in the event the current H5N1 avian virus were to develop the capability to efficiently spread from human to human.

❑ SWINE INFLUENZA

Outbreaks of influenza in swine are common and cause significant economic losses in industry primarily by causing stunting and extended time to market. Swine flu has already been reported numerous times as a zoonosis in humans usually with limited distribution, rarely with a widespread distribution. Now since 26th April 2009 the outbreak has occurred in humans in a large scale.

As of 17 October 2009, worldwide, there have been more than 414,000 laboratory confirmed cases of pandemic influenza H1N1 2009 and nearly 5,000 deaths have been reported to WHO. Mongolia, Rwanda and Sao Tome and Principe have reported pandemic influenza cases for the first time in October 2009.

As of 16th September 2012, India had 51,665 cases and 2,997 deaths since 2009 (27,236 cases and 981deaths in 2009; 20,604 cases and 1,763 deaths in 2010 and 603 cases and 75 deaths in 2011). There was a spurt in the incidence of cases and deaths recently. From 1st January 2012 to 16th September 2012 India recorded 3,222 cases and 178 deaths.

Now since August 2010 the H1N1 influenza virus has moved into the postpandemic period. WHO recommends that surveillance during the postpandemic period should include maintaining routine surveillance including for influenza-like illness and cases of severe acute respiratory infections and monitoring the H1N1 2009 virus for important genetic, antigenic or functional changes such as antiviral drug sensitivity.

Causative Agent

A new strain of influenza A virus subtype H1N1, the pandemic H1N1 2009, a mix of pig, bird and human genes, has caused the present pandemic.

There is a concern that this virus may combine with the seasonal H1N1 virus that was resistant to Tamiflu. If the two virus strains combine, it is possible the swine flu will become resistant to Tamiflu, the current first-line defense against the new swine flu.

Incubation Period

The estimated incubation period is unknown and could range from 1–7 days and more likely 1–4 days.

Mode of Transmission

Droplet infection-swine influenza A (H1N1) virus spreads person to person mainly through coughing or sneezing. Sometimes people may become infected by touching something (such as a surface like a desk) with flu viruses on it and then touching their mouth or nose. Some viruses and bacteria can live 2 hours or longer on surfaces like cafeteria tables, door knobs and desks. It passes with apparent ease from human to human, an ability attributed to an as yet unidentified mutation.

Swine influenza viruses are not spread by eating pork or pork products; properly handled and cooked pork products are safe. Cooking pork to an internal temperature of 71°C kills the swine flu virus along with other bacteria and viruses.

Period of Communicability

Infected people may be able to infect others beginning 1 day before symptoms develop and up to 7 or more days after becoming sick.

Factors Facilitating Transmission

People who work with swine, especially people with intense exposures, are at risk of catching swine influenza if the swine carry a strain able to infect humans. However, swine influenza virus(SIV) rarely mutates into a form able to pass easily from human to human.

Clinical Features

Swine flu in humans can vary in severity from mild to severe. The symptoms of swine flu are similar to those of influenza and of influenza-like illness in general. The strain in most cases causes only mild symptoms and the infected person makes a full recovery without requiring medical attention and without the use of antiviral medicines. Groups at increased risk of severe illness from the pandemic H1N1 virus includes young children, pregnant women and people with underlying respiratory or other chronic conditions, including asthma and diabetes. People with existing cardiovascular disease, respiratory disease, diabetes and cancer are at higher risk of serious complications from the new flu virus.

Prevention and Control

World Health Organization strongly recommends vaccination of high-risk individuals in countries, where influenza vaccines are available using monovalent H1N1 vaccine, especially where trivalent seasonal influenza vaccine is not available.

One can prevent getting infected by avoiding close contact with people who show influenza-like symptoms trying to maintain a distance of about 1 m if possible and taking the following measures:

1. Avoid touching one's mouth and nose.
2. Washing hands thoroughly with soap and water or cleansing them with an alcohol-based hand rub on a regular basis; hands should be washed for 15–20 seconds with soap.
3. Avoiding close contact with people who might be ill.
4. Avoiding crowded places.
5. Improve airflow in living space by opening windows.
6. Get adequate sleep and rest.
7. Eat nutritious food and drink plenty of water.

8. Should not shake hands or hug.
9. Should not spit in public.

Sick persons should:

1. Cover their cough and sneezing with a kerchief.
2. Stay home and limit contact with others as much as possible.
3. Rest and take plenty of fluids.
4. Seek medical advice.

For the control of cases oseltamivir or zanamivir is recommended. These drugs can be used for the prevention of infection also. These drugs work best if started within 2 days of symptoms. However, antiviral drugs are reserved only for those at high risk such as pregnant women and patients with underlying health conditions like cardiovascular disease or diabetes. Pregnant women are more likely to develop pneumonia when they catch the flu. Pneumonia in pregnancy from the infection is much more serious than the unknown risks to the fetus from these antiviral drugs.

WHO is not recommending travel restrictions related to the outbreak of the influenza A (H1N1) virus. Individuals who are ill should delay travel plans and travelers from endemic countries who fall ill should seek appropriate medical care.

❑ SEVERE ACUTE RESPIRATORY SYNDROME

Severe acute respiratory syndrome (SARS) reported for the first time in Asian countries during 26th February 2003 is a disease primarily affecting the respiratory system and causing widespread morbidity and significant mortality. From Guangdong Province in China, SARS virus spread to 30 countries. China, Taiwan, Hong Kong, Hanoi, Bangkok and Singapore were affected seriously killing many. As of July 2003, 8,439 people have been affected with 812 deaths. It was also reported in USA, Canada, UK, Italy, Ireland, Spain, France and Switzerland. The pandemic has died down since July 2003. But the world is not SARS free according to WHO, which warns that continued global vigilance for SARS is crucial for the foreseeable future. Intense investigations into a possible animal reservoir are needed.

Causative Organism

The SARS virus is the causative agent (WHO). It is a new pathogen, a member of the corona virus family never before seen in humans.

Host Factors

The SARS affects mainly adults 25–70 years of age. Few suspected cases in children aged ≤ 15 years have also been reported.

Reservoir and Source

Human cases form the reservoir and there is no knowledge about carrier state. But the latest studies during the subsequent occurrence of SARS cases in December to January 2004 in China indicate the possibility of animal reservoir in civet cats. The earlier view that any product or animal arriving from regions affected by SARS does not pose a risk to public health has to be viewed with caution. Respiratory secretion is the source of infected material.

Period of Communicability

Patients are infectious to others when they have symptoms—such as fever and cough. But the exact period of communicability has not been established.

Incubation Period

The incubation period is 2–7 days, occasionally up to 10 days.

Mode of Transmission

Droplet infection is the main mode of transmission. Aerosals and fomites may also transmit the infection. Some unidentified routes of transmission are also suspected.

Factors Facilitating Transmission

Overcrowding and close contact facilitate transmission. Medical personnel and close family contacts are at risk of contracting SARS. 20% of all cases were in healthcare workers.

Clinical Features

Fever with chills and rigor, headache, muscular stiffness, body aches, loss of appetite, confusion and diarrhea are the initial features. Then, dry cough and shortness of breath (difficulty in breathing) follow. Severe cases may need intubation and mechanical ventilation. Chest examination may show evidence of consolidation. Case fatality is approximately 4%.

Laboratory Investigations

Serum antibody test and viral isolation are done to confirm the diagnosis. Acute and convalescent blood for serology, stool fresh or in viral transport medium, throat and nasopharyngeal swabs in viral transport medium, bronchial, alveolar lavage or tracheal aspirate in sterile containers for viral isolation are the specimens used for identification of the SARS virus.

Prevention and Control

Notification, isolation of cases and suspect cases, preventing travelers from and to endemic regions, wearing of personal protective devices like gloves, goggles and masks by health staff and masks by patients, barrier nursing, use of disposable equipments, wherever possible all will help in preventing transmission.

Treatment is only supportive care. However antiviral agents like oseltamvir and ribavirin are being used. Severe cases receive steroids—oral or IV. Follow-up of close contacts to see whether they develop the disease or not will be useful for taking remedial measures quickly.

❑ DIPHTHERIA

Diphtheria is a childhood disease occurring worldwide. Despite the availability of an effective vaccine sporadic attacks of the disease in unprotected groups are still seen in developed nations. In developing countries, it is an important public health problem. Studies demonstrate an age shift in incidence 40% of the cases have occurred above the age of 5 years. No data about disease in adults is available.

The last decade has seen resurgence of diphtheria in both developed and developing countries, where it was previously well controlled. An epidemic that began in 1990 in the newly created Independent States of the former Soviet Union caused more than 150,000 reported cases and 5,000 deaths by the end of 1996. Most of the cases (60%–77%) and fatalities occurred in adults.

Globally, in 2009 and in 2010, 4,386 cases and 4,234 cases respectively were reported while in 2011, 4,887 cases have been reported (WHO).

In India, it is an endemic disease, but shows a declining trend. The number of reported cases in 2009, 2010 and 2011 were 3,529, 3,123 and 3,485 respectively (WHO). In 2008, the cases reported were 6,081. The figures quoted above may possibly be a gross underestimate due to lack of a good surveillance system and facilities for microbiologic diagnosis.

Causative Organism

Corynebacterium diphtheriae, a gram positive, non-motile bacterium is the causative organism. It is non-invasive, but it causes the disease symptoms by producing an exotoxin. Specific bacteriophage can make a non-toxigenic strain to toxigenic.

Reservoir and Source

Cases and carriers form the reservoir and the secretions of nose and throat are the sources of infective material. Skin lesion (cutaneous diphtheria) also may be a source for transmission. Asymptomatic carriers play an important role in transmission.

Mode of Transmission

Transmission occurs through droplet infection and droplet nuclei. Fomites like toys, pencils and towels may carry the organism for short periods and therefore have some role in transmission. Cutaneous diphtheria occurs due to secondary infection of minor trauma, ulcer or chronic dermatitis. Diphtheria is also transmitted through milk from udder infection of cows.

Incubation Period

The incubation period is 2–6 days.

Factors Facilitating Transmission

Low socioeconomic conditions, low level of herd immunity due to inadequate immunization coverage, lack of medical facilities and ignorance all favor transmission.

Evolution of Disease

The bacilli multiply locally at the site of implantation (commonly fauces), elaborate an exotoxin and cause pseudomembrane. Systemic absorption of toxin produces toxemia, which may cause myocarditis and circulatory failure either cardiac or peripheral.

Clinical Manifestation

Local pseudomembrane that bleeds on peeling is the characteristic lesion of diphtheria infection. The local lesion may be faucial, laryngeal, nasal, otitic, conjunctival, genital or cutaneous. Carditis and postdiphtheritic paralysis of palatine muscles manifested as nasal regurgitation also may be caused by diphtheritic toxin. Death is usually due to respiratory obstruction or myocarditis or respiratory failure caused by paralysis of respiratory muscles.

Schick Test

Schick test is done to detect the immune status of individuals against diphtheria. 0.2 mL of diluted diphtheria toxin (containing 1/50 MLD for guinea pig) is injected intradermally into a forearm. If the individual has immunity due to presence of antitoxin the test becomes negative that is no skin reaction is produced and if susceptible, that is when antitoxin is absent, positive reaction is produced in the form of a red flush at the site of injection within 24–36 hours reaching its maximum size in 4–7 days. Currently, use of this test is limited and antitoxin levels can be measured directly by hemagglutination tests.

Prevention and Control

Diphtheria can be prevented by primary immunization of infants with diphtheria toxoid, which is usually combined with tetanus toxoid and pertussis vaccine (DPT). 3 doses at 1½, 2½ and 3½ months followed by booster doses at 1½–2 years and at school going age are recommended. Non-immunized children above 6 years and adults may be immunized with 2 doses of DT (tetanus and diphtheria toxoid) at 4–6 weeks interval followed by a booster dose 12 months after the 2nd dose.

Control can be achieved by early diagnosis and treatment of cases and carriers, isolation of all suspected cases and carriers until proved non-infectious and protection of contacts with a booster dose of the vaccine or with 500–1,000 units of antitoxin depending upon the immune status of the contact.

Treatment of cases should be started as soon as a clinical diagnosis is made without waiting for laboratory confirmation. 20,000–80,000 units of antitoxin (depending upon the severity and the weight of the patient) are administered to neutralize the toxin on admission. A course of antibiotics (penicillin or erythromycin) is also provided for clearing the infection. Carriers already immunized should receive only a booster dose of the toxoid. Non-immunized carriers receive 1,000–2,000 units of antitoxin who are also simultaneously actively immunized. Carriers should also receive a course of antibiotic treatment to eliminate the diphtheria bacilli from their throats. Clinical surveillance of contacts should continue for a week after exposure and bacteriological surveillance for several weeks by repeated swab testing at weekly intervals. Those with positive culture should be treated with antibiotics.

❑ WHOOPING COUGH (PERTUSSIS)

Whooping cough, also called the 100 days' cough in some countries, occurs in all parts of the world, but the severity has declined in industrialized countries due to good vaccine coverage. In tropical countries, it occurs both as an endemic and epidemic disease. Whooping cough is predominantly a pediatric disease affecting infants and preschool children. But in developed nations, the disease now has become common in older preschool and school age children as a result of efficient immunization coverage of infants.

Despite an effective vaccine and generally high coverage with this vaccine, pertussis is one of the leading causes of vaccine-preventable deaths worldwide. Most deaths occur in young infants who are either unvaccinated or incompletely vaccinated. Cases reported globally in 2004, 2005 and 2006 were 238,119, 109,710 115,924 respectively.

About 111,833 cases have been reported in 2008. In 2009, 166,592 cases were reported while in 2010 and 2011 some reduction is observed (2010-158, 695; 2011-139, 382 cases). The incidence is high in India, USA and Australia.

In India, while the incidence is still high, it is showing a declining trend. Marked decline in the incidence has been observed since 1999. Cases reported have come down to 60,385, 38,493 and 35,217 in 2009, 2010 and 2011 respectively. Some 1.69 lakh cases were seen during 1987.

Causative Organism

Bordetella pertussis and *Bordetella parapertussis,* the gram negative coccobacilli cause whooping cough (95% by *Bordetella pertussis* and the other 5% by *Bordetella parapertussis).*

Reservoir and Source

Whooping cough cases are the only reservoir and no extra human reservoir is known. Infants below 6 months are also susceptible since maternal antibody does not seem to give protection and the disease is more severe in them causing increased mortality. Asymptomatic infection is rare and carrier state is absent. Nasopharyngeal and bronchial secretions are the source of infective material. The disease is more infectious during the catarrhal stage and the infectivity may extend up to 3 weeks after the onset of the paroxysmal stage.

Mode of Transmission

Transmission of this disease occurs mainly through droplet infection. Fomites like freshly contaminated toys or towels may have some role in the transmission. Whooping cough is a highly infectious disease. Secondary attack rate may be as high as 90% in unimmunized household contacts.

Factors Facilitating Transmission

Overcrowding, low socioeconomic conditions, inadequate immunization coverage and ignorance all favor transmission of this disease.

Incubation Period

Usually 7–10 days, but may vary from 4 to 16 days or even 21 days.

Clinical Manifestation

The characteristic feature is the spasmodic cough associated with whoop ending in vomiting. Initially it starts as a catarrh of the upper respiratory tract and gradually develops into paroxysmal cough. The severity of the paroxysmal coughing increases a week or so after the onset of paroxysms and then gradually subsides. The disease is more severe in young infants and lasts for 1–2 months.

Bronchopneumonia, bronchiectasis, subconjuctival hemorrhages and encephalopathy are the complications caused by pertussis infection. The diagnosis is confirmed by demonstration of the bacilli in the sputum. Specimens are collected by cough plate method, prenasal and postnasal swab. The organisms are grown in Bordet and Gengou medium.

Evolution of Disease

Whooping cough is a superficial infection of the lower respiratory tract. The bacilli are attached to the cilia and the ciliary function is inhibited. The infection causes inflammation and necrosis of the mucosal epithelium leading to secondary infection.

Prevention and Control

Active immunization of infants with 3 doses of the vaccine (whole cell preparations) in monthly intervals at 1½, 2½ and 3½ months followed by a booster dose at 1 year is recommended. Vaccination is started as early as 6 weeks because maternal antibodies do not seem to protect the babies and whooping cough in young infants is serious. Control is achieved by early diagnosis, isolation and treatment of cases and concurrent disinfection of sputum and nasal secretions. The antibiotic of choice is erythromycin, but alternatively ampicillin, tetracycline or cotrimoxazole can be administered. Contacts can be given a course of antibiotics for 10 days to prevent the development of the disease. Immunoglobulin is of no use in contacts.

❑ TUBERCULOSIS

Tuberculosis (TB) is a chronic respiratory infection, which causes significant morbidity and mortality. The global burden of TB remains enormous mainly because of poor control in Southeast Asia, subsaharan Africa and Eastern Europe and high rates of *Mycobacterium tuberculosis* and HIV coinfection in some African countries. TB problem is acute in developing countries. They have 95% of total cases in the world. In 2011, 8.7 million people fell ill with TB and 1.4 million died of TB. Over 95% of TB deaths occur in low- and middle-income countries and it is among the top three causes of death for women aged 15–44.

According to WHO, there are 22 high burden countries most of which are in Africa and South-East Asia, that account for much of the world's TB burden (approximately 80% of new TB cases each year). India ranks number one among the high burden countries with 26% of the global cases (WHO-2012).

About 5% of all TB cases are caused by multidrug-resistant tubercle bacilli (MDR-TB). Every year, an estimated 490,000 new MDR-TB cases occurs causing more than 130,000 deaths. The former Soviet Union countries and China account for the highest rates of MDR-TB. There are an estimated 40,000 new extremely drug resistant-TB (XDR-TB) cases annually. By March 2008, XDR-TB cases had been confirmed in more than 45 countries and in all regions of the world.

Though there have been major improvements in TB care and control, TB killed an estimated 1.7 million people in 2009 and 9.4

million people developed active TB last year. TB kills roughly 1.8 million people each year (WHO), i.e. 4,500 deaths a day.

In India, TB is a major public health problem. India has declared TB as a notifiable disease. India accounts for one fifth of the global TB incident cases. Each year nearly 2 million people in India develop TB, of which around 0.87 million are infectious cases, i.e. sputum positive cases. Every day, more than 20,000 people become infected with TB bacilli.

Tuberculosis is one of the leading causes of mortality in India—killing two persons every 3 minutes, nearly 1,000 everyday. It is estimated that annually around 330,000 Indians die due to TB. TB kills more people in India than HIV, STD, malaria, leprosy and tropical diseases combined. However, death rates from TB are declining.

Causative Organism

Mycobacterium tuberculosis is the causative agent of TB in man. Both the human and bovine strains are involved. However, majority of the cases in India are caused by the human strain. Atypical mycobacteriae are increasingly found to cause human disease in developed countries where TB caused by human strains has been controlled. TB may stage a comeback in developed countries because of the situation created by AIDS pandemic.

Multidrug-resistant tubercle bacilli (MDR-TB) and extremely drug-resistant tubercle bacilli (XDR-TB) are now reported in many developed countries. XDR-TB is virtually untreatable.

Reservoir and Source

Tuberculosis patients are the reservoir of infection. The sputum containing the acid-fast bacilli (AFB) from open cases of TB is the source. Milk is the source for bovine TB.

Mode of Transmission

Pulmonary TB is transmitted through droplet infection and droplet nuclei generated by sputum positive (open) cases. A single patient can infect 10 or more people in a year.

Incubation Period

Incubation period may be weeks, months or years depending upon the closeness of the contact and sputum positivity of the source case.

Factors Facilitating Transmission

Low socioeconomic status, malnutrition, overcrowding, ill ventilated housing, large families, ignorance, lack of medical facilities and dusty occupations like mining all favor transmission. TB is an occupational hazard for doctors, nurses and laboratory workers.

Evolution of Disease

Infection occurs early in life in endemic countries. Primary infection may cause features of primary complex in children or heal after sometime. Adult TB is caused either due to reactivation of primary focus or due to exogenous reinfection. Initially the characteristic lesion of TB is formed in the lung. Later it develops into an acute exudative type of lesion, which may resolve and then give rise to productive type of lesion that undergoes caseation necrosis.

Clinical Manifestation

Chronic cough with expectoration of more than 15 days duration, evening rise of temperature, loss of appetite and loss of weight are the early features of pulmonary TB. Later the patient may develop chest pain, hemoptysis and anemia. Fingers and toes may show clubbing. Death may occur due to massive hemoptysis.

Investigations

Mantoux test is done to find out the presence of tuberculous infection in individuals and also the prevalence in the community. Purified protein derivative (PPD) is injected intradermally in the forearm and the reaction at the site of injection is read after 72 hours. The induration at the injection site is measured with a scale. Induration of 10 mm and above is taken as positive reaction while 6 mm or less is considered negative. Positive reaction indicates infection by tubercle bacilli but negativity does not rule out the infection.

The important test to diagnose pulmonary TB is sputum examination for AFB. Tubercle bacilli appear as pink rods occurring singly. Concentration methods aid to increase the positivity of slides and fluoroscopy is used to process and examine large number of slides in a short period.

Xpert MTB/RIF Test

A new test, the Xpert MTB/RIF test [developed by the Foundation for Innovative New Diagnostics (FIND)], Cepheid and the University of Medicine and Dentistry of New Jersey using automated DNA (of the TB bacterium) amplification technology identifies TB in 98% of active cases in 90 minutes and also detects resistance to rifampicin. But the two disadvantages of the test are the need for well-equipped laboratories and the prohibitive cost.

Mantoux test, radiography and blood tests like total and differential counts of white blood cells and erythrocyte sedimentation rate (ESR) estimation are all corroborative and are also helpful in prognosis.

Prevention and Control

The efficacy of the available live attenuated vaccine, BCG, in preventing TB is controversial. Different field trails put the efficacy from nil to 80%. But WHO advises the continuation of BCG vaccination to infants and children on the ground that it may give protection against the more serious forms of TB such as skeletal, meningeal and miliary TB. Chemoprophylaxis with isoniazid (INH) can prevent the development of TB in infected individuals but it cannot be applied at community level. Early diagnosis, effective chemotherapy and health education all will help to prevent the spread. Control of TB is done by means of:

1. Early diagnosis with the help of sputum examination, mass miniature radiography and mantoux text.
2. Chemotherapy.
3. Rehabilitation.
4. Surveillance.

Revised National Tuberculosis Control Program (RNTCP) started in 1993 as pilot projects was launched as a centrally sponsored program in 1997. It aims:

1. To achieve 85% cure rate amongst infectious cases through short course chemotherapy.
2. To detect 70% of estimated cases through sputum microscopy.
3. To involve NGOs.
4. To provide directly observed treatment short course (DOTS).

Now domiciliary treatment is given to all except those who may need temporary hospitalization as in the event of severe hemoptysis. Two types of drugs are being used in the treatment of TB—the bactericidal drugs (rifampicin, INH, streptomycin, pyrazinamide) and the bacteriostatic drugs (ethambutol, thiacetazone, ethionamide, prothionamide, para amino salicylic acid (PAS), cycloserine, kanamycin, viomycin and capreomycin).

Antituberculous drugs are also classified into first-line drugs and second-line drugs. First-line drugs used in treatment of TB are ethambutol, isoniazid, pyrazinamide and rifampicin and the second line drugs are:

1. Aminoglycosides, e.g. amikacin (AMK), kanamycin (KM).
2. Polypeptides, e.g. capreomycin, viomycin, enviomycin.
3. Fluoroquinolones, e.g. ciprofloxacin (CIP), levofloxacin (LVF), moxifloxacin (MXF).
4. Thioamides, e.g. ethionamide, prothionamide.

Directly Observed Treatment Short Course

This strategy devised by WHO is adopted in India. The entire country is covered under directly observed treatment short course (DOTS) since March 2006. In the initial intensive phase health worker watches as the patient swallows the tablets; in continuation phase medicines are issued for 1 week. Different drug regimens used are detailed in Table 3.2.

Any patient treated with category I or category II who has a positive smear at 5, 6 or 7 months of treatment should be considered a failure and started on category II treatment afresh (Table 3.3). Dosage for children is mentioned in Table 3.4.

TABLE 3.2: Different drug regimens

Category	Regimen
Category I patients	
Newly diagnosed sputum positive pulmonary tuberculosis	$2(HRZE)_3$ $4(HR)_2$
Sputum negative pulmonary tuberculosis with extensive parenchymal involvement.	
Severe form of extrapulmonary tuberculosis	
Category II patients	
Treatment failure cases	$2(HRZES)_3$ $1(HRZE)_3$ $5(HRE)_3$
Relapse cases	
Return after interruption	
Category III patients	
Sputum negative pulmonary tuberculosis with minimal involvement	$2(HRZ)_3$ $4(HR)_3$
Less severe form of extrapulmonary tuberculosis	

Note: The number before the letters, e.g. 2(HRZE), etc. refers to the number of months of treatment. The subscript after the letters refers to the number of doses per week; H: Isoniazid (600 mg); R: Rifampicin (450 mg); Z: Pyrazinamide (1,500 mg); E: Ethambutol (1,200 mg adults) 30 mg/kg body weight in children; not given to children below 6 years of age; Patients who weigh more than 60 kg receive additional rifampicin 150 mg; Patients more than 50 years old receive streptomycin 500 mg; Patients in categories I and II who have positive sputum smear at the end of the initial intensive phase receive an additional month of intensive treatment.

TABLE 3.3: Duration of treatment

Category	Duration		Total
	Intensive phase	Continuation phase	
Category I	8 week (24 doses)	18 week (54 doses)	26 week (78 doses)
Category II	12 week (36 doses)	22 week (66 doses)	34 week (102 doses)
Category III	8 week (24 doses)	18 week (54 doses)	26 week (78 doses)

Latent Tuberculosis Infection

Latent tuberculosis infection (LTBI) can be detected with immune based tests such as the tuberculin skin test (TST) or interferon gamma release assays (IGRA). Therapy for those with positive

TABLE 3.4: Dosage for children

Drug	Dosage
Isoniazid: 10–15 mg/kg	Thrice a week
Rifampicin: 10 mg/kg	
Pyrazinamide: 35 mg/kg	
Streptomycin: 15 mg/kg	
Ethambutol: 30 mg/kg	

tests can reduce the subsequent risk of reactivation and development of active TB. Current standard therapy is INH, which reduce the risk of active TB by as much as 90% if taken daily for 9 months. However, this lengthy duration of therapy discourages patients and the risk of serious adverse events such as hepatotoxicity, discourages both patients and providers. As a result, completion of INH therapy is less than 50% in many programs. However, programs that offer close follow-up with supportive staff, who emphasize patient education have reported much better results. The problems with INH have stimulated development and evaluation of several shorter regimens. One alternative was 2 months daily rifampin and pyrazinamide; this regimen has been largely abandoned due to unacceptably high rates of hepatotoxicity and poor tolerability. The combination of INH and rifampin taken for 3 or 4 months, has efficacy equivalent to 6 months INH albeit with somewhat increased hepatotoxicity. 4 months rifampin has efficacy at least equivalent to 6 months INH, but there are inadequate trial data on efficacy. The safety of this regimen has been demonstrated repeatedly. Most recently, a regimen of 3 months INH rifapentine taken once weekly under direct observation has been evaluated in a large scale trial. Results have not yet been published, but if this regimen is as effective as INH, this may be a very good alternative. However, close monitoring and surveillance is strongly suggested for the first few years after its introduction. Evidence from several randomized trials has shown that the benefits of LTBI therapy is only in individuals who are TST positive even among those with HIV infection. Hence, LTBI therapy should be given only to those with positive tests for LTBI. We conclude that LTBI therapy is considerably underutilized in many settings, particularly in low- and middle-income countries.

Directly observed treatment short (DOTS) plus strategy is adopted for the management of drug resistant MDR-TB. The diagnosis is made in intermediate reference laboratories. Qualified staff treat using category IV regimen (second line drugs) in DOTS Plus sites in tertiary care institutions (Table 3.5). At the end of 2008, DOTS plus is available in 7 states, viz. Gujarat, Maharashtra, Andhra Pradesh, Haryana, Delhi, West Bengal and Kerala.

TABLE 3.5: Regimen for category IV MDR-TB

Category	Regimen
Category IV MDR-TB	Initial/intensive phase: 6 (9) Km Ofx (Lfx) Eto Cs Z E
	Continuation phase: 18 Ofx (Lfx) Eto E

Category IV regimen: 6 (9) Km Ofx (Lfx) Eto Cs Z E/18 Ofx (Lfx) Eto E; intensive phase: 6–9 months, 6 drugs; continuation phase: 18 months, 3 drugs. The drugs and dosages are given below:

1. Kanamycin (Km): 750–1,000 mg daily deep 1M.
2. Ofloxacin (Ofl): 600–800 mg daily (one or two divided doses).
3. Levofloxacin (Lfx): 750 mg daily (one or two divided doses).
4. Ethionamide (Eto): 500–750 mg daily (one or two divided doses) (maximum 1 g/day).
5. Cycloserine (Cs): 500–750 mg daily (one or two divided doses).
6. Pyrazinamide (Z): 500 mg for 16–25 kg body weight; 250 mg for 26–45 kg and 1,500 mg for > 45 kg, respectively.

The Stop TB Partnership, the erstwhile 'the Stop TB Initiative' was established in 1998. It comprises a network of international organizations, countries, donors from the public and private sectors, governmental and non-governmental organizations and individuals that have expressed an interest in working together to achieve this goal.

WHO has developed a new six point 'Stop TB Strategy', which builds on the successes of DOTS while also explicitly addressing the key challenges facing TB. Its goal is to dramatically reduce the global burden of TB by 2015 by ensuring all TB patients, including those coinfected with HIV and those with drug-resistant TB, benefit from universal access to high-quality diagnosis and patient-centered treatment. The strategy also supports the development of new and effective tools to prevent, detect and treat TB.

❑ MENINGOCOCCAL MENINGITIS

Meningococcal meningitis (cerebrospinal fever), which carries a high mortality, occurs sporadically in small clusters all over the world with seasonal variations. It is predominantly a disease of children and young adults. Fatality is 50% in untreated cases.

The highest burden of meningococcal disease in the world occurs in the 'African meningitis belt', which extends across the dry, savannah parts of Sub-Saharan Africa from Senegal in the west to Ethiopia in the east. In the 2009 epidemic season, 14 African countries implementing enhanced surveillance, reported 88,199 suspected cases, including 5352 deaths, the largest number since a 1996 epidemic. From 1 January to 17 April 2012, 10 of the 14 countries of the African meningitis belt reported 11,647 cases and 960 deaths.

Outbreaks have occurred also in other countries such as Brazil, Mongolia, Scandinavian countries, etc.

In India, outbreaks have occurred in 1966 (616 cases with 20.9% case fatality rate) and in 1985 (6,133 cases with 799 deaths) in Delhi and adjoining areas besides isolated cases in several parts of India in 1985. During 2005, a total of 405 cases and 48 deaths were reported.

Causative Organism

Neisseria meningitidis, a gram-negative diplococci, is the causative organism. *N. meningitidis* serogroups B and C are the most common cause of disease in Europe, America, Australia and New Zealand and tend to occur more frequently in winter and spring. Serogroup A is the main cause of disease in Africa and Asia.

Reservoir and Source

Cases and carriers form the reservoir pool. 5%–30% of normal population may harbor the organism in the nasopharynx during interepidemic periods. Temporary carrier state may last for 10 months. Nasopharyngeal secretion is the source of infective material.

Mode of Transmission

Droplet infection.

Incubation Period

The incubation period is 3–4 days usually, but may vary between 2 and 10 days.

Factors Facilitating Transmission

Overcrowding, low socioeconomic status and dry, cold months favor transmission.

Clinical Manifestation

Meningococcal meningitis illness begins with intense headache, vomiting and stiff neck. In a few hours coma sets in. Fatality is 50% in untreated cases.

Prevention and Control

Penicillin, if started within 2 days of the illness, can save 95% of patients. If allergic to penicillin chloromphenical can be used as substitute. Isolation is of limited value as carriers outnumber cases. Treating carriers with rifampicin and chemoprophylaxis for close contacts with either rifampicin or sulfadiazine are useful in the control of the spread.

Mass chemoprophylaxis of close communities also can be advocated to prevent the spread. Vaccination of high-risk population with the polysaccharide vaccine and booster every 3 years can prevent the disease. But this vaccine is not recommended for infants below 2 years and contraindicated in pregnancy. Well-ventilated houses and avoiding overcrowding will help to prevent the spread.

❑ ACUTE RESPIRATORY INFECTIONS

Acute respiratory infections (ARIs) continue to be the leading cause of acute illnesses worldwide and the most important cause of mortality in infants and young children accounting for about 2 million deaths globally each year. On an average a child has 5–8 attacks of ARI annually. ARI accounts for 30%–40% of the hospital visits by children in office practice.

Acute lower respiratory infections (severe pneumonia and bronchitis commonly) often do not respond to therapy. Complicating this picture is the increasing number of children infected by HIV/AIDS, which makes them not only more vulnerable to lower respiratory infections, but also more likely to succumb to these infections. Pneumonia is responsible for about 21% of all deaths in children aged less than 5 years (5,000 childhood deaths everyday). It is pertinent to know that hospital-acquired pneumonia is a major public health problem. Pneumonia is the second most common type of all nosocomial infections.

The incidence of ARIs in children aged less than 5 years is estimated to be 151 million and 5 million new episodes each year in developing and industrialized countries respectively. Most cases occur in India (43 million), China (21 million), Pakistan (10 million), Bangladesh, Indonesia and Nigeria (56 million each).

Causative Organisms

Streptococcus pneumoniae or pneumococci is a leading cause of morbidity and mortality among children worldwide and particularly in developing countries. Children become nasopharyngeal carriers during first few years of life. Many children will go on to develop otitis media and a few will eventually develop invasive pneumococcal disease including bacteremic pneumonia and/or meningitis.

Respiratory syncytial virus (RSV) is the most important cause of viral lower respiratory tract illness in infants and children worldwide.

The main etiological agents that cause ARIs in children include the following:

1. *Streptococcus pneumoniae.*
2. *Haemophilus influenzae* type b (Hib).
3. *Staphylococcus aureus* and other bacterial species.
4. Respiratory syncytial virus.
5. Measles virus.

6. Human parainfluenza viruses type 1, 2 and 3 (PIV-1, PIV-2 and PIV-3).
7. Influenza virus.
8. Varicella virus.

Mode of Transmission

Droplet infection: Transmission is by airborne droplets mainly through direct person-to-person contact during the acts of coughing sneezing, etc.

Factors Facilitating Transmission

The populations most at risk for developing a fatal respiratory disease are the very young, the elderly and the immunocompromised. Low birth weight, malnourished and non-breastfed children and those living in overcrowded conditions are at higher risk of getting pneumonia. These children are also at a higher risk of death from pneumonia.

Clinical Features

Acute respiratory infections are of two types based on the site of infection—acute upper respiratory infections (AURI) and acute lower respiratory infections (ALRI). AURI includes nasopharyngitis, pharyngotonsillitis and otitis. ALRI includes epiglottitis, laryngitis, laryngotracheitis, bronchitis, bronchiolitis and pneumonia.

Fever, fast breathing, chest indrawing, stridor, wheezing, abnormally sleepiness, cyanosis, inability to drink, convulsions, nasal flaring, etc are seen in ALRI.

Prevention and Control

Primary prevention involves reduction of major risk factors like low birth weight, malnutrition, indoor air pollution and parental smoking habits.

Interventions

Interventions to control ARIs can be divided into four basic categories:

1. Immunization against specific pathogens.
2. Early diagnosis and treatment of disease.
3. Improvements in nutrition.
4. Safer environments.

The last two fall under public health and require multisectoral involvement.

Adequate primary healthcare services with better facilities for early detection and treatment of ARIs is very important in reducing the morbidity and mortality. Proper treatment of pneumonia with antibiotics can bring down the mortality due to it. Development of the skills in the health personnel will help in early detection of pneumonia. Health education to mothers in this regard is very vital so that they will seek treatment early.

Effective immunization coverage against vaccine preventable diseases is known to reduce the incidence of ARI. Use of Hib conjugate vaccines has resulted in a truly remarkable decline in Hib disease in the areas used. Though WHO has recommended the global implementation of the Hib conjugate vaccines, it is not yet routinely made available to a majority of children worldwide. Similarly, the introduction of the conjugate pneumococcal vaccine in routine infant immunization should have a major impact on pneumonia in children less than 5 years of age worldwide as already documented in the USA.

Guidelines

Practical guidelines issued by WHO for the management of ARI:

1. Case management of ARI in young infants 0–2 months.
   a. Signs of pneumonia, sepsis and meningitis are difficult to differentiate in a young infant less than 2 months of age.
   b. Young infants with fast breathing or chest indrawing should be suspected to have serious bacterial infection.

These infants should be referred to a hospital and treated with IM ampicillin/penicillin and gentamicin for 10 days. In situations where referral is not possible, oral amoxicillin or cotrimoxazole twice daily with IM gentamicin once daily should be given for 10 days.

c. Supportive measures include frequent breastfeeding and keeping the young infant warm.

2. Case management of ARI in children 2 month to 5 years.
   a. All children presenting with cough or difficulty in breathing should be assessed.
   b. Children with non-severe pneumonia should be given antibiotics for 5 days. Cotrimoxazole, a low-cost broad spectrum antimicrobial or oral amoxicillin can be given.
   c. All children should also be assessed for signs of severe malnutrition—visible severe wasting and edema of both foot. Children with any of these signs must be referred to a hospital as they are at a very high-risk of death from pneumonia.
   d. Children with danger signs should be referred to a hospital after a single dose of IM chloramphenicol. In situations where referral is not possible, twice daily injections of IM chloramphenicol should be continued for 5 days, followed by oral antibiotic therapy for another 5 days.
   e. Children with severe pneumonia should be referred to a hospital for treatment with IM ampicillin/penicillin. In situations where referral is not possible, these children can be treated with oral amoxicillin given thrice daily for 7 days. Oral amoxicillin has recently been shown to be effective in treatment of severe pneumonia.
   f. Supportive measures include increased oral fluids to prevent dehydration, continued feeding to avoid malnutrition and antipyretics to reduce high fever.

CHAPTER

4

Intestinal Infections

Intestinal tract of man has to bear the brunt of diseases when his/her food and water is contaminated. More than 60% of diseases that affect man in developing countries are due to infections of the intestinal tract. Important infections acquired through intestinal tract route are the following:

- Poliomyelitis: Food poisoning
- Hepatitis A, E: Amebiasis
- Cholera: Ascariasis
- Acute diarrheal diseases: Hookworm infestation
- Typhoid fever: Dracunculiasis
- *Escherichia coli*: Diarrhea.

❑ POLIOMYELITIS

Poliomyelitis, a childhood disease; is a primary infection of the alimentary tract. But it does not cause any significant abdominal symptoms. In a small percentage of cases (about 1%) the infection spreads to the nervous system and causes acute flaccid paralysis (AFP).

An estimated 350,000 cases were reported in more than 125 endemic countries in 1988. But after the launching of the Global Polio Eradication Initiative in 1988, polio cases have decreased by over 99%.

Globally in 2011, 650 wild polio cases were reported. Most recent cases, in 2012, occurred in Pakistan (43), Afghanistan (21), Nigeria (93) and Chad (5), totally 162 cases.

Causative Organism

Poliovirus, an ribonucleic acid (RNA) virus, which has three serotypes—type 1, type 2 and type 3 causes poliomyelitis. This virus can survive for 4 months in water and 6 months in feces in cold weather conditions. A higher dose of chlorine is needed to kill this virus. But boiling readily kills it.

Reservoir and Source

Man is the only reservoir of infection. Most infections are subclinical, which play an important role in transmission. The feces and oropharyngeal secretion are the source of infective material. The cases are communicable for 7–10 days before the onset and for a similar period after the onset of symptoms.

Mode of Transmission

Main mode of spread is by feco-oral transmission from contaminated water, milk, foods, flies and articles of daily use or from contaminated fingers. Droplet infection by means of secretion from throat can also occur during acute viremia stage.

Incubation Period

Incubation period is usually 7–14 days.

Factors Facilitating Transmission

Overcrowding, filthy environment due to poor sanitation, unsafe water, lack of personal hygiene all favor transmission of polio.

Clinical Manifestation

The main clinical feature of polio is the asymmetrical AFP of limbs after a bout of fever. Recovery takes place slowly leaving some residual paralysis.

Not all poliovirus infected children develop paralytic poliomyelitis. 95% of infections are subclinical. Only about 1% of infected children develop paralysis. During epidemics, injections like diphtheria-tetanus-pertussis (DPT) vaccine may precipitate paralytic poliomyelitis (provocative poliomyelitis). Fatigue, trauma, intramuscular injections, operative procedures such as tonsillectomy are the other risk factors that may provoke paralytic polio.

Prevention and Control

Control of polio is difficult because of the large number of subclinical cases seen (iceberg phenomenon). However notification, isolation, disinfection of feces and articles of daily use, personal hygiene, sanitary disposal of excreta and protected water supply all will help in the control of spread. Boiling drinking water is a simple measure to prevent the spread.

Dramatic progress has been made since the Global Polio Eradication Initiative (GPEI) was formed in 1988. The four pillars of polio eradication are:

1. Routine immunization.
2. Supplementary immunization.
3. Surveillance.
4. Targeted 'mop-up' campaigns.

Cases have plummeted by 99%. Polio is on course to become the second disease after smallpox, to be wiped from the face of the earth. This rapid success has been achieved through a global campaign to immunize every child with the oral polio vaccine (OPV).

The National Polio Surveillance Project, which was launched in 1997, provides technical and logistic assistance to the Government of India and works closely with state governments and a broad array of partner agencies to achieve the goal of polio eradication in India.

Potent live attenuated and killed vaccines are available for prevention. Live attenuated OPV is used in the Indian National Immunization Program. 5 doses at birth, 1½ months, 2½ months and 3½ months and at 1½–2 years of age are administered now for primary immunization. Parents should be advised not to give hot fluids for half an hour after the vaccine administration. However, breast milk can be given. Vaccine droppers are advisable for oral administration of the vaccine. When spoons are used, they should not be cleaned with disinfectants, but should be sterilized by boiling and then cooled with ice water. The vaccine should be kept in ice, while administering it in the field centers and it is preferably administered in a cool room. In PHCs it should be stored in subzero temperature [ice-lined refrigerator (ILR)], but frequent freezing and thawing of the vaccine is not advisable as it would affect the potency of the vaccine. The color of the vaccine vial monitor (VVM) should be noted before administration of the vaccine. OPV can be used only when the inner square is lighter than the outer circle. If the inner square is of the same color as or darker than the outer circle, it should not be used. Advantages of OPV are:

1. It can be easily administered.
2. Induces antibody production quickly.
3. Induces both humoral and local immunity.
4. Useful to control epidemics.
5. It helps to improve the herd immunity as the vaccine virus excreted by the vaccines infects unvaccinated persons also.

However, OPV should not be administered to children with severe acute infectious disease and to those suffering from leukemias and malignancy and those on corticosteroid therapy. Fever, diarrhea and dysentery when mild are not a contraindication for OPV administration.

Inactivated polio vaccine (IPV) has the advantage that it can be safely administered to persons with immune deficiency diseases and it has no serious adverse reactions. However IPV cannot be used during epidemics as it, being an injectable preparation, would cause provocative poliomyelitis. No injection should be given to children during an epidemic of polio for fear of causing provocative poliomyelitis. IPV is not used in the Indian immunization program.

Polio is considered amenable for eradication. With this in view pulse polio immunization program has been launched in India. In December and January, 2 doses of OPV, 1 dose in each month, at 1 month interval, are administered to all children below 5 years throughout the country. Consequent to this program, the incidence of polio has declined significantly and India is polio free for 1 year since January 2011.

Consequent to the declaration by WHO that India is polio free on 13-2-2014, India has made OPV Vaccination Certificate mandatory for travelers from and to seven polio reporting countries namely Afghanistan, Ethiopia, Syria, Kenya, Somalia, Nigeria and Pakistan.

However, the confirmation in 2000 that the vaccine-derived polioviruses can circulate and cause polio outbreaks after interruption of wild poliovirus transmission makes the use of OPV incompatible with a polio-free world.

❑ HEPATITIS A

Hepatitis A is an acute infectious disease commonly known as jaundice. The virus multiplies in the liver and cause disease. The hepatitis A virus (HAV) has a worldwide distribution and causes about 1.5 million clinical cases of each year. HAV is one of the main causes of hepatitis in humans accounting for 20%–40% of acute hepatitis in adults. The incidence in the developed countries is declining. But there is a high incidence in developing countries and rural areas.

Very high incidence is seen in Africa, parts of South America, the Middle East and of South-East Asia. High incidence is seen in Brazil's Amazon basin, China and Latin America. Intermediate incidence is observed in Southern and Eastern Europe and some regions of the Middle East. Low incidence in Australia, USA and Western Europe and very low incidence in Northern Europe and Japan are reported. In India, it occurs in sporadic as well as epidemic form.

Causative Organism

Hepatitis A virus, which causes this hepatitis, is a non-enveloped, spherical, positive-stranded RNA virus. It is an enterovirus (type 72 of the picornaviridae family). It is fairly resistant to disinfectants like chlorine. But boiling for 5 minutes can inactivate it readily.

Reservoir and Source

Man is the only reservoir. Feces containing the virus are the source of infective material.

Mode of Transmission

Feco-oral transmission, from person-to-person directly by contaminated fingers or indirectly by contaminated water, food or milk is the main mode of transmission. Very rarely parenteral and sexual transmission can take place.

Incubation Period

The incubation period varying with the dose of virus ingested 15–45 days.

Factors Facilitating Transmission

Open air defecation, poor sanitation, lack of personal hygiene, overcrowding and heavy rainfall, all favor transmission of this virus.

Clinical Manifestation

The infection may be asymptomatic or may manifest as mild to severe jaundice. Infection is common in children in whom it tends to be mild. However, all ages are susceptible to the infection, if there is no previous immunity. Clinically the disease is characterized by fever, loss of appetite, vomiting and yellow discoloration of conjunctiva and urine. Enlarged and tender liver may be present. Most of the cases recover without any sequelae. Very low mortality (0.1%) is seen.

Prevention and Control

Control of reservoir poses problem because the virus is excreted even during incubation period. Besides, the infection is seen in subclinical form and there is no specific treatment. However, strict bed rest and disinfection of feces and fomites should be advised besides notification. Personal and community hygiene, protected water supply, sanitary disposal of human excreta all will help to interrupt transmission. Ordinary chlorination does not affect the virus, but chlorination at 1 mg/L of residual chlorine (after 30 minutes at pH < 8.5) can destroy the virus. Boiling water can kill it readily.

Human normal immunoglobulin preparation can be advised for persons going to highly endemic areas, for close personal contacts and for the control of institutional outbreaks. But widespread use of immunoglobulins is not desirable. Four inactivated vaccines against hepatitis A are available (2 doses at 6–18 months interval). A combined vaccine with inactivated hepatitis A vaccine and recombinant hepatitis B vaccine is also available for children aged 1 year or older (3 doses at 0, 1 and 6 months).

❑ HEPATITIS E

Hepatitis E virus (HEV) can cause large waterborne epidemics as well as sporadic cases. Most outbreaks have occurred following monsoon rains, heavy flooding, fecal contamination of well water or massive surges of untreated sewage into city water treatment plants.

Hepatitis E is common in many parts of the world, outbreaks being common in parts of the world with hot climates and rare in temperate climates.

Hepatitis E virus was first identified in India in 1955 and has since been recognized in the Middle and Far East, in Northern and Western Africa, the central Asian Republics of the former Soviet Union in China and Hong Kong. More than 50% of acute viral hepatitis in developing countries is due to HEV. It has become an endemic disease in parts of Asia, Mexico, Central America and Africa. Globally, there are approximately 20 million incident hepatitis E infections every year with 70,000 deaths. Over 60% of all hepatitis E infections and 65% of all hepatitis E deaths occur in East and South Asia.

In India, 12%–50% of hepatitis cases are due to HEV. Outbreaks have occurred in Delhi (1955–56), Ahmedabad (1975–76), Pune (1978) and Kashmir (1980). The largest outbreak (over 79,000 cases) occurred in Kanpur, Uttar Pradesh in 1991 due to contaminated water from Ganges.

Causative Agent

Hepatitis E virus is a non-enveloped, spherical, positive-stranded, 27–34 nm RNA virus. HEV is now unclassified.

Reservoir and Source

Man is the reservoir. Feces are the source of infective material. Possible animal reservoirs of HEV are monkeys, pigs, cows, rodents, sheep or goats. All these species are susceptible to infection with HEV.

Mode of Transmission

Hepatitis E virus is spread by the oral-fecal route, implicated in several food and waterborne outbreaks. Fecal excretion of intact HEV is low and therefore secondary attack rate from infected individuals is generally lower (2%) as compared 10%–20% with hepatitis A. No sexual or bloodborne transmission is known. Vertical transmission of HEV from mothers to their infants has been reported.

Incubation Period

Incubation period is longer than that of HAV: 2–9 weeks, average 6 weeks.

Clinical Features

Hepatitis E infection occurs in sporadic and epidemic form. Acute symptomatic HEV infection is most common in young adults aged 15–40 years and is uncommon in children. Though frequent, it is mostly asymptomatic and anicteric in children.

The clinical spectrum of the disease may range in severity from subclinical to fulminant cases. Typical signs and symptoms include jaundice, anorexia, hepatomegaly, abdominal pain and tenderness, nausea and vomiting and fever. No chronic or carrier state has been demonstrated. Generally, a low mortality rate (0.5%–4%) is associated with HEV infection. But in pregnant women HEV can be serious and cause fulminant hepatitis with a case fatality rate of 10%–42%. An Ethiopian study found that 35% of HEV-infected hospitalized pregnant women had premature delivery.

Prevention and Control

In 2011, the first vaccine to prevent hepatitis E infection was registered in China. But it is not available for global use.

Recently, swine HEV was found to be immunologically cross-reactive with human HEV and might thus prove useful as an attenuated 'Jennerian' vaccine for immunization against human hepatitis E.

No specific treatment is available. The usual control measures adopted for hepatitis A can very well be used against HEV also. Washing hands with soap after using a bathroom or changing a diaper and before preparing and eating food is important to prevent the spread. Water with ice of unknown purity, uncooked shellfish, uncooked vegetables and fruits that are not washed are to be avoided. Travelers from non-endemic countries should be careful.

❑ CHOLERA

Cholera is one of the three diseases requiring WHO notification, the others being plague and yellow fever. It is an acute diarrheal disease with a propensity to cause rapid dehydration and shock. It is known to occur as epidemics and pandemics. Six pandemics have already occurred in the world and the seventh pandemic is still continuing.

In 2011, cholera cases have been reported from all regions of the world. A cumulative total of 589,854 cases with 7,816 deaths were reported from 58 countries. The case fatality rate was 1.3%.

In India, there were 37,783 cases with 84 deaths between 1997 and 2006 and in 2006 the country reported 1939 cases with 3 deaths. In Punjab and Haryana, during July–September 2007, there were 745 cases with 4 deaths. Latest outbreaks have occurred in Jammu and Kashmir (238 cases), Karnataka (102 cases) and West Bengal (87 cases) during the week ending 23rd 2012.

Causative Organism

Cholera is caused by *Vibrio cholerae* 01. Two biotypes are classical and El Tor. Both the types are further divided into three serotypes—Inaba, Ogawa and Hikojima. The current pandemic is caused by El Tor biotype. A new strain *Vibrio cholerae* 0139 has also been reported. The vibrios produce an exotoxin (enterotoxin), which causes the severe diarrhea seen in cholera. Boiling kills it in a few seconds. Bleaching powder is also a good disinfectant against *Vibrio.*

Reservoir and Source

Man is the only reservoir known cases and carriers. Carrier state is usually temporary, but may be chronic also. Stool and vomit of cases are the source of infective material. Cholera is dose dependent. Normally very high dose (1,011 organisms) is needed to produce clinical disease.

Mode of Transmission

Transmission is by fecal-oral route through contaminated water, food and drinks. Bottle feeding may be a risk for infants. Transmission from person to person can also occur through contaminated fingers, linen and other fomites. Flies also may be involved in the transmission.

Incubation Period

Incubation period is few hours to 5 days; commonly 1–2 days.

Clinical Manifestation

Cholera affects all ages and both the sexes. In endemic areas, attack rate is highest in children. The onset of the disease is abrupt with profuse, painless, watery diarrhea and vomiting. The stools have the characteristic 'rice water' appearance. The patient develops shock and collapses quickly due to loss of large quantity of water and salts from the body. The signs of dehydration are sunken eyes, scaphoid abdomen, loss of skin elasticity, dry tongue, intense thirst, oliguria, cold and clammy extremities and weak or absent pulse. The patient may complain of cramps in legs and abdomen and even die due to dehydration and acidosis. Most mild cases recover slowly in 1–3 days.

Confirmation of Diagnosis

Laboratory tests are needed to confirm the diagnosis of cholera. Stool samples, using a rubber catheter, are directly collected in a bottle containing the transport medium [Venkataraman Ramakrishnan (VR) medium]. Alternately rectal swabs dipped into the holding medium also can be used to collect the stool sample. Vomitus is usually not collected for laboratory test. Using a microscope with dark field illumination, diagnosis of cholera can be established quickly on the bed side. Suspected water source and food article are also tested for *Vibrio cholerae.*

Suspected water should be collected in sterile bottles (1–3 L) or 9 volumes of sample water added to 1 volume of 10% peptone water is sent to laboratory by the quickest mode of transport for identification of cholera bacilli. Suspected food article (1–3 g) collected in transport media is also sent for isolation of the bacilli.

Prevention and Control

The usefulness of cholera vaccine as a preventive measure is doubted. Currently available vaccine is a killed vaccine and it is administered in 2 doses of 0.5 mL each at 4 weeks interval. Children below 1 year of age are not given cholera inoculation. The protective value of the vaccine is only 50% for a period of 3–6 months. Boosters are required every 6 months. Advice to boil drinking water should be an important health education message in prevention.

In the control of cholera, verification of diagnosis is to be done quickly by laboratory tests. Cholera is a notifiable disease locally, nationally and internationally. All national governments are obliged to notify WHO within 24 hours of the occurrence under International Health Regulations (IHR). All cases should be identified by aggressive search (early diagnosis) and promptly treated. Mildly dehydrated patients can be treated with oral rehydration salt (ORS) solution. But severely dehydrated cases should be treated with intravenous fluids by establishing treatment centers in the community or by transferring to a nearby hospital. However transporting to a long distance is not advisable as it may facilitate transmission. The antibiotic of choice against *Vibrio cholerae* is tetracycline. It is administered in a dose of 500 mg 6th hourly for 3 days. Erythromycin, furazolidone and cotrimoxazole are also effective against *Vibrio.*

After identifying all the cases and initiating prompt treatment, epidemiological investigation to ascertain the extent of the outbreak and the mode of transmission should be carried out to control the epidemic effectively. Disinfection of water sources, food sanitation and sanitary disposal of human excreta, concurrent disinfection of patient's stools, vomit and soiled linen and terminal disinfection of the rooms are very important to contain the epidemic. Chemoprophylaxis with tetracycline can be advised for household contacts. But this method is not suitable for mass community application. Educating people to wash hands with soap after attending to a cholera patient and to boil water for drinking during epidemics is also important in the control of the epidemic.

❑ ACUTE DIARRHEAL DISEASES

Acute diarrheas are a group of diseases characterized by episodes of diarrhea, which usually last for 3–7 days, but sometimes may last up to 10–14 days.

Diarrheal disease is the second leading cause of death in children under 5 years old. It is both preventable and treatable. Diarrheal disease kills 1.5 million children every year. Globally, there are about 2 billion cases of diarrheal disease every year. Diarrheal disease mainly affects children under 2 years old. Diarrhea is a leading cause of malnutrition in children under 5 years old. Being a major public health problem in developing countries diarrheal diseases consume a significant amount of health budget. About 15% of all pediatric beds in some developing countries are occupied by admissions due to gastroenteritis.

In India, diarrhea is one of the most common causes of death in under 5 children. Up to a third of the total pediatric admissions are due to diarrheal diseases. Water pollution and the failure of proper management of sewage in both urban and rural areas are responsible acute diarrheal disease in India.

Causative Organisms

Acute diarrheas are caused by a number of organisms. Viruses like *Rotavirus,* adenovirus, coronavirus and *Enterovirus,* bacteriae like enterotoxigenic *Escherichia coli, Shigella, Salmonella, Bacillus cereus* and *Campylobacter jejuni* and others like *Entamoeba histolytica, Giardia lamblia* and intestinal worms are all incriminated in causing acute diarrheas. *Rotavirus* is the leading cause of diarrhea in infants and young children worldwide.

Reservoir and Source

Man is the principal reservoir (e.g. *E. coli, Shigella* species, *Giardia).* Animals also are important reservoirs (e.g. *E. coli* 0157:H7, *Campylobacter jejuni, Salmonella* species and *Yersinia enterocolitica).*

Most *E. coli* illnesses have been associated with eating undercooked, contaminated ground beef. *Escherichia coli* bacteria live in the intestines of healthy cattle.

Mode of Transmission

Feco-oral transmission through contaminated water, food or through contaminated fingers, fomites or dirt is the primary or exclusive mode of transmission. Meat becomes contaminated with *E. coli* during slaughter and organisms can be thoroughly mixed into beef when it is ground. Contaminated beef looks and smells normal. Bacteria present on a cow's udders or on equipment, may get into raw milk and cause the infection. Infection may occur after swimming in or drinking sewage-contaminated water. Unpasteurized juices such as apple cider, may also cause the infection.

Factors Facilitating Transmission

Poverty, malnutrition, lack of personal and domestic hygiene, bottle feeding and the unhygienic practices associated with it, open air defecation all favor transmission of acute diarrhea.

Clinical Manifestation

Acute diarrheas are common among children specially those between 6 months and 2 years of age. Infants below 6 months who are fed on formula foods are also affected. Acute diarrheas are manifested as diarrheal episodes and the incidence may be 6–12 episodes per child per year. The diarrhea is watery, but may be stinged with blood in dysentery. Mild fever may also be present.

Prevention and Control

Immunization against measles, protected water supply, sanitary disposal of human excreta, improved food hygiene at home and hotels, antifly measures and health education stressing the importance of hygienic preparation of weaning foods and hand washing before eating all will help in the prevention of diarrheal diseases.

Rotavirus vaccine will prevent about 74% of all rotavirus cases, about 98% of severe cases and about 96% of hospitalizations due to rotavirus. The vaccine is given by mouth. The 1st dose of rotavirus vaccine should be given between 6–12 weeks of age and two additional doses are given at 4–10 week intervals. Children should get all three doses before they are 33 weeks old.

In diarrheal diseases, ORS solution has assumed a primary role in preventing mortality due to dehydration. ORS are dispensed in packets, which are provided to all primary healthcare institutions for distribution to the needy.

Slight hypertonicity of hitherto used standard ORS solution combined with transient partial glucose malabsorption may cause worsening diarrhea and increasing serum sodium concentrations in some children when given only small amounts of plain water additionally.

In May 2004 WHO and UNICEF recommended low osmolarity ORS along with zinc supplementation. Zinc ($\geq$ 5 mg/day) is supplemented as dispersible tablets or as syrup for children above 6 months of age for a period of 10–14 days as an adjunct therapy and it should not contain other micronutrients that may compete for absorption.

The entire powder is to be dissolved in 1 L of potable water and fed to the patient within 24 hours. The reduced osmolarity ORS solution was equally as effective as the standard WHO; ORS solution among adult cholera patients, but that the incidence of asymptomatic hyponatremia was higher in those who received the reduced osmolarity ORS solution (Tables 4.1 and 4.2).

Parents should be educated to give home available foods like rice kanji, coconut water or butter milk and also to continue breastfeeding during diarrheal episodes.

Antibiotics are indicated only when the cause of diarrhea is established. Unnecessary administration of antibiotics is known to cause more harm than good.

As a long-term measure, maternal nutrition and supplementary feeding to children should be improved. Breastfeeding and proper weaning practices should be promoted.

❑ TYPHOID FEVER

Typhoid fever, also known as enteric fever, is a bacterial disease caused by the bacterium *Salmonella typhi*. As it is seen wherever there is poor sanitation and lack of safe water, typhoid is still common in the developing world. WHO identifies typhoid as a serious public health problem. Its incidence is highest in children and young adults between 5 and 19 years old.

The disease remains an important public health problem in developing countries. In 2008, it was estimated that annual global incidence was 21 million cases worldwide, resulting in 216,000 deaths. More

TABLE 4.1: Composition of reduced osmolarity ORS

Ingredient	g/L
Sodium chloride	2.6
Trisodium citrate, dihydrate	2.9
Potassium chloride	1.5
Glucose, anhydrous	13.5

TABLE 4.2: Composition of reduced osmolarity ORS

Ingredient	mmol/L
Sodium	75
Potassium	20
Chloride	65
Citrate	10
Glucose	75
Total osmolarity	245

(*Adapted from* WHO Drug Information, Volume 16, Nov 2002)

than 90% of this morbidity and mortality occurred in Asia. It has been virtually eliminated in many areas of industrialized countries because of the availability of proper sanitary facilities. Most cases in developed countries are imported from endemic countries.

In India, typhoid fever is endemic. It may also occur as a sporadic or an epidemic disease. Typhoid is the 5th most common communicable disease in India. About 69% of hospitalized typhoid patients in India are children.

Causative Organism

The bacterium *Salmonella enterica* serovar *typhi* is the major cause of enteric fever. *Salmonella paratyphi* A and B also cause this disease infrequently. The *S. typhi* is a very sensitive organism and it is readily killed by drying, sunlight, boiling and disinfection with bleaching powder.

Reservoir and Source

Man is the only reservoir cases and carriers. Typhoid is known for its occurrence in chronic carrier state in 2%–5% of cases who may excrete the bacilli for many years. Colonization of the bacilli in gallbladder is responsible for this chronic carrier state. Typhoid carriers excrete the bacilli not only in feces, but also in urine. Therefore the sources of infective material are the feces and urine.

Mode of Transmission

Fecal-oral or urine-oral transmission through contaminated water, food and milk or through flies and soiled finger is the mode of transmission of typhoid bacilli.

Incubation Period

The incubation period is usually 10–14 days usually, but may vary from 3 days to 3 weeks depending upon the dose of bacilli ingested.

Factors Facilitating Transmission

Open defecation and urination, lack of food hygiene and personal hygiene at homes and hotels, bad environmental sanitation leading to fly breeding, lack of protected water supply all facilitate transmission of typhoid. This disease is observed more during rainy season (July–September).

Clinical Manifestation

In virtually all endemic areas, the incidence of typhoid fever is highest in children 5–19 years of age. Typhoid fever manifests as continuous fever for 3–4 weeks with involvement of lymphoid tissues and constitutional symptoms. If untreated, mortality may be significant due to septicemia and intestinal perforation. Carrier state: 2%–5% of cases may become chronic carriers in whom the gallbladder (with an alkaline pH) gets infected. The story of 'Typhoid Mary', who had been transmitting the disease to more than 1,300 inmates of households where she worked as a cook is a classic case of chronic carrier state in typhoid.

Prevention and Control

The occurrence of *S. typhi* strains that are resistant to fluoroquinolones emphasizes the need to use safe and effective vaccines to prevent typhoid fever. WHO recommends vaccination for people travelling in endemic areas. People living in such areas, people in refugee camps, microbiologists, sewage workers and children should be the target groups for vaccination. Vaccination is also indicated to household contacts, school children, hospital staff and those attending melas and yatras.

Two safe and effective vaccines are now licensed and available—the Vi polysaccharide and the live oral vaccine Ty2la. An efficacy trial is being planned for a new *S. paratyphi* A vaccine composed of the surface O-specific polysaccharide (OSP) conjugated with tetanus toxoid.

In routine immunization, either Vi or Ty21a vaccine should be used where typhoid fever is endemic in children aged over 2 years.

Oral typhoid vaccine is indicated for adults and children above 6 years. One capsule on days 1, 3 and 5 is the dose irrespective of age. It is administered 1 hour before meal with cold or lukewarm milk or water. Antibiotics should be avoided for 7 days before or after the immunization series. Protection is for 3 years and therefore boosters are necessary once in 3 years. But it is not recommended in immune deficiency whether congenital or acquired and acute febrile and intestinal infections. The Vi vaccine is recommended for use in immunocompromised hosts.

Before or during an outbreak situation, if the community in question cannot be fully immunized, persons aged 2–19 years should be the target group for vaccination in addition to children in nursery schools.

Advice to boil drinking water should also be stressed to prevent the spread.

Control of the reservoir is important to contain the spread of the disease. Typhoid cases are to be notified. All cases should be diagnosed early, isolated in hospitals and put on complete treatment. Blood culture and stool or rectal swab culture can detect the organisms. New rapid diagnostic tests such as Typhidot detects IgM and IgG antibodies to *S. typhi* much early (in hours) when compared to blood culture reports, which take 1 day. Typhidot-M test would be useful in areas of high endemicity. IgM dipstick test, another serological test provides a rapid and simple alternative for the diagnosis of typhoid fever particularly in situations where culture facilities are not available.

Attendants of typhoid patients should be advised to wash their hands with soap and disinfectant. Chloramphenicol is now not used in the treatment of typhoid because of its propensity to cause aplastic anemia. Amoxicillin or trimethoprim + sulfamethoxazole or 4-fluoroquinolone such as ciprofloxacin or ofloxacin is the latest drugs employed. Multidrug resistant cases are treated with ceftriaxone or ciprofloxacin. Disinfection of stools and urine of typhoid cases with 5% cresol for at least 2 hours, disinfection or steam sterilization of soiled linen and cleaning of hands after attending to a typhoid patient are important to arrest the spread. Identification of carriers of typhoid and their effective treatment is another important step to contain the disease.

❑ FOOD POISONING

Acute gastroenteritis, caused by the ingestion of food contaminated with bacteria or their toxins, inorganic chemical substances like arsenic and other poisons derived from plants and animals, is called food poisoning.

Food poisoning cases may be mistaken for cholera or arsenic poisoning. The differentiating points are:

1. Food poisoning starts with vomiting, while cholera starts with purging.
2. There is history of the partaking of a common meal in food poisoning.
3. No secondary cases occur in food poisoning, while it occurs in cholera.
4. Dehydration and collapse will be marked in cholera, while it is not so in food poisoning.

Food poisoning can be caused by organisms such as *Staphylococcus aureus, E. coli, Salmonella, Shigella, Campylobacter, Clostridium botulinum, Listeria, Bacillus cereus* and *Yersinia* and foods like mushroom and fish.

Infants and elderly people have the greatest risk for food poisoning. Adults are also at higher risk when they have a serious medical condition like kidney disease or diabetes or a weakened immune system.

Common food poisonings affecting man are:

1. *Salmonella* food poisoning.
2. Staphylococcal food poisoning.
3. Botulism.
4. *Clostridium perfringens* food poisoning.
5. *Bacillus cereus* food poisoning.
6. Listeriosis.

Salmonella Food Poisoning

The organisms that cause this food poisoning are *S. typhimurium, S. cholerasuis* and *S. enteritidis.* Farm animals, poultry, rats and mice are the reservoir and man gets the infection through ingestion of contaminated meat, milk and milk products, sausages, custards, eggs and egg products and through the foods contaminated by rat feces or its urine. Incubation period is 12–24 hours. There is sudden onset of chills, fever, nausea and vomiting. The diarrhea is watery, which may last 2–3 days.

Staphylococcal Food Poisoning

The enterotoxin of *Staphylococcus aureus* causes this food poisoning. Foods like salads, custards, milk and milk products get contaminated with staphylococci from the skin, throat and nose of humans and animals and from the boils in the hands of food handlers. Milk can get contaminated from the mastitis of cows. The staphylococci multiply in foods and elaborate the toxin. Since the toxin is preformed, the incubation period is short (1–6 hours) and therefore the food poisoning symptoms develop quickly. There is sudden onset of vomiting, abdominal cramps and diarrhea. Heating foods before consumption will not prevent this food poisoning as the toxin is thermostable. Therefore prevention of contamination during preparation of foods is essential for preventing this food poisoning.

Botulism

Botulism is a serious disease having high mortality, but rare. It is caused by the exotoxin of *Clostridium botulinum,* an anaerobic organism, which is abundantly present in soil, dust and intestinal tract of animals as spores. Water can also carry spores as well as the toxin. Foods like home canned vegetables, smoked or pickled fish, homemade cheese and tinned foods get contaminated with the spores from the soil or dust. Honey and dust are incriminated as sources for infant botulism in infants. Gastrointestinal infection of adults after broad spectrum antibiotic treatment and intestinal surgery or inflammatory bowl disease has been reported. Under anaerobic conditions, the spores germinate and elaborate the toxin. Incubation period is 12–36 hours. Unlike the other food poisoning, botulism causes no gastrointestinal symptoms like vomiting and diarrhea, but causes dysphagia, diplopia, ptosis, dysarthria, blurring of vision, muscle weakness and even quadriplegia.

Heating foods before consumption can prevent this food poisoning since the toxin is thermolabile. Antitoxin and toxoid are available for control and prevention of botulism. Poisoning also can result from wound infection (wound botulism) though very rare. Growth of the organism and the toxin formation takes place in the wound and the toxin reaches other parts via bloodstream. Wound botulism occurs in horses through procedures like injections, castration and umbilical infections in foals.

Clostridium perfringens Food Poisoning

This food poisoning is caused by *C. perfringens (C. welchii),* which is found in soil, water, feces of humans and animals and air. Foods like meat and poultry get contaminated with the spores of the organism during preparation. The spores survive cooking and when the dish is allowed to cool slowly at room temperature, germinate at optimum temperatures (between 30°C and 50°C) and produce toxins, which cause food poisoning. Incubation period is 6–24 hours. The clinical features are diarrhea and abdominal cramps. This food poisoning can be prevented by consuming the food immediately after cooking or by rapidly cooling it after preparation to prevent the germination of the spores.

Bacillus cereus Food Poisoning

This is caused by *B. cereus,* an aerobic, spore-bearing, motile gram positive rod, which is present in soil and in raw, dried and processed foods. The spores survive cooking, germinate at favorable temperature, while the food is allowed to cool slowly at room temperature and elaborate enterotoxins. Clinically it causes two types of symptoms, one characterized by predominantly vomiting and the other by diarrhea. The toxin of *B. cereus* is heat stable.

Listeriosis

Listeriosis is relatively a rare disease associated predominantly with ready-to-eat food products. The importance of this disease lies in the fact that it has the propensity to cause severe and serious infections in pregnant women and immunocompromised patients.

Listeriosis is caused by *Listeria monocytogene,* a gram-positive facultative anaerobic, non-spore forming rod. The organism is ubiquitous in the environment-widely distributed in soil, vegetables, silage, fecal material, sewage and water. It is resistant to high salinity and acidity. But it is killed by pasteurization and cooking. However, in certain ready-to-eat foods such as hot dogs and deli meats, contamination may occur after cooking, but before packaging.

The main mode of transmission is through contaminated food. Ready-to-eat foods are the main sources of infective material. Contamination occurs from soil, vegetables, silage, fecal material, sewage and water. Hot dogs, luncheon meats or deli meats, refrigerated pâtés or meat spreads, refrigerated smoked seafood, contaminated raw vegetables, unpasteurized (raw) milk or foods made from unpasteurized milk are the foods involved.

The incubation period is 1–2 days and the illness lasts 1–3 days. It manifests in two forms, viz.

1. Febrile gastroenteritis.
2. Severe or invasive listeriosis.

Febrile gastroenteritis patients present with fever, muscle aches, gastrointestinal nausea or diarrhea, headache, stiff neck, confusion, loss of balance or convulsions.

Invasive listeriosis manifests as perinatal listeriosis, meningitis or septicemia with 20%–30% mortality. Babies may be born with listeriosis if their mothers eat contaminated food during pregnancy.

Prevention needs hygienic practices in the kitchen such as washing hands, knives and cutting boards after handling uncooked food, thorough cooking of all meat, thorough washing of all vegetables and keeping raw meats separately from other foods during preparation to avoid cross-contamination. Pregnant women and immunocompromised patients should avoid soft cheeses such as Feta, Brie, blue cheese, Mexican-style cheese, Camembert and deli foods unless thoroughly heated. Thorough reheating of leftovers will make them safe for consumption.

Severe cases are treated for 2–6 weeks with intravenous Ampicillin. Gentamicin is added frequently for its synergistic effects. Trimethoprim-sulfamethoxazole is used as an alternative therapy.

Investigation of Food Poisoning

Investigation of food poisoning is important to ascertain the cause. The entire list of persons who consumed the suspected food should be collected. Particulars such as the list of foods eaten during the previous 2 days, time of onset of symptoms and their order of occurrence, age, sex, residence and occupation should be collected by using questionnaires. Samples of stool, vomit and remaining food should be collected and sent for identification of the organisms involved. Stool samples of food handlers should also be investigated. Animal experiments and antibody studies may be needed to confirm the diagnosis.

Kitchens and eating places should also be inspected and the food handlers questioned regarding food preparation. The data collected should be analyzed with reference to time, place and person. Food specific attack rates are calculated to fix the food responsible for poisoning.

Prevention and Control

Meat inspection, personal hygiene of food handlers, hotel sanitation, health education, refrigeration facilities to prevent bacterial proliferation and continuous surveillance of food preparation units and eating establishments by taking samples periodically are all necessary to control food poisoning outbreaks.

❑ *ESCHERICHIA COLI* (DIARRHEA)

Enterotoxigenic *E. coli* (ETEC) is an under-recognized, but extremely important cause of diarrhea in the developing world where there is inadequate clean water and poor sanitation. They are the most commonly isolated bacterial enteropathogen in children below 5 years of age in developing countries and account for several hundred million cases of diarrhea and several 10 of thousand deaths each year. *Escherichia coli* infection is an emerging food-borne illness. 10%–20% of acute diarrheas in developing countries are due to *E. coli*. ETEC was thought to account for approximately 200 million diarrhea episodes and 380,000 deaths annually. A more conservative estimate, about 170,000 deaths every year, was more recently suggested.

Causative Organism

Most of the strains of *E. coli* are harmless. But the ETEC causes disease in man. It is non-invasive, but elaborates two toxins that induce extreme fluid secretion from the small intestine and causes diarrhea.

Reservoir and Source

Human or animal wastes (e.g. feces) are the main source of infective material.

Mode of Transmission

Through food, drinks, water or ice contaminated with the bacteria.

Clinical Features

Enterotoxigenic *E. coli* (ETEC) colonize the small intestine and cause severe diarrhea, dysentery, abdominal cramps and fever. ETEC is often the cause of traveler's diarrhea.

Prevention and Control

Treatment for ETEC infection includes rehydration therapy and antibiotics although ETEC is frequently resistant to common antibiotics. Fluoroquinolones have been found to be effective in treating ETEC infection. ETEC is frequently resistant to common antibiotics including trimethoprim/sulfamethoxazole and ampicillin.

Presently there is no vaccine to prevent this infection. Therefore improved sanitation is important to prevent infection. Another simple prevention of infection is by drinking factory bottled water. This is especially important for travelers.

❑ AMEBIASIS

Harboring *Entamoeba histolytica* with or without clinical manifestations is termed amebiasis. It is a common intestinal infection in man.

Amebiasis occurs worldwide, but is more common in areas of poor sanitation and nutrition particularly in the tropics. The disease is prevalent throughout the developing nations of the tropics, at times reaching a prevalence of 50% of the general population and is estimated to cause 50 million cases of invasive *Entamoeba histolytica* disease and more than 100,000 deaths per year.

However, only 10%–20% of infected individuals become symptomatic. 15% of Indian population is supposed to suffer from amebiasis.

Causative Organism

A protozoan parasite called *Entamoeba histolytica* causes amebiasis. It occurs in the intestine in two forms: vegetative and cyst forms. Cysts can survive for several days in feces, water, sewage and soil. Ordinary chlorination is not enough to destroy amebic cysts, but boiling kills them readily.

Reservoir and Source

Man is the only reservoir, feces is the source of infective material. Carrier state is common in amebic infection.

Mode of Transmission

Fecal-oral transmission of amebic cysts from person to person takes place through contaminated food, water and hands. Sewage contaminated vegetables can readily transmit the infection. Flies and cockroaches may also transfer the cysts to food articles.

Incubation Period

The incubation period is 2–4 weeks or longer.

Factors Facilitating Transmission

Poor sanitation, open air defecation, low socioeconomic status, lack of personal hygiene practice like washing hands with soap after defecation, use of night soil for agriculture purposes all favor transmission.

Clinical Features

The cysts after entering the colon become invasive trophozoites, which cause the signs and symptoms. Amebiasis manifests as diarrhea or dysentery, acute as well as chronic. Sometimes liver also may be invaded by ameba causing amebic hepatitis. Many people with the infection remain symptom free carriers passing cysts in their stools and transmit to others.

Prevention and Control

Sanitary disposal of excreta, washing hands with soap after ablution and before eating, safe water supply, food hygiene practices like washing raw vegetables and fruits (grapes) before eating them and health education all can help in the prevention of the disease. Going for boiled water especially in hotels will be a sound practice in prevention.

Control of the reservoir is done by diagnosing all cases early, detecting all carriers and putting them on effective treatment. For symptomatic intestinal infection and extraintestinal disease (e.g. liver abscess), treatment with metronidazole or tinidazole should be immediately followed by treatment with paromomycin or iodoquinol. For asymptomatic, but proven *E. histolytica* infections iodoquinol or paromomycin are the drugs of choice.

❑ ASCARIASIS

Presence of adult roundworms *(Ascaris lumbricoides)* in the intestinal tract is termed as ascariasis. This is the most common helminthic infection. It is found worldwide. Infection occurs with greatest frequency in tropical and subtropical regions and in any areas with inadequate sanitation.

Worldwide, ascariasis causes about 1,000,000 new cases annually and severe *Ascaris* infections cause approximately 60,000 deaths per year, mainly in children.

Causative Agent

Ascaris lumbricoides, a nematode parasite, causes ascariasis. Adult worms live in small intestine. Female worms lay up to 240,000 eggs per day, which are passed in the stools. The eggs in the stools become embryonated in 2–3 weeks and become infective and they may remain viable for months or years under favorable conditions. Such embryonated eggs on ingestion, hatch in the intestine and the resultant larvae penetrate the intestinal wall, reach the bloodstream and are then carried to the liver and to the lungs. In the lungs, they moult twice and then migrate to the bronchioles. From there, they are coughed up and swallowed. After reaching the small intestine, they grow into adult worms in 60–80 days. Adult worms live for 6 months to 1½ years.

Reservoir and Source

Man is the only reservoir and feces are the source of infective material. However, studies have demonstrated the role of dogs as a significant disseminator and environmental contaminator of *A. lumbricoides* in communities where promiscuous defecation practices exist.

Mode of Transmission

Transmission of *A. lumbricoides* is by fecal-oral route through contaminated food, drinks and vegetables and fruits eaten raw. Children may get infected through fingers soiled with embryonated eggs while playing in contaminated soil around the houses.

Incubation Period

Incubation period is about 2 months.

Factors Facilitating Transmission

Open defecation around dwelling houses, lack of personal hygiene, unsafe water and poor sanitation are factors that facilitate transmission of ascariasis.

Clinical Features

Ascariasis may manifest as abdominal pain, loss of appetite or mere passing of adult worms in the feces. When a child harbors hundreds of worms inside the intestinal tract, the worms coil up and block the passage causing intestinal obstruction, which may necessitate emergency surgical removal of the worms. According to WHO, intestinal obstruction, usually of the terminal ileum in children, is the most commonly attributed fatal complication, resulting in 8,000–100,000 deaths per year. Penetration of intestinal wall by the worms causing acute abdomen is also reported. Besides direct obstruction of the bowel lumen, toxins released by live or degenerating worms may result in bowel inflammation, ischemia and fibrosis.

Prevention and Control

Sanitary disposal of human excreta, safe water supply, personal hygiene measures like washing hands with soap before eating and health education are necessary to prevent the transmission.

All cases should be identified and treated adequately. Mebendazole 100 mg twice a day for 3 consecutive days irrespective of age is the treatment. Mass periodic deworming may be undertaken at 2–3 months interval in high prevalence areas to reduce worm load.

❑ HOOKWORM INFESTATION

Human hookworm infection is a soil-transmitted helminthic infection caused by the nematode parasites *Necator americanus* and *Ancylostoma duodenale. Necator americanus* is the most common hookworm worldwide, while *A. duodenale* has restricted geographical distribution.

Hookworm infection is a leading cause of anemia and protein malnutrition affecting an estimated 740 million people in the developing nations of the tropics. Very high loads of the parasite coupled with poor nutrition (inadequate intake of protein and iron) eventually lead to iron deficiency anemia.

Hookworm infestation affects almost one fourth of world population. The largest numbers of cases occur in impoverished rural areas of sub-Saharan Africa, Latin America, South-East Asia and China. In China and Vietnam where human excreta is used for agriculture there is heavy infection. 29%–70% of the Vietnam population is infected. On the other side, it has been almost eradicated in developed nations.

In India it is widely prevalent. 534 million are at risk of contracting the infection. 71 million had hookworm infection with a prevalence of 7% in 2003.

Causative Agent

Two nematode worms namely *Ancylostoma duodenale* and *Necator americanus* cause infection in man. Female worms lay thousands of eggs (*A. duodenale*—30,000 eggs per day; *N. americanus* – 9,000 eggs per day), which are passed in the stools. In a warm moist soil, the larvae develop and hatch out in 1–2 days. These larvae moult twice in the soil and become infective larvae in 5–10 days. These larvae can survive up to 1 month in shaded moist soil. Adult worms are capable of living up to 1–4 years in the intestine.

Mode of Transmission

Hookworm infective larvae in the soil penetrate the skin of foot, migrate and reach lungs via bloodstream or lymphatics. From the lungs they are coughed up and swallowed. In the small intestine, they become sexually mature. *Ancylostoma duodenale* is also transmitted through oral route from contaminated fruits and vegetables.

In the case of *A. duodenale,* translactational transmission of infection is found to occur. The newborn baby can receive a large dose of infective larvae through its mother's milk. This has been seen in places such as China, India and Northern Australia.

Reservoir and Source

Man is the only reservoir and soil contaminated with hookworm larvae is the source of infective material. Damp and sandy soil with decaying vegetation is essential for the survival of hookworm larvae.

Incubation Period

Ranges between 5 weeks and 9 months.

Factors Facilitating Transmission

Open defecation, walking bare footed in feces contaminated soil and lack of food hygiene practice like washing vegetables and fruits before eating them raw favor transmission of hookworms.

Clinical Features

The most important feature of hookworm infestation is the iron deficiency anemia. Adult worms attach to the intestinal wall and suck blood and thereby cause anemia. The presence of between 40 and 160 adult hookworms in the human intestine results in blood loss sufficient to cause anemia and malnutrition.

Prevention and Control

Sanitary disposal of human excreta is the most important preventive step against hookworm disease. People should be advised to wear footwears while going for defecation in the open fields through health education. Cases should be identified and treated with mebendazole at a dose of 100 mg bid for 3 consecutive days. Anemia also should be corrected after deworming the patients. Attempts are being made to make a vaccine against this disease.

❑ GUINEA WORM DISEASE (DRACUNCULIASIS) ON THE VERGE OF ERADICATION

Dracunculiasis, more commonly known as Guinea worm disease is a parasitic infection caused by the nematode, *Dracunculus medinensis.*

An estimated 3 million cases in more than 20 countries were reported in the early 1980s. But by the end of 2008, the number of cases has dropped to fewer than 5,000 and the number of reporting countries has came down to just six (Sudan, Ghana, Mali, Ethiopia, Nigeria and Niger). Guinea worm disease is expected to be the next disease after smallpox to be eradicated. India has been declared free of dracunculiasis since February 2000.

Man is the reservoir. Water containing the infected cyclops is the source of infective material. Infected *Cyclops,* when swallowed, transmits the disease. Use of step wells or ponds to collect drinking water is an important factor facilitating transmission of Guinea worm disease.

The adult worms live in the subcutaneous tissues of different parts of body. The gravid female penetrates the skin and induces inflammation. The inflamed area develops a blister, which ruptures through which the worm protrudes out to discharge larvae into water sources. The worms come out through the skin usually from areas, which come into contact with water such as leg.

Abolition of step wells, provision of safe drinking water, control of *Cyclops,* health education, continuous surveillance and treatment of all cases are necessary to control the disease. Guinea worm disease can be eradicated. It is on the verge of eradication globally.

CHAPTER

5

Arthropod-borne Infections

Arthropod vectors like mosquitoes, which share man's environment frequently, are responsible for causing diseases in man. The important arthropod-borne diseases are:

1. Arbovirus diseases.
   - Dengue syndrome.
2. Arbo parasitic diseases.
   - Filariasis
   - Malaria.

❑ ARBOVIRUS DISEASES

There are many arboviruses, but only a small number of them are known to infect man. They are classified into:

1. Group A (alphaviruses): For example, sindbis and chikungunya.
2. Group B (flaviviruses): For example, dengue, Kyasanur forest disease (KFD), Japanese encephalitis (JE), West Nile.
3. Others: For example, sandfly fever virus.

The arbovirus diseases of importance in India are the dengue syndrome, JE, KFD, chikungunya fever, West Nile fever and sandfly fever. Yellow fever is another important arbovirus disease in Africa, but it is not seen in India.

Dengue Syndrome

The incidence of dengue has grown dramatically around the world in recent decades. Some 2.5 billion people, two-fifth of the world's population, are now at risk of contracting dengue in over 100 countries across the globe. Dengue has become one of the most important emerging disease problems among international travelers. World Health Organization (WHO) currently estimates that there may be 50–100 million dengue infections worldwide every year. Before 1970, only nine countries had experienced dengue hemorrhagic fever (DHF) epidemics. Now the disease is endemic in more than 100 countries in Africa, America, Eastern Mediterranean, Southeast Asia and Western Pacific. Southeast Asia (293,868 cases with 1,896 deaths in 2010) and the Western Pacific (354,000 cases with 1,075 deaths in 2010) are the most seriously affected ones, which bear nearly 75% of the current global disease burden due to dengue. Not only the number of cases are increasing as the disease is spreading to new areas, but explosive outbreaks are also occurring.

Dengue became a serious public health problem in India during 2010, having 28,292 cases. The disease was prevalent in most of the metropolitan cities and towns. Outbreaks were also reported from rural areas of Haryana, Maharashtra and Karnataka; all age groups and both sexes are affected.

Now dengue trend is one of decline in India. In 2010 there were 28,292 cases with 110 deaths. In 2011, India reported 18,860 cases with 169 deaths, while in 2012 there were 17,104 cases with 100 deaths.

Causative Organisms

Dengue is caused by any of the four antigenetically and genetically distinct viruses of the family flaviviridae named dengue 1, 2, 3 and 4. It can occur both as an endemic and epidemic.

Reservoir

The reservoir of infection is man, the main amplifying host of the virus.

Mode of Transmission

Transmission of dengue fever from person-to-person is by the bite of infected *Aedes aegypti* mosquito (man-mosquito-man cycle). Travelers play an essential role in the global epidemiology of dengue infections, as viremic travelers carry various dengue serotypes and strains into areas with mosquitoes that can transmit infection. Once infected, the mosquitoes remain infective for life. After a bloody meal from a case, the mosquito becomes infective to another person after an extrinsic incubation period of 8–10 days.

Incubation Period

The incubation period in man is 3–10 days.

Clinical Characteristics

Zoonotic cycle involving mosquitoes and monkeys are also suspected.

Dengue syndrome comprises three distinct clinical entities namely classical dengue fever, DHF and dengue shock syndrome.

Dengue fever: Manifests as sudden onset of high fever with chills, intense headache, muscle and joint pains, which incapacitate the individual. Case fatality is very low. All age groups and both the sexes are affected.

Dengue hemorrhagic fever: A severe illness, which is caused when more than one dengue virus infect the individual at the same time. First infection sensitizes the patient and the second infection produces an immune reaction. Transmission is by the bite of infected *A. aegypti.* Children below 15 years are the victims of this disease. It causes significant mortality. Clinically it is seen as acute fever lasting 2–7 days with hemorrhagic manifestations like petechiae, purpura, ecchymosis, epistaxis, gum bleeding, hematemesis, melena and enlargement of liver.

Dengue shock syndrome: It is yet another clinical form characterized by all the features of DHF with shock manifested as weak pulse, hypotension and cold and clammy extremities.

Control Measures

Currently, vector control is the available method for the dengue and DHF prevention and control. Live attenuated vaccines, live chimeric virus vaccines, live recombinant, DNA and subunit vaccines are undergoing different phases of clinical trials.

The vector *A. aegypti,* a peridomestic mosquito can be controlled by antilarval and antiadult measures. The patients should be isolated and kept under mosquito nets. Individual protection against mosquitoes is also important. As of 2008, there were no antiviral drugs designed to treat dengue and no drug candidates in late-stage development.

The endosymbiotic bacterium *Wolbachia* inhibits viral replication and dissemination in the main dengue vector, *A. aegypti.* The virus transmission potential of *Wolbachia*-infected *A. aegypti* was significantly diminished when compared to wild type mosquitoes that did not harbor *Wolbachia.* This underscores the potential usefulness of *Wolbachia*-based control strategies in dengue.

Six Nations Initiative to Fight Dengue

Indian Council of Medical Research (ICMR) had embarked upon a new research initiative, 'Eco-Bio-Social aspects of dengue in Asia', project to eradicate dengue; assisted by the Special Program for Research and Training in Tropical diseases, Geneva and the International Development Research Center (IDRC), Canada. The initiative focuses on better understanding of ecological, biological and sociological aspects to prevent dengue. Scientists from India, Thailand, Sri Lanka, Philippines, Indonesia and Myanmar will develop and evaluate community-based ecosystem management interventions in 2008–2009 to reduce transmission below threshold level for epidemic outbreak. WHO, World Bank, UNICEF and UNDP fund the program.

ARBO PARASITIC DISEASES

❑ LYMPHATIC FILARIASIS

Lymphatic filariasis is an infection with the filarial worms, *Wuchereria bancrofti* and *Brugia malayi.* Microfilariae (Mf) of these parasites transmitted to humans through the bite of infected mosquitoes develop into adult worms in the lymphatic vessels causing severe damage and swelling (lymphedema). Elephantiasis, the disfiguring swelling of the legs and genital organs, is a classic late-stage manifestation of the disease. Lymphatic filariasis is the world's second leading cause of long-term disability. Although filariasis does not kill, it causes debility and imposes severe social and economic burden to the affected individuals, their families and the endemic communities.

More than 1.3 billion people are at risk of the infection globally; 120 million people in 73 countries are actually infected, with more than 40 million incapacitated or disfigured. One-third of the people infected with the disease live in India, one-third are in Africa and most of the remainders are in South Asia, in Pacific and in America. In tropical and subtropical areas where lymphatic filariasis is well-established, the prevalence of infection is continuing to increase. A primary cause of this increase is the rapid and unplanned growth of cities, which creates numerous breeding sites for the mosquitoes that transmit the disease.

The disease has been eliminated in countries like Japan, Taiwan, South Korea and Solomon Islands and a marked reduction of transmission has been achieved in China. Egypt is on the verge of eliminating lymphatic filariasis with the fifth annual mass drug administration (MDA) to 2.5 million people in 2004 under the WHO Global Alliance to Eliminate Lymphatic Filariasis.

In India, filariasis is endemic in 250 districts in 20 States/Union Territories with about 454 million people (120 million in urban areas) at risk of infection. There are 29 million filariasis cases and 22 million microfilaria carriers. Hyperendemic areas are found in Tamil Nadu, Andhra Pradesh, Uttar Pradesh, Bihar, Odisha, Kerala and Gujarat.

Causative Organism

The disease is caused by three species of thread-like nematode worms, known as filariae—*W. bancrofti, B. malayi* and *Brugia timori.* Male worms are about 3–4 cm in length and female worms are 8–10 cm.

The nematodes that cause filariasis in India are *W. bancrofti* and *B. malayi.*

Reservoir

Affected persons with microfilaria in their peripheral blood are the reservoir for *W. bancrofti* and *B. malayi* in India. There is no animal reservoir for *W. bancrofti*. But *B. malayi* is found to occur also in monkeys, cats and dogs. Man is the definitive host and the mosquito is the intermediate host for filarial worm.

Mode of Transmission

In India, bancroftian filariasis is transmitted to man by the bite of infected female *Culex* (quinquefasciatus) mosquitoes, which breed in polluted and sewage water. *B. malayi* is transmitted by female mansonoides annulifera and mansonoides uniformis mosquitoes, which breed in water sources having aquatic plants like *Pistia stratiotes* and *Eichornia speciosa*. *B. malayi* is seen commonly in the State of Kerala because of the large number of ponds with these aquatic plants present there.

Incubation Period

Incubation period varies from 1 to 1½ years. Extrinsic incubation period in mosquito is 10–14 days.

Factors Facilitating Transmission

Urbanization, industrialization, migration of people, outdoor sleeping habits, environmental conditions favoring *Culex* breeding like optimum temperature and humidity, stagnant sewage water, lack of medical facilities, rampant quack medical practice, improper town planning, indifferent attitude of people to the problem because of ignorance, all contribute for the transmission in continuity. Improper and inadequate enforcement of public health laws, political interference in the routine administration and lack of collective responsibility also contribute for the transmission.

Evolution of Disease

When a mosquito bites an infected person, it takes in Mf along with the bloody meal. The Mf undergoes development, finally reaches the proboscis of the mosquito and becomes infective to man. When such an infected mosquito bites a susceptible individual, it injects the infective larvae. These larvae develop into adult worms in the lymphatic vessels and block the flow of lymph. This blocking of lymph leads to the development lymphangitis, lymphadenitis and edema. Subsequent infections and reinfections over a long period of time (decades) leads to fibrosis of lymph nodes, cellular infiltration in the edematous areas and permanent tissue enlargement.

Clinical Characteristics

Filarial infection manifests as fever with chills, lymphangitis, lymphadenitis and edema, funiculitis and epididymitis. If untreated, it leads to formation of hydrocele and elephantiasis of extremities, genitals and breast. Chyluria may be late sequelae.

Diagnosis can be confirmed by identification of Mf in peripheral blood. Blood for Mf is taken in the night between 8.30 PM and 12.00 mid night in India, because the Mf here shows nocturnal periodicity. Non-periodic (or subperiodic) form of Mf, which are found in Malaya are absent throughout India except in Nicobar Islands. Administration of diethylcarbamazine (DEC) before taking blood smear will increase the chances of detection of Mf.

Prevention and Control

Personal prophylaxis against mosquito bites by means of mosquito nets, repellants and electric fans, early diagnosis and treatment of microfilarial carriers with DEC, control of mosquito breeding places, improvement of medical facilities, health education will help in the prevention of the disease. Control of filariasis is done by detection and treatment of carriers and by repeated antimosquito measures.

The Mf carriers are treated with DEC at a dosage of 6 mg/kg daily for 2–3 weeks. Treatment must be repeated every 2 years in endemic areas to prevent reinfection. DEC may produce severe adverse reactions like headache, nausea, vomiting, fever, local inflammation around the dead worms, pruritus, etc. and they usually subside with or without symptomatic treatment. Another drug ivermectin also has been found to be effective against Mf.

Wolbachia, bacterial endosymbionts in the adult filarial worms and Mf of both *W. bancrofti* and *B. malayi* is necessary for the development, viability and fertility of the adult parasites. Drug interventions directed against *Wolbachia* cause deleterious effect on the survival of the adult worms.

Antimosquito measures are restricted only to antilarval measures now. Periodic antilarval measures in endemic areas and up to 3 km around the endemic areas are undertaken using mosquito larvicidal oil (MLO) or abate and by minor engineering methods. Removal of aquatic vegetation like *Pistia* and *Eichornia* plants has to be done to control mansonoides. Currently National Filarial Control Program (NFCP) covers only 40 million people (7% of population at risk) in urban areas.

Mass annual single dose treatment with either a single drug (DEC or ivermectin) or in combination with albendazole is recommended by WHO for the control/elimination of filariasis. MDA to eliminate lymphatic filariasis is already in place in 32 out of 83 endemic countries. India, as a signatory to 50th World Health Assembly Resolution (1997) on global elimination of lymphatic filariasis, has launched MDA in the country and it has been put in place in 202 endemic districts. Medical colleges, private sectors and community volunteers are being involved in providing MDA.

❑ MALARIA

Malaria is a serious disease caused by malarial parasites, transmitted from man-to-man by the bite of female *Anopheles* mosquitoes.

According to the World Malaria Report 2011, malaria is prevalent in 106 countries of the tropical and semitropical world with 35 countries in central Africa bearing the highest burden of cases and deaths. There were about 216 million cases, of which 174 million (81%) is contributed from Africa. An estimated 655,000 deaths occurred in 2010.

Malaria mortality rates have fallen by more than 25% globally since 2000 and by 33% in the WHO African region. Most deaths occur among children living in Africa, where a child dies every minute from malaria.

In India, malaria cases declined from 1.76 million in 1995 to 0.99 million in 2007. The annual parasitic incidence (API) also declined from 4.89 in 1995 to 2.18 in 2007. Annual deaths due to malaria were between 400 and 700 during this period. In 2010, 1,310,367 cases with 753 deaths were reported, while in 2011, there were 575,349 cases and 157 deaths.

The problem of malaria is now plagued by vector resistance to insecticides specially in Sub-Saharan Africa and India and parasite resistance to chloroquine and recently to artemisinin.

Causative Organism

Plasmodium vivax, Plasmodium falciparum, Plasmodium malariae and *Plasmodium ovale* are the four species of protozoan parasites that cause malaria. *P. vivax* is the commonest. *P. ovale* is very rare confined to tropical Africa. *P. malariae* has limited distribution in India in Tumkur and Hassan Districts of Karnataka. *P. falciparum* causes severe type of malaria (cerebral malaria).

Plasmodium knowlesi malaria, thought to primarily affect monkeys, can infect and kill humans according to a study published.

Reservoir and Source

Malaria cases with gametocytes both male and female are the reservoir. Higher apes may harbor *P. malariae* in Africa. Mosquito is the definitive host and man is the intermediate host.

Mode of Transmission

The transmission occurs mainly through the biting of certain species of female *Anopheles* mosquitoes, which breed in clear water in unused wells, overhead tanks, etc. They are *A. fluviatilis* (hills), *A. culicifacies* (rural), *A. stephensi* (urban), *A. sundaicus, A. minimus* and *A. philippinensis.* Transmission occurs also through blood transfusion and rarely from the infected mother to the fetus.

Incubation Period

The incubation periods for *P. falciparum* (extrinsic incubation period in mosquitoes 10–29 day) is 12 days, for *P. vivax* and *P. ovale,* is 13–17 days and for *P. malariae* is 28–30 days.

The incubation period may be long in those who are on suppressive drugs for chemoprophylaxis.

Factors Facilitating Transmission

Malaria is more prevalent in underdeveloped countries. Ill-ventilated and ill-lighted houses, migration of people, habit of sleeping outdoors, environmental conditions favoring mosquito breeding like optimum temperature, humidity and rainfall and the availability of natural and man-made water sources, availability of specific vectors (anthropophilic), lack of medical facilities and lack of committed workers all contribute for the transmission of malaria.

Although coinfection with HIV and malaria does cause increased mortality, this is less of a problem than with HIV/tuberculosis coinfection. However, HIV and malaria do contribute to each other's spread. This effect comes from malaria increasing viral load and HIV infection increasing a person's susceptibility to malaria infection.

Evolution of Disease

When the infected mosquito bites a man, sporozoites are injected into the bloodstream. After some time they reach red blood corpuscles in which they undergo development. The red blood cells (RBCs) rupture and release the parasites, which infect fresh RBCs. This cycle goes on for some time. The fever in malaria coincides with the rupture of RBCs. Parasites are carried by blood to the brain (cerebral malaria) and to other vital organs. When large number of RBCs are destroyed as in the case of *P. falciparum* infection (not in others), it leads to shock, renal failure, acute encephalitis and coma. Death can occur if not treated early especially in infants and children.

Clinical Characteristics

Malaria manifests as fever with rigor. Three stages recognized are—the cold stage, the hot stage and the sweating stage. The paroxysms of fever recur every 42–45 hours in pure vivax and falciparum infections and 50 hours and 72 hours in ovale and malariae infections respectively.

Parasitological Diagnosis

In the majority of cases, microscopic examination of thick and thin films of the peripheral blood will reveal malaria parasites. Thick films are more useful than thin films in the detection of a low-density malaria parasitemia.

Plasmodium falciparum

Young, growing trophozoites and/or mature gametocytes are usually seen (Table 5.1).

TABLE 5.1: Different stages of *Plasmodium falciparum* in peripheral blood

Trophozoite	Schizont	Gametocyte
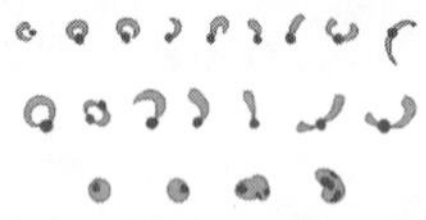	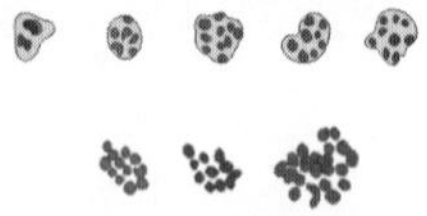	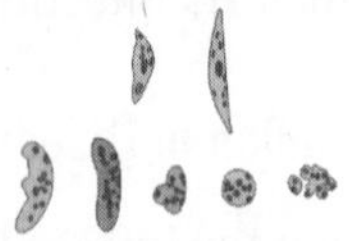
Size: Small-to-medium **Number:** Often numerous **Shape:** Ring and comma forms are common **Chromatin:** Often two dots **Cytoplasm:** Regular, fine to fleshy **Mature forms:** Sometimes present in severe malaria, compact with pigment as few coarse grains or a mass	Usually associated with many young ring forms **Size:** Small, compact **Number:** Few, uncommon, usually in severe malaria **Mature forms:** 12–30 or more merozoites in compact cluster **Pigment:** Single dark mass	Immature pointed-end forms uncommon **Mature forms:** Banana-shaped or rounded **Chromatin:** Single, well defined **Pigment:** Scattered, coarse, rice-grain like, pink extrusion body sometimes present Eroded forms with only chromalin and pigment often seen

Adapted from WHO Publication. Management of severe malaria: A practical handbook, 2nd edition.

Plasmodium vivax

All stages are seen. Schuffner's stippling in 'ghost' of host of red cells, especially at film edge (Table 5.2).

Rapid Diagnostic Tests

Rapid diagnostic tests (RDTs) may be an alternative to light microscopy in situations where normal laboratory services are non-existent or overworked. RDTs are immunochromatographic tests that detect parasite-specific antigens in a finger-prick blood sample. Some tests detect only one species (*P. falciparum*); others detect one or more of the other three species of human malaria parasites (*P. vivax, P. malariae* and *P. ovale).* RDTs are commercially available in different formats, as dipsticks, cassettes or cards. Cassettes and cards are easier to use in difficult conditions outside health facilities.

TABLE 5.2: Different stages of *Plasmodium vivax* in peripheral blood

Trophozoite	Schizont	Gametocyte
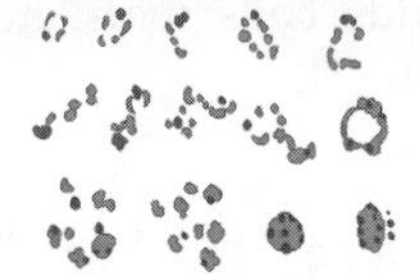	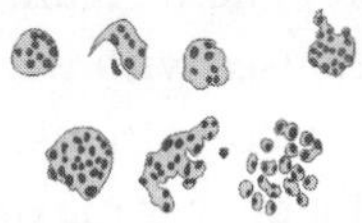	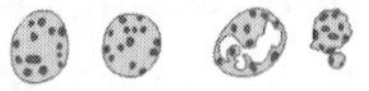
Size: Small-to-large **Number:** Few-to-moderate **Shape:** Broken ring to irregular forms common **Chromatin:** Single, occasionally two **Cytoplasm:** Irregular or fragmented **Mature forms:** Compact, dense **Pigment:** Scattered, line	**Size:** Large **Number:** Few-to-moderate **Mature forms:** 12–24 merozoites, usually 16, in irregular cluster **Pigment:** Loose mass	Immature forms difficult to distinguish from mature trophozoites **Mature forms:** Round, large **Chromatin:** Single, well defined **Pigment:** Scattered, fine Eroded forms with scanty or no cytoplasm and only chromalin and pigment present

Adapted from WHO Publication. Management of severe malaria: A practical handbook, 2nd edition.

Prevention and Control

No preventive vaccine is available now against malaria.

Malaria control strategies followed in India are:

1. Early case detection and prompt treatment.
2. Vector control.
   a. Chemical control.
      i. Use of indoor residual spray (IRS) with insecticides recommended under the program.
      ii. Use of chemical larvicides like Abate in potable water.
      iii. Aerosol space spray, during day time.
      iv. Malathion fogging during outbreaks.

      Note: Recent field studies have shown an added killing effect of ivermectin against malaria vectors.
   b. Biological control.
      i. Use of larvivorous fish in ornamental tanks, fountains, etc.
      ii. Use of biocides.
3. Personal prophylactic measures that individuals/communities can take up.
   a. Use of mosquito repellent creams, liquids, coils, mats, etc.
   b. Screening of the houses with wire mesh.
   c. Use of bed nets treated with insecticide.
   d. Wearing clothes that cover maximum surface of the body.
4. Environmental management and source reduction methods.
   a. Source reduction, i.e. filling of the breeding places.
   b. Proper covering of stored water.
   c. Channelization of breeding source.
5. Community participation.
   a. Sensitizing and involving the community for detection of *Anopheles* breeding places and their elimination.
   b. Involving NGO schemes in program strategies.
   c. Collaboration with Confederation of Indian Industry (CII)/ The Associated Chambers of Commerce and Industry of India (ASSOCHAM)/Federation of Indian Chambers of Commerce and Industry (FICCI).
6. Monitoring and evaluation of the program.

In the control of malaria, parameters like API, annual blood examination rate (ABER) and annual falciparum incidence (AFI) are useful.

Annual parasite incidence is the number of confirmed cases in 1 year for every 1,000 population under surveillance.

Annual parasite incidence is calculated as follows:

$$\frac{\text{Confirmed cases during 1 year}}{\text{Population under surveillance}} \times 1{,}000$$

The ABER gives the number of blood smears examined for every 100 population in the area under surveillance. It is calculated by the formula given below.

$$\frac{\text{Number of slides examined}}{\text{Population}} \times 100$$

Presumptive treatment with chloroquine is no more advocated.

Approved treatment schedule is given below.

All fever cases suspected to be malaria should be investigated by microscopy or RDT.

Treatment of Uncomplicated Malaria

Plasmodium vivax

Plasmodium vivax cases should be treated with chloroquine for 3 days and primaquine for 14 days. Primaquine is used to prevent relapse, but is contraindicated in pregnant women, infants and individuals with G6PD deficiency (chloroquine 25 mg base/kg body weight; primaquine 0.25 mg base/kg body weight) (Table 5.3).

1. Primaquine is contraindicated in infants, pregnant women and individuals with glucose-6-phosphate dehydrogenase (G6PD) deficiency. Primaquine regimen of 14 days should be given under supervision.
2. Patients should be instructed to report back in case of hematuria or high colored urine or cyanosis or blue coloration of lips and primaquine should be stopped in such cases. Care should be taken in patients with anemia.

TABLE 5.3: Age-wise dosage schedule of chloroquine + primaquine

Age (in year)	Tablet chloroquine (150 mg base)			Tablet primaquine (2.5 mg base)
	Day 1	Day 2	Day 3	Day 1–14
< 1	½	½	¼	0
1–4	1	1	½	1
5–8	2	2	1	2
9–14	3	3	1½	4
15 and above	4	4	2	6

Plasmodium falciparum

Plasmodium falciparum cases should be treated with artemisinin-based combination therapy (ACT) [artesunate 3 days + sulfadoxine-pyrimethamine (ASP) 1 day]. This is to be accompanied by single dose primaquine on day 2 (Table 5.4).

TABLE 5.4: Dosage schedule of artesunate + sulfadoxine-pyrimethamine

Age (in year)	Artesunate (number of 50 mg tablet) once daily for 3 day	Sulfadoxine-pyrimethamine (number of 500/25 mg tablet) single dose on day 1
< 1	25 (½ tablet)	125/6.25 (¼ tablet)
≥ 1–4	50 (1 tablet)	500/25 (1 tablet)
≥ 5–8	100 (2 tablet)	750/37.5 (1½ tablet)
≥ 9–14	150 (3 tablet)	1,000/50 (2 tablet)
≥ 15	200 (4 tablet)	1,500/75 (2 tablet)

Adapted from WHO, NVBDCP, 2010

1. National Vector Borne Disease Control Program (NVBDCP) recommends ASP as the ACT of choice for treating *P. falciparum* malaria all across India.
2. The NVBDCP also recommends single dose of primaquine (0.75 mg/kg) on day 2 for all cases of *P. falciparum* malaria.

Under the NVBDCP, artesunate + sulfadoxine-pyrimethamine kits are available for free at all the PHCs.

Dosage schedule of artesunate plus amodiaquine, artesunate plus mefloquine, artemether plus lumefantrine (AL) tablets and artemether plus lumefantrine suspension are given in Tables 5.5 to 5.8 respectively.

Caution

1. In 1st trimester of pregnancy, ACT is not to be given.
2. The SP is not to be given to children of age under 5 months and he/she should be treated with alternate ACT.

TABLE 5.5: Dosage schedule of artesunate + amodiaquine

Age	Dose
5–11 month	½ tablet of each once daily for 3 day
≥ 1–6 year	1 tablet of each once daily for 3 day
≥ 7–13 year	2 tablet of each once daily for 3 day
> 13 year	4 tablet of each once daily for 3 day

(Tablet artesunate, 50 mg each and tablet amodiaquine, 153 mg each)

Adapted from WHO guidelines for the treatment of malaria, 2nd edition. March 2010.

TABLE 5.6: Dosage schedule of artesunate + mefloquine

Age	Artesunate (50 mg) tablet	Mefloquine (250 mg) tablet
5–11 month	½ tablet once daily for 3 day	½ tablet on 2nd day
≥ 1–6 year	1 tablet once daily for 3 day	1 tablet on 2nd day
≥ 7–13 year	2 tablet once daily for 3 day	2 tablet on 2nd day, 1 tablet on 3rd day
> 13 year	4 tablet once daily for 3 day	4 tablet on 2nd day, 2 tablet on 3rd day

Adapted from WHO, 2010

Mefloquine is associated with an increased incidence of nausea, vomiting, dizziness, dysphoria and sleep disturbance in clinical trials, but these are seldom debilitating and in general have been well tolerated.

Fat-containing food (like milk or butter) enhances the absorption of the ACT and is therefore recommended, particularly on the 2nd and 3rd day of treatment.

TABLE 5.7: Dosage schedule of artemether + lumefantrine tablet

Weight (kg)	Age (in year)	Dose number of 20/120 mg tablet twice daily for 3 day
5–14	< 3	20/120 (1 tablet)
15–24	≥ 3–8	40/240 (2 tablet)
25–34	≥ 9–14	60/360 (3 tablet)
> 35	> 14	80/480 (4 tablet)

Adapted from WHO, 2010

TABLE 5.8: Dosage schedule of artemether + lumefantrine suspension

Weight (kg)	Dose of suspension (5 mL containing 15 mg artemether and 90 mg lumefantrine) once daily for 3 day
5	7 mL
> 5–7.5	10 mL
> 7.5–10	14 mL
> 10–15	20 mL

Dihydroartemisinin plus Piperaquine

Dihydroartemisinin plus piperaquine (DHA + PPQ) has now been found to be as effective as other ACTs and therefore recommended for the treatment of uncomplicated falciparum malaria by the WHO. DHA + PPQ is currently available as tablets of fixed-dose combination containing 40 mg of DHA and 320 mg of PPQ. The recommended dose is 4 mg/kg/day dihydroartemisinin and 18 mg/kg/day piperaquine once a day for 3 days.

Uncomplicated P. falciparum Cases in Pregnancy

- 1st trimester: Quinine salt 10 mg/kg 3 times daily for 7 days
- 2nd and 3rd trimester: ACT as per dosage given above.

Note: Quinine may induce hypoglycemia; pregnant women should not start taking quinine on an empty stomach and should eat regularly while on quinine treatment.

Treatment of P. vivax and P. falciparum Cases

All mixed infections should be treated with full course of ACT and primaquine 0.25 mg/kg body weight daily for 14 days (Table 5.9).

In North-Eastern states: Treat with age-specific ACT-AL for 3 days plus primaquine 0.25 mg/kg body weight daily for 14 days.

In other states: SP-ACT 3 days plus primaquine 0.25 mg/kg body weight daily for 14 days.

Treatment of P. ovale and P. malariae Cases

In India these species are very rarely found in few places. *P. ovale* should be treated as *P. vivax* and *P. malariae* should be treated as *P. falciparum*.

Treatment of Mixed Infections

All cases of mixed infection are to be treated as *P. falciparum* as per the drug policy applicable in the area plus primaquine for 14 days.

TABLE 5.9: Dosage chart for treatment of mixed malaria (*P. vivax* and *P. falciparum*) with ACT*-SP†

Age (in year)	Day 1			Day 2		Day 3		Day 4–14
	AS‡ tablet (50 mg)	SP tablet	PQ§ (2.5 mg)	AS tablet (50 mg)	PQ (2.5 mg)	AS tablet (50 mg)	PQ (2.5 mg)	PQ (2.5 mg)
< 1	½	½	0	½	0	½	0	0
1–4	1	1	1	1	1	1	1	1
5–8	2	1½	2	2	2	2	2	2
9–14	3	2	4	3	4	3	4	4
> 15	4	3	6	4	6	4	6	6

*ACT, artemisinin-based combination therapy; †SP, sulfadoxine-pyrimethamine; ‡AS, artesunate + sulfadoxine; §PQ, primaquine.

Severe Malaria

Severe malaria is an emergency and treatment should be given as per severity and associated complications, which can be best decided by the treating physician.

Artesunate: 2.4 mg/kg body weight IV or IM given on admission at 0 hour, then at 12 hours and 24 hours and then once a day.

OR

Artemether: 3.2 mg/kg body weight IM given on admission and then 1.6 mg/kg body weight per day.

OR

Arteether: 150 mg IM daily for 3 days in adults only (not recommended for children).

OR

Quinine: 20 mg/kg* body weight on admission (IV infusion or divided IM injection) followed by maintenance dose of 10 mg/kg body weight 8 hourly. The infusion rate should not exceed 5 mg salt/kg body weight per hour (loading dose of quinine, i.e. 20 mg/kg body weight on admission may not be given if the patient has already received quinine or if the clinician feels inappropriate).

Note: The parenteral treatment in severe malaria cases should be given for minimum of 24 hours once started (irrespective of the patient's ability to tolerate oral medication earlier than 24 hours).

After parenteral artemisinin therapy, patients will receive a full course of oral ACT for 3 days.

Those patients who received parenteral quinine therapy should receive oral quinine 10 mg/kg body weight three times a day for 7 days (including the days when parenteral quinine was administered) + doxycycline 3 mg/kg body weight once a day or clindamycin 10 mg/kg body weight 12 hourly for 7 days (doxycycline is contraindicated in pregnant women and children under 8 years of age) or ACT as described.

Treatment response should be assessed by parasite count daily until clearance of all trophozoites is achieved. Parasitemia may rise during the first 12–24 hours, because available drugs do not inhibit schizont rupture and release of merozoites. Rising parasitemia beyond 36–48 hours after the start of antimalarial treatment indicates treatment failure, usually because of high-level drug resistance. Because non-immune hosts may exhibit a high pretreatment total parasite burden, it may take up to 6 days to achieve complete elimination of *P. falciparum* trophozoites from the blood, even with fast-acting antimalarial agents (e.g. quinine, artemisinin derivatives). A rising gametocyte count does not indicate treatment failure.

Prereferreal Treatment

In most malaria endemic countries arrival of the patient at the appropriate health facility for proper treatment may be delayed resulting in deterioration of the disease or even death. So, WHO recommends that one of the recommended treatments is instituted as a rectal suppository before referral. If referral is not possible, rectal treatment should be continued until the patient can tolerate oral medication. A full course of the recommended ACT for uncomplicated malaria in the locality should be given.

For adult: Dosage for initial (prereferral) treatment in adult patients aged above or equal to 16 are given in Table 5.10.

TABLE 5.10: Dosage for initial (prereferral) treatment in adult patients (aged ≥ 16 years)

Weight (kg)	Artesunate dose	Regimen (single dose)
< 40	10 mg/kg bw*	Use appropriate number of 100 mg rectal suppositories
40–59	400 mg/kg bw	One 400 mg suppository
60–80	800 mg/kg bw	Two 400 mg suppositories
> 80	1,200 mg/kg bw	Three 400 mg suppositories

*bw, body weight

Adapted from WHO guidelines for the treatment of malaria, 2006.

For children: One or more artesunate suppositories inserted in the rectum as indicated in Table 5.11. The dose should be given once and followed as soon as possible by definitive therapy for malaria.

TABLE 5.11: Dosage for initial (prereferral) treatment in children (aged 2–15 year) and weighing at least 5 kg

Weight (kg)	Age	Artesunate dose (mg)	Regimen (single dose)
5–8.9	0–12 month	50	One 50 mg suppository
9–19	13–42 month	100	One 100 mg suppository
20–29	43–60 month	200	Two 100 mg suppositories
30–39	6–13 year	300	Three 100 mg suppositories
> 40	> 14 year	400	One 400 mg suppository

Adapted from WHO guidelines for the treatment of malaria, 2006.

In cases where parasitological diagnosis is not possible due to non-availability of either timely microscopy or RDT, suspected malaria cases will be treated with full course of chloroquine, till the results of microscopy are received. Once the parasitological diagnosis is available, appropriate treatment as per the species is to be administered.

Resistance should be suspected if, in spite of full treatment with no history of vomiting, diarrhea, patient does not respond within 72 hours, clinically and parasitologically. Such cases not responding to ACT should be treated with oral quinine with tetracycline/doxycycline. These instances should be reported to concern District Malaria/State Malaria Officer/Regional Office for Health and Family Welfare (ROHFW) for initiation of therapeutic efficacy studies.

Treatment Failure/Drug Resistance

After treatment patient is considered cured if he/she does not have fever or parasitemia till day 28. Some patients may not respond to treatment, which may be due to drug resistance or treatment failure, especially in falciparum malaria. If patient does not respond and presents with following, he/she should be given alternative treatment.

Early Treatment Failure

Development of danger signs or severe malaria on day 1, 2 or 3 in the presence of parasitemia; parasitemia on day 2 higher than on day 0, irrespective of axillary temperature; parasitemia on day 3 with axillary temperature greater than 37.5°C; and parasitemia on day 3, greater than 25% of count on day 0.

Late Clinical Failure

Development of danger signs or severe malaria in the presence of parasitemia on any day between day 4 and day 28 (day 42) in patients who did not previously meet any of the criteria of early treatment failure; and presence of parasitemia on any day between day 4 and day 28 (day 42) with axillary temperature greater than 37.5°C in patients who did not previously meet any of the criteria of early treatment failure.

Late Parasitological Failure

Presence of parasitemia on any day between day 7 and day 28 with axillary temperature lesser than 37.5°C in patients who did not previously meet any of the criteria of early treatment failure or late clinical failure.

Such cases of falciparum malaria should be given alternative ACT or quinine with doxycycline. Doxycycline is contraindicated in pregnancy, lactation and in children up to 8 years. Treatment failure with chloroquine in *P. vivax* malaria is rare in India.

Chemoprophylaxis

Chemoprophylaxis should be administered only in selective groups in high *P. falciparum* endemic areas. Use of personal protection measures including insecticide-treated bed nets (ITNs)/long-lasting insecticidal nets (LLINs) should be encouraged for pregnant women and other vulnerable population including travelers for longer stay. However, for longer stay of military and paramilitary forces in high *P. falciparum* endemic areas, the practice of chemoprophylaxis should be followed wherever appropriate, e.g. troops on night patrol duty and decisions of their Medical Administrative Authority should be followed. Short-term chemoprophylaxis up to 6 weeks can be given.

Doxycycline

Doxycycline should be administered 100 mg once daily for adults and 1.5 mg/kg once daily for children (contraindicated in children below 8 years). The drug should be started 2 days before travel and continued for 4 weeks after leaving the malarious area.

Note: It is not recommended for pregnant women and children less than 8 years. Chemoprophylaxis for longer stay (more than 6 weeks) can be given.

Mefloquine

Mefloquine, 250 mg weekly for adults and should be administered 2 weeks before, during and 4 weeks after exposure.

Note: Mefloquine is contraindicated in individuals with history of convulsions, neuropsychiatric problems and cardiac conditions. Therefore, necessary precautions should be taken and all should undergo screening before prescription of the drug.

Mass Drug Administration

There is no convincing evidence for the efficacy of MDA. Mass treatment of symptomatic febrile patients is considered appropriate in epidemic and complex emergency situations. Whenever this strategy is adopted, a full treatment dose should be given.

Intermittent Preventive Treatment

Administration of therapeutic courses of an antimalarial to risk populations at predefined times regardless of whether they are infected or not is known as intermittent preventive treatment (IPT). It has been shown to reduce the burden of malaria in pregnant women. Chloroquine should not be taken on empty stomach.

Antimalarials and Lactation

The amounts of antimalarials that enter breast milk and are therefore likely to be consumed by the breastfeeding infant are relatively small.

Antimalarials and HIV

Patients with HIV infection who develop malaria should receive standard antimalarial treatment regimens as recommended in the relevant sections of the guidelines. There is insufficient evidence to recommend any modification to the existing antimalarial treatment regimens.

Sulfadoxine-pyrimethamine (SP) should be avoided for malaria treatment in HIV-infected patients receiving co-trimoxazole prophylaxis.

Antimalarials and Travelers

For travelers returning to non-endemic countries, WHO recommend any of the following:

1. Atovaquone–proguanil (15/6 mg/kg; usual adult dose, 4 tablets once a day for 3 days).
2. Artemether–lumefantrine (adult dose, 4 tablets twice a day for 3 days).
3. Quinine [10 mg salt/kg body weight (bw) every 8 hours] + doxycycline (3.5 mg/kg bw once a day) or clindamycin (10 mg/kg bw twice a day); all drugs to be given for 7 days.

Artesunate or artemisinin-based suppositories used as prereferral treatment for severe malaria should be deployed where parenteral prereferral treatment is difficult or not possible at peripheral health institutions and at the community level in the context of home management of malaria.

Amodiaquine + sulfadoxine-pyrimethamine may be considered as an interim option where ACTs cannot be made available provided that efficacy of both is high.

The ACTs ensure the highest cure rates and have the potential to reduce the spread of drug resistance. Artemisinin monotherapy is not recommended as it will promote resistance to artemisinins.

The most common toxic effects that have been identified are nausea, vomiting, anorexia and dizziness; these are probably due, in many patients, to acute malaria rather than to the drugs. More serious toxic effects including neutropenia, anemia, hemolysis and elevated levels of liver enzymes have been noted rarely. Two cases of severe allergic reactions to oral artesunate have been reported.

Artemether or arteether, the two oil-based derivatives, which are released relatively slowly from the IM injection site are more toxic than the rapidly absorbed water-soluble artesunate. Neurotoxicity from the artemisinin derivatives with short-course oral treatment is unlikely.

Because of the limited safety data, artemisinin compounds are contraindicated in 1st trimester pregnancy and they should be used only in the 2nd and 3rd trimesters when other treatments are considered unsuitable (WHO).

Resistance to Artemisinins

Delayed parasite clearance after artemisinin treatment has been found in Cambodia, Myanmar, Thailand and Vietnam, which has raised some concern about the emergence and spread of falciparum resistance to artemisinins. Routine monitoring must be carried out to ensure that the first-line treatments are effective and to detect artemisinin resistance.

Vaccines Against Malarial Parasites

There are currently no licensed vaccines. Several groups are working on malaria vaccine development.

CHAPTER

6

Zoonoses

Man contracts diseases not only from fellow human beings, but also sometimes from animals with which he/she comes into contact. Important zoonoses are the following:

1. Viral.
   a. Rabies.
   b. Japanese encephalitis.
   c. Kyasanur forest disease.
   d. Chikungunya fever.
   e. West Nile fever.
   f. Yellow fever.
   g. Ebola hemorrhagic fever.
2. Bacterial.
   a. Brucellosis.
   b. Leptospirosis.
   c. Plague.
   d. Anthrax.
   e. Salmonellosis.
3. Rickettsial.
   a. Scrub typhus.
   b. Murine typhus.
   c. Indian tick typhus.
   d. Q fever.
   e. Epidemic typhus.

f. Trench fever.
g. Rickettsialpox.

4. Parasitic.
   a. Teniasis.
   b. Hydatid disease.
   c. Leishmaniasis.
   d. Toxoplasmosis.

VIRAL ZOONOSES

❑ RABIES

Rabies is a vaccine-preventable zoonotic disease caused by a virus. It is still a significant public health problem in many countries of Asia and Africa even though safe and effective vaccines for both human and veterinary use are available.

In humans, rabies is almost invariably fatal once clinical symptoms have developed. Rabies occurs in all parts of the world except Australia and Antarctica. It occurs in more than 150 countries and territories. Even advanced country like USA is not free from this disease. But UK, New Zealand, Cyprus and Hawaii have rid their countries of rabies by stringent measures. Most of the 55,000 deaths from rabies reported annually around the world occur in Asia, Africa and South America. Most of the victims are children. One of the causes of recent high incidence of rabies in East Asia is the pet boom. China introduced the 'one-dog policy' in November 2006 to control the problem.

In India, rabies is endemic. Roughly 36% of the world's rabies deaths occur in India each year. Every year more than 20,000 people die in India due to rabies according to the Association for Prevention and Control of Rabies in India.

Causative Organism

The causative organism is a virus, which belongs to the genus *Lyssavirus* in the family rhabdoviridae. This rhabdovirus causes rabies in man and animals.

Reservoir and Source

Mustelids and viverrids, ermine, skunk, mottled pale cat, civet, mongoose and vampire bats are the natural reservoir of rabies virus. Rabies in dogs is the source of 99% of human infections. The saliva of affected animals is the source of infective material.

Mode of Transmission

From the natural reservoir, wild animals like fox, jackals and wolves acquire the infection by eating carcasses containing the virus. From these animals, infection spreads to domestic animals like the dog. Man acquires the infection usually through the bite of a rabid dog. Transmission among vampire bats occurs through aerosols (in caves of Mexico, Central and South America). Occasionally corneal transplants have transmitted the infection. No man-to-man transmission occurs ordinarily and therefore it is a dead end infection in man.

Incubation Period

In man, usually it is 1–3 months, but may vary from 10 days to 3 years. In dogs it is 3–6 weeks usually, but it may vary from 10 days to 1 year.

Factors Facilitating Transmission

Keeping unvaccinated pet dogs, inadequate implementation of licensing of dogs, non-availability of pre-exposure prophylaxis, stray dogs and lack of knowledge about carrier state sometimes seen in dogs all favor transmission to man.

Evolution of Disease

From the site of bite or lick, the virus reaches the spinal cord via the peripheral nerves and the brain through axoplasm. Then from the brain it reaches the peripheral tissues including the salivary glands. It multiplies in the salivary glands and is shed in the saliva. The symptoms of rabies are due to encephalitis.

Clinical Characteristics in Man

Neuritic type of pain or paresthesia at the site of bite is followed by prodromal features like low grade fever, headache, fatigue, anorexia, apprehension, anxiety, irritability and insomnia or depression. The autonomic nervous system is affected. This manifests itself as copious salivation and weeping.

Acute neurological phase begins with the onset of seizures, which may be spontaneous or induced by external stimuli like noise. Hydrophobia (fear of water) develops, which is pathognomonic of rabies. Death occurs due to respiratory arrest. Those surviving acute neurological phase develop coma and die due to respiratory arrest or other complications. Some established cases have recovered with intensive treatment.

Prevention and Control

Rabies can be prevented by pre-exposure and postexposure active immunization with antirabies vaccine. Of the three types of vaccines available namely:

1. Nervous tissue vaccine.
2. Duck embryo vaccine.
3. Cell culture vaccines.

The last one is the best because it does not cause serious complications and the number of doses needed is also few.

For immediate protection as in the case of a bite in the face (category III cases), in which case the incubation period is likely to be short, passive immunization can be given using either horse serum [antirabies serum (ARS)] or rabies immunoglobulin (human) along with active immunization. Licensing of pet dogs and destruction of stray dogs are other important measures for prevention.

Local Treatment

After washing well with soap and water the wound should be treated with tincture of iodine or 70% alcohol. Wounds should not be sutured. Tetanus toxoid and antibiotics are also indicated. Hyperimmune serum locally and systemically may be beneficial in non-immunized individuals. The biting animal should not be destroyed but observed for 10 days. If the animal survives, then rabies can be excluded and no antiretroviral (ARV) treatment is needed.

Pre-exposure Immunization

Pre-exposure immunization is advised to veterinarians, animal handlers and the naturalists. Only cell culture based vaccines (e.g. human diploid cell strain vaccine) should be used for pre-exposure immunization.

Dose: 3 doses of 1 mL each intramuscularly (IM) on day 0, 7 and 28.

Postexposure Treatment

Because of long and variable incubation period of rabies, immunization must be started at the earliest to ensure that the individual is immune before the rabies virus reaches the nervous system. The immunization will depend upon the severity of bite. The bites are classified as follows:

Class I: Persons with slight risk.

1. Licks on fresh cuts or abrasions on all parts except head, neck, face or fingers.
2. Licks on mucous membranes or conjunctiva.
3. Bites or scratches without drawing blood on all parts except head, neck, face or fingers.
4. Consumption of unboiled milk or handling raw flesh of rabid animals.

Class II: Persons with moderate risk.

1. Licks on fresh cuts or abrasions on the fingers.
2. All bites or scratches on the fingers without penetration of true skin.
3. Bites or scratches in all parts except hand, face, neck or fingers without much laceration.

Class III: Persons with great risk.

1. Licks on fresh cuts on the head, face or neck.
2. All bites or scratches on head, face or neck.
3. All bites or scratches on fingers with penetration of true skin.

4. All bites penetrating the true skin.
5. All bites on any part of body causing extensive lacerations.
6. All jackal and wolf bites.
7. Any class II patient who has not received ARV within 14 days of exposure.

Vaccination Schedule According to Severity

1. Neural vaccine [beta-propiolactone (BPL) vaccine, which is a sheep brain vaccine].
   a. Class I: 2 mL × 7 days.
   b. Class II: 3 mL × 10 days.
   c. Class III: 5 mL × 10 days.
2. Non-neural vaccine (duck embryo vaccine). 5 dose of 1 mL each IM on day 0, 7, 14, 30 and 60.
3. Tissue culture vaccines: 5 dose of 1 mL each IM on days 0, 3, 7, 14 and 30 and an optional booster dose on day 90.

For rabies-exposed patients who had previous complete pre-exposure vaccination or complete postexposure prophylaxis with a cell culture based vaccine (CCV), 1 dose delivered IM or intradermal (ID) on days 0 and 3 is sufficient. Rabies immunoglobulin is not indicated in such cases.

Because vaccine-induced immunity persists in most cases for years, a booster would be recommended only if rabies virus neutralizing antibody titers fall to < 0.5 IU/mL.

Rabies immunoglobulin should be administered in all people with category III exposure and to those with category II exposure who are immunodeficient.

Replacing IM injections by ID inoculations using 0.1 mL (1/5th of a dose) of vaccine can reduce the cost and duration and postexposure ID vaccination is routinely practiced in India, the Philippines and Sri Lanka.

Vaccination for Dogs and other Animals

Mass vaccination of dogs is the single most cost-effective intervention to control and eliminate canine rabies.

For the vaccination of stray or ownerless dogs, baits containing live vaccinia virus recombinant that expressed the rabies G glycoprotein (Raboral™) could be presented manually in areas where the dogs tend to congregate to eat and/or sleep, e.g. garbage disposal sites. After a certain time period uneaten baits would be removed.

In rabies enzootic areas, vaccines are incorporated in edible baits and distributed by dropping them from aeroplanes over the target areas. Vaccines may also be spread manually, e.g. by farmers and hunters.

❑ JAPANESE ENCEPHALITIS

Japanese encephalitis (JE) is a zoonotic disease affecting man incidentally. It is caused by a group B arbovirus (flavivirus) and the transmission from animals to man is by the bite of infected mosquitoes. Nearly 3 billion people are believed to be at risk for JE virus infection. Approximately 20,000 clinical cases with 6,000 deaths are reported annually.

Sporadic cases are observed in China, Japan, Taiwan, Korea, Philippines, Indonesia, Malaysia, Singapore, Myanmar, Bangladesh and Eastern areas of Russia. Regional, seasonal outbreaks occur in Thailand, parts of India and Sri Lanka. Annual incidence ranges from 6 to 10 cases per 100,000 inhabitants in high endemic areas such as Thailand and Vietnam. It is a leading cause of severe central nervous system (CNS) infection in Asia and Australia where 30,000–50,000 cases are reported annually. In Nepal, till 15 September 2005 a total of 1,540 cases have been reported with a case fatality rate of 17%.

In India, there were 5,167 cases with 679 deaths in 2010 and 8,249 cases with 1,169 deaths in 2011. Till September 2012, 9 states have reported JE cases, with UP (344), Assam (228) and Bihar (275) reporting highest number of cases. Major outbreaks coincided with the heavy rainfall and/or floods.

Causative Organism

The causative agent of JE is JE virus from the family of flaviviridae. It is an enveloped single-stranded RNA virus.

Reservoir

The reservoir of infection is the pigs and birds like herons, egrets and ducks. Pigs are amplifying hosts.

Mode of Transmission

Transmission is through the bite of vector mosquitoes. No man-to-man transmission occurs. Infected humans are therefore dead-end hosts. The vector mosquitoes that transmit the infection to man are *Culex tritaeniorhynchus, C. vishnui* and *C. gelidus;* and also some anopheline mosquitoes. *C. tritaeniorhynchus* is the main vector, which breeds in rice fields, shallow ditches and pools.

Incubation Period

After an incubation period of 5–15 days, some persons develop the disease. Inapparent infections are far more than clinical cases. Children and infants are at high risk developing the disease. Both the sexes are equally affected.

Clinical Characteristics

Clinically it is characterized by prodromal features like fever, headache and malaise followed by encephalitic features like neck rigidity, local CNS signs, convulsions and coma. Case fatality is high, may be up to 58% or more. About 30% of survivors have persistent motor deficits and about 20% have severe cognitive and language impairment.

Control

Control of the vector mosquito is not easy. Aerial or ground fogging with ultra-low volume insecticides (e.g. Malathion, fenitrothion) can kill adult mosquitoes. Besides, indoor residual spraying of all houses in the affected area and the unaffected villages up to a radius of 2–3 km should be undertaken. The spraying should include vegetation around the house, breeding sites and animal shelters. Use of mosquito nets for personal prophylaxis should be promoted. Destruction of pigs in the affected area is also an important control measure.

Vaccination Strategy

Three types of JE vaccines in large-scale uses are:

1. Mouse brain-derived, purified and inactivated vaccine.
2. Cell culture-derived, inactivated JE vaccine based on the Beijing P3 strain.
3. Cell culture-derived, live attenuated vaccine based on the SA 14-14-2 strain of the JE virus.

Government of India has decided to introduce JE vaccination as a component of the National Vaccination Program. Live attenuated SA14-14-2 JE vaccine manufactured in Chengdu Institute of Biological Products, China is recommended. One time campaign targeting all children between 1 and 15 years followed by introducing the vaccine in the routine immunization program targeting children 1–2 years of age (WHO-recommended strategy) is to be followed. Phased implementation of mass immunization strategy is considered suitable in highest risk districts. Boosters are unlikely to be required as most live attenuated vaccines are known to provide lifelong protection.

Killed mouse brain vaccine is best used in the inter-epidemic period. 2 dose of 1 mL each (0.5 mL for children less than 3 years) at 7–14 days interval subcutaneously is indicated for primary vaccination. A booster after few months also is needed for protection and revaccination is indicated once in 3 years.

❑ KYASANUR FOREST DISEASE

Kyasanur forest disease (KFD) is a tick-borne viral hemorrhagic fever endemic in South Asia. It is a zoonotic disease incidentally occurring in man. The disease was first reported in the year 1957 from Kyasanur forest in Karnataka state in India as an epizootic outbreak among monkeys killing several of them.

The KFD is limited to Karnataka State in India. The outbreak during 1983–1984 is the largest with 2,167 cases and 69 deaths. In 1997 the cases came down to 75 and deaths to 4. There are approximately 400–500 cases of KFD per year with a case fatality rate of 3%–5%. From January 1999 through January 2005, an increasing number of KFD cases have been detected in the state despite routine vaccination suggesting insufficient efficacy of the current vaccine protocol.

Causative Organism

The causative agent of KFD is KFD virus, a member of the flaviviridae virus family classified under group B arboviruses. It is an RNA virus. Recently, a virus very similar to KFD virus, the Alkhurma hemorrhagic fever virus (AHFV), was discovered in Saudi Arabia.

Reservoir

The reservoir of infection is mainly rats and squirrels. Monkeys, langur *(Semnopithecus entellus)* and bonnet monkey *(Macaca radiata)* are amplifying hosts. The vectors of KFD are hard ticks, *Haemaphysalis spinigera* and *Haemaphysalis turturis.*

Mode of Transmission

Transmission from animals to man is by the bite of infected ticks (especially nymphal stages).

Incubation Period

The incubation period is 3–8 days.

Clinical Characteristics

Clinically it heralds with sudden onset of fever, headache, severe myalgia and prostration. Gastrointestinal disturbances and bleeding from nose, gums, stomach and intestine may occur. In some cases a second phase of fever with neck stiffness and mental disturbances may be seen. This disease carries a case fatality of 5%–10%.

Control

Control of ticks in the forest area can be done by aerial spraying of carbaryl, fenthion, naled or propoxur concentrating specially in areas where monkey deaths are observed (for 50 meters around the spots of monkey deaths). Restriction of cattle movement in forests also will help to reduce the tick population. Personal protection of people frequenting forests can be done by using tick repellents on their body. People also should be cautioned not to sit or lie down in forest area to prevent tick bites and to look for ticks on their person and remove them immediately. A killed KFD vaccine and an attenuated live vaccine are available for protection of people at risk.

❑ CHIKUNGUNYA FEVER

Chikungunya fever is a viral illness that is spread by the bite of infected *Aedes* mosquitoes. The disease resembles dengue fever. It is rarely life-threatening. Nevertheless widespread occurrence of diseases causes substantial morbidity and economic loss.

Since its discovery in Tanganyika (Tanzania) in Africa in 1952, chikungunya virus outbreaks have occurred occasionally in Africa, South Asia and Southeast Asia. Now after a long gap, chikungunya fever has been reported from several countries including India, Indonesia, Maldives, Thailand and various Indian Ocean Islands including Comoros, Mauritius, Reunion and Seychelles.

In India, after a gap of 32 years since it occurred in 1973 in Maharashtra, Chikungunya has come back and affected 9 states/provinces, viz. Andhra Pradesh, Andaman and Nicobar Islands, Karnataka, Maharashtra, Tamil Nadu, Madhya Pradesh, Gujarat, Kerala and Delhi in 2005. More than 1.38 million suspected cases were reported. In some areas reported attack rates have reached 45%. The resurgence is attributed to mutation of the virus, absence of herd immunity, lack of vector control and globalization of trade and travel. The outbreak is continuing and till September 2012, 11,076 cases have been reported.

Causative Organism

An RNA virus belonging to the togaviridae family is the causative organism. Three genotypes are known the East African, West African and Asian genotypes. The past outbreaks in India were caused by the Asian genotype, but the current epidemic (2005–2006) was caused by the East African genotype.

Mode of Transmission

The disease is transmitted by the bite of *Aedes* mosquitoes. *Aedes aegypti* and *Aedes albopictus* are the vectors in Asia, while

Aedes furcifer, Aedes leptocephalus and *Aedes taylori* are the vectors in Africa. Man-to-man transmission is not known.

Reservoir

Most likely reservoir is the primates, which generate high viremia, but manifest no disease. Other mammals and birds are also the likely reservoirs.

Incubation Period

The incubation period is 2–10 days.

Clinical Characteristics

Chikungunya affects mainly adults. High fever, headache, nausea, abdominal pain, photophobia, conjunctival injection and disabling arthralgia are the features of the disease. Stiff, swollen, painful joints (ankles, wrists) may last for several weeks. An attack is thought to confer life-long immunity. No deaths related to chikungunya infection have been conclusively documented. But chikungunya virus may be a contributing factor in the death of some individuals with underlying health problems.

Prevention and Control

There is no vaccine against this virus. So, preventive measures depend entirely on avoiding mosquito bites, which occur mainly during the daytime and eliminating mosquito breeding sites.

As both the dengue and the chikungunya are transmitted by the same vector, the control measures of dengue can be applied to the control of chikungunya also. Adult control with residual sprays, larvicidal control and environmental sanitation are the important mosquito control measures.

Repellent having 30% N,N-diethyl-meta-toluamide (DEET) can be applied to the exposed skin, which gives protection for 5 hours. Non-immune travelers to the affected areas are advised to take insect bite precautions, particularly during daylight hours as *Aedes aegypti* mosquitoes are active day biters. Cases are treated symptomatically with analgesics like paracetamol and non-steroidal anti-inflammatory drugs. Aspirin is to be avoided.

Travelers from endemic countries should be screened for the virus. There are no specific drugs to cure the disease. Treatment is directed primarily at relieving the symptoms, including the joint pain. There is no commercial chikungunya vaccine. Indian vaccine maker Bharat Biotech has claimed in a recent report that they have successfully developed a vaccine against chikungunya virus.

❑ YELLOW FEVER

Yellow fever (YF) is a viral hemorrhagic fever transmitted by infected mosquitoes. It is found only in parts of South America and Africa. The 'yellow' tag in the name is because it manifests as jaundice in some patients. Although an effective vaccine has been available for 60 years, the number of people infected over the last 2 decades has increased. There has been a dramatic re-emergence of YF in Africa and South America since the 1980s.

There are 2 lakh estimated cases of YF with 30,000 deaths per year. However, it is probable that only a small percentage of these cases are identified. 44 countries (33 in Africa and 11 in South America) are considered to be at risk. Bolivia, Brazil, Colombia, Ecuador and Peru are considered to be at greatest risk. Small numbers of imported cases also occur in countries free of YF.

Yellow fever has never been reported from Asia including India. Presence of a related virus—the dengue virus in the region is cited as the reason for the absence of YF in India (due to cross immunity).

Causative Organism

Yellow fever is caused by the YF virus, which belongs to the flavivirus group. It causes disease in both monkeys and human beings. Man and monkey are the principal reservoirs.

Mode of Transmission

The transmission is through the bite of the vector mosquitoes. Vectors—several different species of the *Aedes* and *Haemagogus* (South America only) mosquitoes transmit YF. Vertical transmission is seen in the mosquito, the virus being passed via infected eggs to its offspring.

Jungle YF in the tropical rain forests is transmitted among monkeys by the vector mosquitoes. Accidentally the infected mosquitoes bite people who venture into the forests and transmit the infection. The infected individuals spread the disease among people (Urban YF) and the transmission from man to man is by the vector mosquitoes. Once man-to-man transmission is established, epidemics occur.

Incubation Period

The incubation period is 3–6 days.

Clinical Characteristics

Clinically, the first, acute phase is normally characterized by fever, muscle pain (with prominent backache), headache, shivers, loss of appetite, nausea and/or vomiting. Often, the high fever is paradoxically associated with a slow pulse. After 3–4 days most patients improve and their symptoms disappear.

However, in 15% of patients a 'toxic phase' develops with jaundice, bleeding and kidney failure. Half of the patients in the 'toxic phase' die within 10–14 days. Others recover without significant organ damage.

Prevention and Control

There is no specific treatment for YF. Intensive supportive care may improve the outcome for seriously ill patients.

Vaccination is the single most important measure for preventing YF. A single dose of a live attenuated virus vaccine—the 17D vaccine provides protection for 10 years and probably for life. Serious side effects are extremely rare. However, recently a few serious adverse outcomes, including deaths, have been reported in Brazil, Australia and the United States. The 17D vaccine is contraindicated in infants below 6 months, pregnant women and anyone with a diminished immune capacity including those taking immunosuppressant drugs. To prevent an epidemic in a country, at least 80% of the population must have immunity to YF.

For prevention and control of YF, priority is placed on vaccination programs. Emergency vaccination campaigns are conducted during an epidemic.

Mosquito Control

Spraying of insecticides to kill adult mosquitoes during epidemics may help to interrupt virus transmission and this will protect people till they develop immunity from vaccination.

A vaccination certificate is required for entry to many countries particularly for travelers arriving in Asia from Africa or South America.

Yellow Fever Initiative

Twelve countries, viz. Benin, Burkina Faso, Cameroun, Côte d'Ivoire, Ghana, Guinea, Liberia, Mali, Nigeria, Senegal, Sierra Leone and Togo are taking part in the YF initiative backed by a US $ 58 million contribution from the Global Alliance for Vaccines and Immunization (GAVI) Alliance.

West Nile fever and sandfly fever are the other arbovirus diseases transmitted to man by the bite of vectors like mosquitoes and sand flies.

❑ EBOLA HEMORRHAGIC FEVER

Ebola hemorrhagic fever (EHF) is a zoonotic disease affecting monkeys and gorillas, but the causative virus can infect humans as well, similar to the YF virus. This fever outbreak occurs primarily in remote villages in Central and West Africa, near tropical rainforests. Since its discovery 30 years ago in 1976, ebolavirus has struck repeatedly in several epidemics breaking out mainly in Central Africa causing more than 2,400 cases with case fatality rate of 90% till 2012.

Ebola hemorrhagic fever is a febrile hemorrhagic illness caused by ebolavirus belonging to filoviridae family (4 subtypes—Zaire, Sudan, Côte d'Ivoire and Reston). Fruit bats of the pteropodidae family are considered to be the natural host of the ebolavirus.

The virus is believed to be transmitted to humans via contact with infected animal hosts. Man-to-man transmission then occurs via contact with blood and body fluids of the infected person. Contact with contaminated medical equipment such as needles also may transmit the infection.

Prevention and Control

No specific treatment or vaccine is yet available for ebola hemorrhagic fever.

Routine cleaning and disinfection of pig or monkey farms (with sodium hypochlorite or other detergents), culling of infected animals with close supervision of burial or incineration of carcasses and restricting or banning the movement of animals from infected farms to other areas can reduce the spread of the disease. If an outbreak is suspected, the premises should be quarantined immediately.

RICKETTSIAL ZOONOSES

Rickettsial diseases contribute substantially to the preventable acute febrile illness of many populations. *Rickettsia* is gram-negative, cocci-shaped or rod-shaped bacteria. Unlike other bacteria, but like viruses, they require a living cell to survive. The different rickettsial fevers and the countries reporting them are given in Table 6.1.

TABLE 6.1: Different rickettsial fevers and their geographical distribution

Types of fever	Geographical distribution
Typhus fever	
Epidemic typhus	Africa, Asia and Central and South America
Murine typhus	Worldwide
Spotted fever	
Rocky mountain spotted fever	Mexico, Central and South America
Mediterranean spotted fever	Africa, India, Europe, Middle East and Mediterranean

Contd...

Contd...

Types of fever	Geographical distribution
African tick-bite fever	Sub-Saharan Africa
North Asian tick typhus	Russia, China and Mongolia
Oriental spotted fever	Japan
Rickettsialpox	Russia, South Africa and Korea
Tick-borne fever	Europe
Aneruptive fever	Old World
Cat flea rickettsiosis	Europe and South America
Queensland tick typhus	Australia and Tasmania
Flinders island spotted fever, Thai tick typhus	Australia and Thailand
Orientia infection	
Scrub typhus	India, Central, Eastern and Southeast Asia and Australia
Coxiella infection	
Q fever	Worldwide
Bartonella infection	
Cat scratch fever	Worldwide
Trench fever	Worldwide
Oroya fever	Peru, Ecuador and Colombia

Rickettsial diseases reported in India are Scrub typhus, Murine typhus, Indian tick typhus and Q fever.

❑ SCRUB TYPHUS (MITE-BORNE TYPHUS)

Scrub typhus struck as an epidemic in Assam and West Bengal during World War II. Later it was found throughout India. It is caused by *Rickettsia tsutsugamushi.* Reservoir of infection is trombiculid mite, field mice, rats and shrews. It is transmitted to man by the bite of infected larval mites. The mites pick up the infection from small mammals like field mice and rats and transmit to man. The incubation period is 10–12 days, but may vary from 6 to 21 days. Clinically the onset is acute with chills and fever, headache, malaise, prostration and macular rashes appearing around the 5th day of fever. Generalized lymphadenopathy is commonly seen. At the site of mite bite there is the typical punched-out ulcer covered with a blackened scab.

Control

Treatment with tetracycline, clearing the scrub vegetations where rats and mice live, application of insecticides like lindane to the ground and vegetation and personal prophylaxis from the bite of mite using repellents are the control measures.

❑ MURINE TYPHUS (ENDEMIC TYPHUS OR FLEA-BORNE TYPHUS)

Murine typhus is observed in areas where rats infest. In India, the causative organism has been found in rats, fleas and bandicoots in Simla hills, Bombay, Jabalpur, Kashmir, Lucknow, Pune, etc. This disease is caused by *Rickettsia typhi* and the reservoir of infection is rat (*Rattus rattus, Rattus norvegicus*). Transmission from rats to man is by rat flea *(Xenopsylla cheopis).* The actual transmission takes place not by the bite of flea but by inoculation of feces of flea into the skin and possibly by inhalation of rat feces. Incubation period is 1–2 weeks. Clinically it is a mild disease.

Control

Control is achieved by treatment of cases with tetracycline and by control of the vector (fleas) and rat population.

❑ INDIAN TICK TYPHUS

Tick typhus disease is widespread in India. It has been reported from Nagpur, Jabalpur, Kanpur, Sagar, Pune, Lucknow, Bengaluru, Secunderabad, etc. It is caused by *Rickettsia conorii.* Tick, rodents and dogs are the reservoir of infection. Transovarial and transstadial transmission is seen in ticks.

Transmission to man is by the bite or by inoculation of the feces or tissues of infected tick into the skin. Incubation period is 3–7 days. The disease heralds as an acute fever with malaise and headache and the fever may last 2–3 weeks. Maculopapular rash appears on the 3rd day in the extremities, which moves centripetally to involve other parts. This fever may be mistaken for measles.

Control

Control is by treatment of cases with broad-spectrum antibiotics, control of tick population by disinfestation of dogs, personal protection from tick bite and health education.

❑ Q FEVER

Q fever is a disease observed in people who deal with sheep, goats and cattle. In India, it has been reported in animals and humans in Haryana, Punjab, Delhi, Rajasthan and other places.

Causative Organism

The causative agent is *Coxiella burnetii.* Ticks, cattle, sheep and goat constitute the reservoir of infection. Camels, horses and dogs are also known to act as maintenance hosts. Transmission to man occurs not through any vector, but by:

1. Inhalation of infected dusts from soil contaminated by urine or feces of diseased animals.
2. By gaining entry through abrasions in the skin or conjunctivae.
3. by ingestion of contaminated meat or milk. Placenta of infected cows and sheep contains the organism and during parturition, may generate infectious aerosols. Incubation period is 2–3 weeks. The disease manifests as an acute fever with headache and malaise. It resembles influenza rather than a typhus fever. While complications like endocarditis, pneumonia and hepatitis may occur, inapparent infections have also been observed.

Control

Control is effective by treating cases with tetracycline for 5 days, pasteurization or boiling of milk, by providing sanitary cattle sheds and by disinfection and sanitary disposal of products of conception. An inactivated vaccine is available for prevention and it is indicated for people who deal with cattle, sheeps or goats.

❑ OTHER RICKETTSIAL INFECTIONS

Epidemic typhus (louse-borne typhus) is reported from Europe, Asia and Africa. In the last 2 decades African countries, especially Ethiopia and Nigeria, have reported most cases. It had caused devastating epidemics among military and refugee populations and in famine affected areas. It is caused by *Rickettsia prowazekii.* Transmission from man to man is by louse *(Pediculus corporis* and *Pediculus capitis).* Louse feces, in which the organism is excreted gets inoculated into the skin, while scratching or it is inhaled. Control of louse, improvements in personal hygiene and surveillance (under IHR) are the control measures.

Brill-Zinsser disease is usually milder and is caused by reactivation of the organism from a latent state (up to decades) after primary infection.

Trench fever caused by *Bartonella quintana* is also transmitted from man to man by human body louse and it occurs worldwide. Fever, headache, pain in the shins, splenomegaly and disseminated rash are the clinical features.

Rickettsialpox caused by *Rickettsia akari* is transmitted from the reservoir of infection (house mice) to man by the bite of infected mites. Fever, eschar, adenopathy and disseminated vesicular rash are the clinical features. It is reported from Russia, South Africa and Korea.

Prevention and Control

With the exception of the louse-borne diseases, travelers and healthcare providers are generally not at risk of becoming infected via exposure to an ill person. Infections result primarily from exposure to an infected vector or animal reservoir. Limiting these exposures remains the best means for reducing the risk for disease. Travelers should be advised that prevention is based on avoidance of vector-infested habitats, use of repellents and protective clothing (see protection against mosquitoes and other arthropods), prompt detection and removal of arthropods from clothing and skin and attention to hygiene. Disease management should focus on early detection and proper treatment to prevent severe complications of these illnesses.

BACTERIAL ZOONOSES

❑ BRUCELLOSIS

Mainly a zoonotic disease in cattle, pigs, goats and sheep, brucellosis occasionally affects human beings. While animal brucellosis is observed in all states of India, incidence in man is difficult to estimate. This disease is seen wherever large number of domestic animals is reared without proper standards of hygiene.

Syria reports the highest incidence (1,603.4 cases per million people). Other nations reporting high annual incidence are Mongolia, Kyrgyzstan, Iraq, Turkey, Iran, Saudi Arabia, Tajikistan, Macedonia, Kazakhstan, Algeria, Albania, Azerbaijan, Turkmenistan, Lebanon, United Arab Emirates, Oman, Peru, Tunisia), Kuwait, Armenia, Mexico, Georgia, Jordan, Greece and Bosnia/ Herzegovina. Formerly endemic areas such as Israel, France and much of Latin America have achieved control of the disease. South Korea may have experienced resurgence.

For India, Pakistan and Afghanistan where the disease is undoubtedly endemic, no reliable data is available.

Causative Organism

Causative agent is an intracellular gram-negative coccobacilli, viz. *Brucella melitensis, Brucella abortus, Brucella suis* and *Brucella canis. Brucella melitensis* infects goats and sheep; *B. abortus* infects cattle; *B. suis* infects pigs and *B. canis* infects dogs. Brucellosis is much more common during summer than winter months. *B. abortus* accounts for the largest number of human and veterinary cases worldwide.

Reservoir and Source

The cattle, sheep, goats, swine, buffaloes, horses and dogs constitute the reservoir, while urine, milk, placenta, uterine and vaginal secretions of infected animals are the sources of infective material for transmission. Farmers, shepherds, butchers, abattoir workers, veterinarians and laboratory workers are occupationally exposed to this infection.

Mode of Transmission

Transmission is through contact with the infected tissues of animals like blood and aborted fetuses and with their urine or vaginal discharge. Abraded skin, mucous membrane and conjunctiva may be the route of entry of the pathogen. Ingestion of raw milk or dairy products from infected animals and drinking contaminated water also can transmit the infection. Airborne transmission in the form of aerosols can take place in slaughter houses, laboratories and cow sheds. Transmission to infants may occur through breast milk or ingestion of raw milk, but it is quite uncommon in infants.

Clinical Characteristics

After an incubation period of 1–3 weeks, patients develop sudden acute fever with rigor, arthritis, hepatosplenomegaly and leucopenia. In some patients symptoms may recur and prolong. Overall mortality is very low, probably less than 2% and it is usually due to endocarditis or severe CNS involvement. Diagnosis is made by isolating the organism from culture of blood, bone marrow and biopsy specimens.

Prevention and Control

Early diagnosis and treatment with streptomycin and tetracycline (doxycycline 100 mg twice a day for 45 days + streptomycin 1 g daily for 15 days), pasteurization of milk and protective measures for handlers of animals and animal products are important in the control of brucellosis in man.

Destruction of infected animals, vaccination of young animals on a yearly basis, providing clean and hygienic environment for animals, sanitary disposal of urine and dungs of cattle and health education all will help in the control of brucellosis among animals.

The Mediterranean Zoonoses Control Project has steadily reduced the prevalence of brucellosis in that region. Implementation of similar projects in other parts of the world has been inadequate because of expense, warfare, lack of concern and other reasons. There is currently no licensed vaccine for brucellosis in humans.

❑ LEPTOSPIROSIS

Essentially an animal infection, leptospirosis (also known as Weil's disease) affects man sometimes. It was first described by Adolf Weil in 1886. It may be a mild disease or a very severe and fatal one.

It is an occupational hazard for people who work outdoors or with animals, such as rice and sugarcane field workers, farmers, sewer workers, veterinarians, dairy workers and military personnel. It is also a recreational hazard to those who swim or wade in contaminated waters. In endemic areas the number of leptospirosis cases may peak during the rainy season and even may reach epidemic proportions in case of flooding.

Leptospirosis occurs worldwide, in both rural and urban areas and in temperate and tropical climates. During epidemics and in high risk groups, the incidence may reach 100 per 1 lakh per year. The disease is underreported for many reasons, including difficulty in distinguishing clinical signs from those of other endemic diseases and a lack of appropriate diagnostic laboratory services. Major outbreaks have been reported notably from India, Indonesia, Sri Lanka and Thailand.

In India, there is no national data on leptospirosis. However, Indian Council of Medical Research (ICMR) has reported a high prevalence. Several epidemics of leptospirosis have occurred on Andaman and Nicobar Islands (50 per 1 lakh population) and in Southern and Western parts of India. In 1997, leptospirosis outbreak was reported from Surat district in Gujarat state. The diseases have been reported for many years in Valsad district south of Surat.

Causative Organism

The causative organism is *Leptospira interrogans,* a light motile spirochete.

Reservoir and Source

Rodents and other animals like dogs, cattle, sheep, goats, pigs, etc. are the reservoir for this organism and they excrete the spirochetes in their urine. Infection spreads from wild animals to domestic livestock and thence to man.

Mode of Transmission

Percutaneous route: The spirochete voided in the urine of rats and other animals is transmitted to man through skin abrasions or though intact mucous membrane.

Droplet infection: Can also occur by means of breathing air polluted with droplets of urine, while milking infected cows or goats. Direct man-to-man transmission is rare.

Incubation Period

Incubation period is about 10 days.

Factors Facilitating Transmission

Contact with contaminated soil, water or vegetation can transmit the infection.

Clinical Features

The disease manifestations range from mild febrile illness to fatal disease with kidney and liver involvement. So it is difficult to diagnose leptospirosis clinically. Diagnosis is made only after isolation of the organism in blood and urine. The organism can be identified early by dark-field examination of blood, but blood culture takes 1–6 weeks to become positive. Urine culture may be done from 10th day onwards up to 6 weeks. Serological tests like the IgM enzyme-linked immunosorbent assay (ELISA) is useful for early diagnosis as it is positive as early as 2 days of illness.

Prevention and Control

Control is achieved by chemotherapy with penicillin. Tetracycline or doxycycline also is effective. Measures to prevent exposure to contaminated water, rodent control, protection of workers in hazardous occupations, health education are all important in the prevention of leptospirosis. A killed vaccine is available for humans in Asia (China, Japan and Vietnam).

Rodent Control

Rodents are recognized as the most important reservoirs in the transmission of leptospirosis. The use of rodenticides, entrapment of animals and improved sanitation has been shown to successfully diminish the risk of leptospirosis transmission. In India, rodent control measures in the premonsoon period would bring better vector control.

❑ PLAGUE

Primarily a zoonotic disease involving rodents and fleas, plague is transmitted to man accidentally. Plague bacilli survive in its natural foci in many areas such as Central Asia, Central and South Africa, Myanmar, Vietnam, Indonesia, South America and Western USA.

Although epidemics of urban plague have dramatically waned, plague still is a significant public health problem especially in Africa, Asia and South America. Worldwide, 1,000–2,000 cases of plague with 5%–15% fatality are reported each year. Recently plague has attracted a considerable attention because of its possible use as a biological weapon.

Historically, the first major epidemic of plague was recorded in China in 224 BC. Plague in Europe came in long-lasting pandemic waves. The first documented pandemic, the Justinian plague, killed several million people in the Byzantine Empire during the 6th–8th centuries. The second pandemic, the 'Black Death', caused some 25 million deaths (more than 30% of the European population) starting in the mid 14th century and culminating with the Great Plague of London in 1665. The third pandemic started in China in the middle of the 19th century and caused 10 million deaths in India alone.

In 2003, 2,118 cases and 182 deaths were reported from 9 countries. 98.7% of cases and 98.9% of deaths were from Africa.

India was plague free from 1966 until 1994. Plague staged a comeback in 1994 after a gap of 28 years. During August to October in 1994, a total of 693 suspected bubonic or pneumonic plague cases with 56 deaths were reported by India to the WHO. Cases were reported from Maharashtra (488 cases), Gujarat (77 cases), Karnataka (46 cases), Uttar Pradesh (10 cases), Madhya Pradesh (4 cases) and the federal district of New Delhi (68 cases).

Again in 2002, 16 cases of pneumonic plague, which included 4 deaths, were reported in Hatkoti village, Shimla district, Himachal Pradesh.

Causative Organism

Causative agent is *Yersinia pestis,* a gram negative, non-motile coccobacillus. It produces exotoxin, endotoxin, fraction I and some other toxins.

Reservoir and Source

Wild rodents like field mice, gerbils and other small animals are the reservoir in the nature. *Tatera indica* (bandicoot) is the main reservoir in India. Infected rodents and fleas and the sputum of pneumonic plague cases are the sources for transmission.

Mode of Transmission

1. By the bite of an infected flea.
2. By direct contact with the tissues of infected rodents.
3. By droplet infection from pneumonic plague.

Vectors

Out of 3 species of fleas involved in transmission of plague, *Xenopsylla cheopis* is the most efficient vector. *Xenopsylla astia* and *Xenopsylla brasiliensis* are the other two. Rarely human flea (*Pulex irritans*) is also involved in transmission.

Rapidly multiplying plague bacilli in the gut of flea block its proventriculus. Such a flea called `blocked flea' frantically bites more number of people and in the process becomes an efficient transmitter of plague. Partially blocked flea transmits much more efficiently than fully blocked flea.

Incubation Period

- Bubonic plague: 2–7 days
- Septicemic plague: 2–7 days
- Pneumonic plague: 1–3 days.

Factors Facilitating Transmission

Hunting, grazing, agricultural activities, construction activities and outdoor recreational activities expose man to flea bites. Wars and movement of people and cargo in ships also facilitate man flea contact. Poor housing favors rat infestation.

Clinical Manifestation

Bubonic Plague

Sudden fever, chills, headache, prostration and painful lymphadenitis (bubo) are the features in bubonic plague.

Pneumonic Plague

In this type, plague bacilli are excreted in sputum. Therefore pneumonic plague is highly infectious and is transmitted from person to person by droplet infection. Respiratory distress will be present and fatality is 100% if untreated.

Septicemic Plague

Bubonic plague may give rise to septicemia when the infection is overwhelming. Unless treated promptly, it has 50% mortality.

Plague is diagnosed by identifying the coccobacilli with bipolar staining in bubo fluid or sputum. Culture of blood, bubo fluid or sputum may reveal the bacilli. Cary-Blair transport medium is used to transport the specimens. Serological studies for specific antibody detection, immunofluorescent microscopic test and inoculation test using guinea pigs or mice are also done to diagnose plague.

Prevention and Control

Human Cases

Early diagnosis, notification to local health authority and WHO under International Health Regulation (IHR), isolation of cases and suspected cases, treatment without waiting for laboratory confirmation and disinfection of sputum, discharges and articles soiled by the patient are the control measures pertaining to human cases. Dead bodies should be handled with aseptic precautions.

Fleas

Control of fleas is important in breaking the chain of transmission. Flea control should precede or coincide with rat control. After ensuring the removal of all foodstuffs, cooking and eating utensils from the households, spraying of either dichlorodiphenyltrichloroethane (DDT) or hexachlorocyclohexane (HCH) covering the entire floor area, walls up to 3 feet above floor level, back of the door, roof of thatched houses, crevices of walls, rat runs, clothing, bedding, cats, dogs and other pets, is done. Spraying of insecticides should be done up to a radius of 5 miles around each infected locality.

Rodent

Rodent control is an important plague-preventive measure. Cyanogas is pumped into rat burrows to kill rats as well as fleas.

Vaccination

A killed vaccine is available for prevention and it is given in 2 doses of 0.5 mL and 1.0 mL at 7–14 days interval. Booster dose every 6 months is needed for persons at risk of infection (geologists, biologists, anthropologists). Vaccinations should be done prior to an epidemic and vaccine is not recommended for the control of plague epidemic.

Subunit vaccines and a candidate DNA vaccine expressing a secreted form of the V antigen are being developed.

Chemoprophylaxis with tetracycline is a valuable preventive measure. Continuous surveillance of natural foci of plague and health education to the community are essential for the control of plague.

❑ ANTHRAX

Anthrax, also known as woolsorters' disease and malignant pustule, is an occupational disease of man caused by *Bacillus anthracis.* Farmers, butchers, dealers in hides, hair, wool and bone meal are affected. Making use of the nature of anthrax bacilli, ironically, it is suspected to be used in biological warfare against enemies.

Domestic animals are the natural reservoir and they get infected by inhaling or ingesting the spores of the organism from the soil.

Man gets infected by means of inoculation into the skin commonly. At the site of inoculation, a vesicle (malignant pustule) is formed after an incubation period of 1–3 days. Regional lymph nodes may be enlarged. Fever, toxemia and fatal septicemia may develop. Inhalation of spores causes acute laryngitis or hemorrhagic bronchopneumonia (woolsorters' disease). Ingestion of infected meat causes fatal gastroenteritis.

Anthrax cases are treated with penicillin 1,200 mg 6 hourly. Erythromycin, tetracycline, chloramphenicol and streptomycin are also useful in the treatment.

Prevention

Prevention involves vaccination of animals, deep burial of dead animals with quick lime and vaccination of persons at risk.

❑ SALMONELLOSIS

Salmonellosis is an acute food poisoning caused by *Salmonella typhimurium, Salmonella enteritidis* and *Salmonella choleraesuis.* It manifests as nausea, vomiting and diarrhea after an incubation period of 6–72 hours from the ingestion of the contaminated food or drink. Man-to-man transmission by feco-oral route also occurs either from cases or carriers. Unhygienic food handling and processing methods and insanitary condition of premises favor transmission. The foods involved are usually foods of animal origin, viz. meat, poultry and egg products. As the organisms are killed at temperatures above 70°C, boiling will make foods safe.

Cattle, swine, rats and fowl form the natural reservoir. Intestinal tract of these animals harbor the organisms. The sources of infective material are the excreta, eggs or the meat of infected animals. Dust, water, soil, sewage and vegetables may also contain the organism.

Keeping farm animals free from *Salmonella* infection, use of hygienic animal feeds, pasteurization of milk, hygienic slaughtering of animals, cold storage facilities and health education are all necessary for prevention.

PARASITIC ZOONOSES

❑ TENIASIS (TAPEWORM INFESTATION)

Teniasis is cyclozoonoses needing two vertebrate hosts for completion of their life cycle. Two tapeworms namely *Taenia solium* and *Taenia saginata* cause disease in man. While *T. saginata* is moderately reported, *T. solium* is widely prevalent in India.

Man gets *T. solium* infestation by eating undercooked pork in which the larvae remain alive. After reaching the intestine the larvae develop into adults. Man is the definitive host. When *T. solium* eggs are ingested through contaminated water or food, larval forms develop in man in various parts of the body. These cyst-like structures are called cysticercus cellulosae and the condition is called cysticercosis. Cysticerci in the brain may cause epilepsy, hydrocephalus and psychiatric diseases and even death.

Taenia saginata infestation is acquired by eating undercooked beef. Adult worms in the intestine may cause abdominal discomfort and loss of appetite. Rarely appendicitis and cholangitis may be caused by the straying proglottids. Proglottids may also be passed in the stool.

Incubation Period

Incubation period is 8–14 weeks.

Prevention and Control

Control of teniasis can be effective by early detection of cases and their treatment with praziquantel or niclosamide, meat inspection, health education and adequate sewage treatment and disposal. Proper cooking of beef and pork is the most effective method to prevent this infestation. Personal hygiene and avoiding open defecation are important to prevent transmission of proglottids to pigs or cattle.

❑ HYDATID DISEASE

Hydatid disease is seen in all sheep-raising countries. In India, the highest prevalence is observed in Andhra Pradesh and Tamil Nadu.

Echinococcus granulosus (the dog tapeworm) causes hydatid disease in man. Man gets infected through ingestion of contaminated food, water and unwashed vegetables with dog feces containing the eggs of the worm. Hand-to-mouth transfer and inhalation of eggs also can take place while playing with pet dogs.

Dogs harbor adult worms and pass eggs in their feces. Eggs can survive for several months in pastures, gardens and around households. Sheep and cattle get infected while grazing on the contaminated grass and vegetation. The eggs hatch in the intestine of cattle, penetrate its wall and migrate to organs like liver, lungs and brain and become hydatid cysts. Dogs get the infection by eating organs with hydatid cysts thrown around slaughter houses. In dogs, the cysts develop into adults. Man is an accidental intermediate host.

In man, the hydatid cysts develop in liver, lungs, brain, peritoneum, long bones and kidney. Small cysts are symptomless. But large cysts can cause pressure symptoms requiring surgical removal and may even cause death.

Prevention and Control

The disease can be controlled by preventing dogs from having access to raw offal at the slaughter houses, proper meat inspection and destruction of infected viscera, control of dog population and their treatment with praziquantel if infected and by health education, particularly to butchers, dog owners, animal breeders and shepherds regarding transmission and control.

❑ LEISHMANIASIS

Leishmaniasis is a group of diseases caused by several species of flagellated protozoan parasites, *Leishmania* species, which are transmitted by the bite of a female phlebotomus sandfly. The disease is found in many areas of the world, particularly in Africa, the Mediterranean Basin, South and Central Asia, the Middle East and Latin America. Number of similar parasites cause different varieties of clinical diseases. One parasite may cause different clinical features in the same areas. In most areas of the world leishmaniasis is a zoonotic disease. But, in India, it is only a human disease.

Visceral leishmaniasis (kala-azar) occurs in Asia, Mediterranean countries, South America and Africa. An estimated 500,000 deaths are caused by visceral leishmaniasis each year worldwide. Cutaneous leishmaniasis (oriental sore) is distributed over Central Asia, Middle East, North West Africa, Central and South America. Mucocutaneous leishmaniasis (espundia) is seen in Brazil.

In India, kala-azar was a big problem in 1940s. The disease almost disappeared during 1958-1964 as a result of the insecticidal spraying operations undertaken under the National Malaria Eradication Program (NMEP). Again it reemerged in 1970s. At present kala-azar is present in Bihar and West Bengal, which account for 90% and 9% respectively of the total cases. Sporadic cases are also reported from Gujarat, Kashmir, Himachal Pradesh, Uttar Pradesh and Tamil Nadu.

Kala-azar

Kala-azar (visceral leishmaniasis, donovanosis) is caused by some intracellular protozoan parasites namely *Leishmania donovani, Leishmania infantum* and *Leishmania chagasi*. In India only *L. donovani* causes kala-azar.

Mode of Transmission

Kala-azar is transmitted by the bite of female sandfly phlebotomus argentipes. Kala-azar transmission has also been reported to occur from blood transfusion.

Factors Facilitating Transmission

Poor maintenance of houses, presence of animal reservoirs, lack of medical facilities and ignorance of people all favor transmission.

Reservoir

In India, man is the only reservoir and no extra human reservoir is known. But in Africa and the America, the main reservoirs are dogs, foxes and rodents.

Incubation Period

Incubation period is generally 1–3 months, but may vary from less than 2 weeks to many years. Extrinsic incubation period in the vector is 6–9 days.

Evolution of Disease

Leptomonad form of the parasite is injected into the blood by the biting sandfly. These leptomonad forms develop into Leishman-Donovan (LD) bodies in the reticuloendothelial system of alimentary canal, bone marrow, liver and spleen. Lymph nodes may also be involved. They multiply and increase in number. When the cell is packed, it bursts and the released parasites infect fresh cells and thus cause widespread destruction of reticuloendothelial cells specially those in the liver and spleen.

Clinical Manifestation

Young adults and teenagers are more affected by kala-azar in India. Fever starts insidiously, which goes on for months. Double peak of fever in 24 hours is characteristic of kala-azar. The liver and spleen are enlarged and tender. Untreated cases progress to emaciation and severe anemia with edema of extremities. Death may occur. Post kala-azar dermal leishmaniasis (PKDL) is a late sequelae seen only in India.

Prevention and Control

Prevention of sandfly bites by using mosquito nets with fine mesh and repellant creams, and health education are the preventive measures.

Control involves:

1. Treatment of cases with antimony compounds.
2. Eradication of breeding places of the vector-like cracks and crevices in the walls and floors by plastering and removal of dust accumulations inside the houses.
3. Destruction of adult vectors by indoor spraying with 5% DDT.

Animal studies demonstrate that protection can be achieved through immunization with purified proteins or DNA vaccines. There is, however, no effective vaccine for prevention of any form of leishmaniasis.

Oriental Sore and Espundia

Oriental sore (cutaneous leishmaniasis) is caused by *L. tropica, L. guyanensis, L. panamensis* and *L. mexicana.*

Espundia (mucocutaneous leishmaniasis) is caused by *Leishmania braziliensis.*

Mode of Transmission

Cutaneous and mucocutaneous leishmaniasis is transmitted by *Phlebotomus papatasi* and *Phlebotomus sergenti.*

Factors Facilitating Transmission

Poor maintenance of houses, presence of animal reservoirs, lack of medical facilities and ignorance of people all favor transmission.

Reservoir

Man is the main reservoir known in India, but in Africa and America, the main reservoirs are dogs, foxes and the rodents.

Incubation Period

Incubation period is generally 1–3 months, but may vary from less than 2 weeks to many years. Extrinsic incubation period in the vector is 6–9 days.

Evolution of Disease

Oriental sore: The organism is restricted to skin causing ulcers in the legs, arms and face.

Espundia: The agent invades skin and mucosa causing ulcers around the margins of mouth and nose.

Clinical Manifestation

Oriental sore: Manifests as an ulcer which does not heal for a long time (a year or more). When it heals, it leaves a disfiguring scar.

Espundia: Manifests as ulcers around the margins of the nose and mouth and cause disfigurement.

Prevention and Control

The preventive measures are: using mosquito nets with fine mesh and repellant creams to avoid sandfly bites and health education.

The control involves—treatment of cases with antimony compounds; eradication of breeding places of the vector-like cracks and crevices in the walls and floors by plastering and removal of dust accumulations inside the houses; destruction of adult vectors by indoor spraying with 5% DDT.

❑ *TOXOPLASMA GONDII*

Toxoplasmosis is usually a minor and self-limiting disease, but can have serious or even fatal effects on the fetus when a pregnant woman contracts the disease for the first time during pregnancy and on immunocompromised individuals.

The causative organism is *Toxoplasma gondii*. The definitive host of *T. gondii* is the cat, in which sexual cycle takes place and the asexual cycle in many warm-blooded animals including humans.

Mode of Transmission

Oocysts from cats are shed in their feces, which become infective to others after 1–5 days. Animals and humans ingest oocysts through unwashed vegetables, etc. or tissue cysts in improperly cooked meat and get infected.

Clinical Manifestation

The organism enters macrophages in the intestinal lining and is distributed via the bloodstream throughout the body. Toxoplasmosis in immunocompromised patients can cause deadly toxoplasmic encephalitis. During pregnancy, for the first time, the organism crosses the placental barrier and causes hydrocephalus, intracranial calcification and chorioretinitis. Even spontaneous abortion or intrauterine death can result. Most people recover from toxoplasmosis without treatment.

Prevention and Control

Toxoplasmosis can be treated with a combination of drugs such as pyrimethamine and sulfadiazine plus folinic acid. Pregnant women, newborns and infants can be treated, but the parasite is not eliminated completely. Immunocompromised individuals need treatment until they show improvement in their condition. AIDS patients may need medication for the rest of their lives.

Prevention of Risk from Food

Cooking food to safe temperatures (145°F–180°F), not sampling meat until it is cooked, peeling or washing fruits and vegetables thoroughly before eating, washing cutting boards, dishes, counters, utensils and hands with hot soapy water after contact with raw meat, poultry, seafood or unwashed fruits or vegetables and freezing meat for several days before cooking are important to prevent risk of toxoplasmosis from food.

Prevention of Risk from the Environment

Avoiding drinking untreated water, wearing gloves when gardening and during any contact with soil or sand because it might be contaminated with cat feces that contain *Toxoplasma,* washing hands thoroughly after gardening or contact with soil or sand, keeping outdoor sandboxes covered, feeding cats only canned or dried commercial food or well-cooked table food and not raw or undercooked meats and changing the litter box daily if there is a cat around are the important measures to prevent risk of toxoplasmosis from the environment.

Prevention of Risk in Pregnant or Immunocompromised Individuals

Pregnant or immunocompromised individuals should avoid changing cat litter if possible. Wearing disposable gloves and washing hands thoroughly with soap and water afterwards is necessary. Cats should be kept indoors. Stray cats, especially kittens should not be adopted or handled. A new cat should not be adopted during pregnancy.

CHAPTER

7

Surface Infections

In some diseases, pathogens are present in skin, genital tract or eye of the affected individuals and these organisms are transmitted to others by close physical contact. Below is the list of some surface infections described here.

1. Trachoma.
2. Tetanus.
3. Leprosy.
4. Pediculosis.
5. Parenterally transmitted hepatitis B, C, D and G.
6. Sexually transmitted diseases (STDs).
7. AIDS.
8. Scabies.

❑ TRACHOMA

Trachoma is a chronic eye infection, which can cause blindness if not treated adequately. Trachoma is more prevalent in developing countries. The greatest burden of trachoma is found in Sub-Saharan Africa, particularly in countries along the Sahel belt and in East Africa. Prevalence of trachoma is patchy throughout Asia and the Western Pacific; 14 countries in these regions are considered endemic. In Latin America, trachoma burden is concentrated in the northern states and indigenous populations of Brazil. Trachoma is the cause for about 6 million blindness cases in Africa and Asia. However, it shows a decreasing trend now in endemic countries due to improvement in sanitation, water supply, housing and control measures.

Causative Organism

Chlamydia trachomatis, an intracellular filterable microbe, is the causative agent of trachoma.

Mode of Transmission

Trachoma is transmitted from eye to eye through fingers and fomites. Flies also may transmit this disease mechanically.

Factors Facilitating Transmission

Poor hygiene, poverty and crowded living conditions, fly breeding, dry and dusty atmosphere, and the practice of applying kajal or surma to the eyes, all favor transmission of this disease.

Reservoir and Source

Affected persons mainly children below 10 years and women act as reservoirs and the discharge from the eyes is the source for transmission.

Incubation Period

Incubation period is variable, which is influenced by the dose of infection, and it is 5–12 days in experimental volunteers.

Clinical Characteristics

Trachoma is a chronic inflammatory disease of eye. Follicular hypertrophy over the tarsal conjunctiva, papillary hyperplasia and pannus formation occur. Later stage is characterized by cicatrization leading to ectropion or entropion. If untreated, may lead to blindness.

Prevention and Control

Prevention is mainly by observing personal hygiene. Health education to the community is of vital importance in this respect.

Control is achieved by mass therapy using sulfonamide or tetracycline orally and locally in the eyes for several weeks.

National Trachoma Control Program by Government of India started in 1963 has been integrated with the National Program for Prevention and Control of Visual Impairment and Blindness.

With improved environmental sanitation, access to water and economic development, trachoma can be eliminated according to World Health Organization (WHO). The WHO leads an international alliance of interested parties to work for the global elimination of trachoma, the Alliance for Global Elimination of Trachoma, by the year 2020 (GET 2020).

❑ TETANUS

Tetanus, commonly called lockjaw, is a disease manifested by uncontrolled muscle spasms. It is an occupational hazard for agricultural laborers. Tetanus in the newborn (tetanus neonatorum) can occur when delivery is not conducted following aseptic precautions. It is frequently fatal, specially in the very old or very young. However, it is preventable by immunization.

Tetanus occurs worldwide, but is more common in developing countries; more common in hot, damp climates with soil rich in organic matter. Globally, 14,132 cases and 4,213 neonatal cases of tetanus were reported in 2011.

Tetanus is an endemic disease in India occurring more in rural areas than in the urban. India reported 3,714 tetanus cases out of which 811 were neonatal tetanus cases during 2008.

Causative Organism

Clostridium tetani, a spore bearing anaerobic bacilli, causes tetanus. Tetanus spores are widely distributed in the intestines and feces of many animals such as horses, sheeps, cattle, dogs, cats, rats, guinea pigs and chickens. Consequently, soil contaminated by fecal matter will be harboring tetanus spores.

Mode of Transmission

From the soil, the organism gains entry into injuries like thorn prick, glass prick, road accidents and the like. Picking the ear affected by chronic suppurative otitis media (CSOM) with dirty sticks picked up from road, cutting the umbilical cord of the newborn with unsterilized instruments during delivery and rarely surgical procedures may also transmit the spore. Ordinarily no man-to-man transmission occurs and therefore it is a dead end infection.

Factors Facilitating Transmission

Ignorance, superstition, lack of medical facilities, lack of immunity due to inadequate immunization coverage and unhealthy practices like application of cow dung to the cut end of the umbilical cord are the factors responsible for its occurrence as an endemic disease.

Evolution of Disease

At the site of entry, the spores germinate when anaerobic condition is created by other contaminated organisms and elaborate an exotoxin known as tetanospasmin. This powerful toxin acts on motor end plates of skeletal muscles and on the spinal cord, and blocks the inhibition of reflexes and thereby causes spasms and rigidity.

Incubation Period

The incubation period is usually 6–10 days, but may be shorter or longer.

Reservoir and Source

Soil is the reservoir and source. The spores are present in the alimentary canal of cattle, goat and sheep.

Clinical Characteristics

Inability to open the mouth (lockjaw) due to spasm of masseter muscle is the earliest manifestation. Painful spasm of other muscles ensues later. Noise and bright light may provoke paroxysmal convulsions. History of injury within the incubation period may or may not be available. History of an operation or the presence of CSOM (middle ear infection) may help in the diagnosis. Inability to suckle breast milk is the feature in newborn babies (neonatal tetanus).

Prevention and Control

Active immunization with tetanus toxoid can prevent tetanus. Infants are immunized with 3 doses of DPT at 1½, 2½ and 3½ months followed by booster doses at 2 years and 5 years. Those who have not received any immunization during childhood should receive 2 doses of tetanus toxoid at 4–6 weeks interval followed by a 3rd dose after 1 year. Herd immunity cannot protect the susceptibles in the community, as it is not transmitted from man to man.

Neonatal tetanus (tetanus neonatorum) can be prevented by immunizing expectant mothers with 2 doses of tetanus toxoid at 20 and 24 weeks of gestation and by observing aseptic precautions while cutting the umbilical cord during delivery. Health education about the mode of transmission and the preventive measures is important to reduce the incidence of this disease. Passive immunization may be needed for a susceptible wounded person to give immediate protection. Tetanus human Ig is available for this purpose. It gives protection for a longer period. The dose of human Ig is 250–500 IU intramuscularly irrespective of age. Antitetanus serum (ATS) prepared from horse serum is not being used now.

The patients' wound should be cleaned and dressed with antiseptic lotion and the patient should also receive a course of antibiotics like penicillin or erythromycin to control the tetanus infection in the wound with a view to prevent further production of the toxin. For the treatment of tetanus, human Ig should be given according to the severity of the symptoms. Expert nursing in dim lit rooms helps to reduce muscular spasms.

❑ LEPROSY

Leprosy is a chronic disease caused by bacilli called *Mycobacterium leprae*. It affects the skin and nerves leading to disfigurement. Leprosy is also called Hansen's disease, named after Armauer Hansen of Norway who discovered that leprosy was caused by a bacterium in 1873.

Prevalence of leprosy globally in 2011 and 1st quarter of 2012 is 181,941 cases from 105 countries and territories. The number of new cases detected annually (219,075) continues to increase in all regions except the American and the African regions.

Cases of leprosy in India have decreased dramatically from 5,000,000 cases in 1985 to 21,300 in 2009. India achieved the elimination goal at the national level in December 2005; 32 States/Union territories have achieved elimination goal. As on April 2011, 0.83 lakh cases were on record in India and 1.27 lakh new cases were detected. The States which showed an increase in cases were Maharashtra, Odisha, Madhya Pradesh, Assam, Jammu and Kashmir, Himachal Pradesh, Dadra and Nagar Haveli, and Kerala.

Causative Organism

Mycobacterium leprae, an acid and alcohol fast bacilli, causes leprosy. It is an intracellular aerobic rod-shaped bacillus surrounded by the characteristic waxy coating, unique to mycobacteriae. This organism has been grown only in footpads of mice and armadillos, but has not been successfully grown either in bacteriological media or in tissue culture, so far. The generation time of leprosy bacilli is 12–13 days usually, but may vary from 18 to 42 days and so it is a slowly multiplying organism.

Nasal and skin smears will show lepra bacilli, which appear as pink rods in groups (cigar bundle appearance).

Reservoir and Source

All patients with active leprosy form the reservoir. Asymptomatic (inapparent) infections are also important sources for transmission. Extra human reservoir exists in armadillos, mangabey monkeys and chimpanzees, but it is not certain whether these transmit leprosy to man.

Nasal secretions and the discharge from the superficial lesions of lepromatous patients are the main source of infective material. Leprosy bacilli may be discharged from intact skin through hair follicles also.

Incubation Period

Incubation period is long because *M. leprae* is a slowly growing organism. It may be between 2 and 5 years, but may vary from few months to 30 or 40 years or more.

Mode of Transmission

The transmission occurs by means of droplet infection and direct contact due to intimate and prolonged contact. Contact during childhood is more likely to result in disease. Transmission can also occur through mother's milk as lepra bacilli are excreted in it. Some workers suggest that insect vectors like bedbug may play some role in leprosy transmission. Discharges from the superficial lesions of lepromatous leprosy cases are highly contagious. The opinion that tuberculoid type of leprosy is not communicable is controversial. It is better to assume that all active cases of leprosy are communicable. Indirect transmission from soil is also considered now as a possibility.

Factors Facilitating Transmission

Low standard of living, begging by leprosy patients and their migration to different areas, overcrowding, lack of personal hygiene, social stigma, which leads to its concealment, the belief that it is a curse and therefore incurable, ignorance of the fact that it is also a communicable disease like other diseases and therefore can be cured if proper treatment is taken, lack of adequate medical facilities and lack of health education, all leads to its endemic occurrence.

Evolution of Disease

The leprosy bacilli have a predilection for nerve tissue, skin and mucosa of upper respiratory tract and the signs and symptoms are caused by the affection of nerve and skin. The status of cell-mediated immunity (CMI) in individuals exposed to the organism decides the type of the disease that results. Individuals with adequate CMI develop tuberculoid type of leprosy, while those deficient in CMI develop lepromatous leprosy. So, leprosy is clinically classified into two broad categories namely the tuberculoid type and the lepromatous type. In between these two forms, leprologists include two more types namely borderline tuberculoid and borderline lepromatous depending on the clinical presentation of cases.

Clinical Characteristics

The earliest manifestation is a hypopigmented anesthetic patch. The patches commonly occur over the extensor surface of elbow, face and skin over the buttock. As the disease progresses, the patches may become numerous and the edges of the patches may become raised. Patients have thickened peripheral nerves. Loss of eyebrow and loss of hair over the patches are characteristic. High stepping gait may be present. In advanced cases, contractures develop leading to claw hand formation. Fingers and toes may be lost because of repeated trauma and resorption. In lepromatous leprosy, the patient has nodular granulomas over the face and breast. Nodules ulcerate and produce purulent discharge (because of secondary infection), which are highly contagious.

Prevention and Control

No specific vaccine is available now for prevention, but bacille Calmette-Guérin (BCG) is supposed to offer some protection against leprosy.

Health education, early diagnosis, effective chemotherapy, chemoprophylaxis, prevention of contact and selective isolation may help to prevent the disease. Compulsory isolation has been abolished. Chemical isolation is now resorted to prevent the spread of leprosy.

The emphasis now is on active search for cases and effective chemotherapy. Follow-up of cases till it is declared cured is important. Rehabilitation services for the crippled are also provided (medical reconstructive surgery and physiotherapy; social helping to lead a normal social life after cure; emotional—improving the patient's self-confidence and vocational preparing to earn the bread).

Multidrug Regimen Therapy

Multidrug regimen therapy (MDT) is being given since 1995. This has helped to reduce the disease prevalence appreciably according to latest evaluation report. At present, more than 99% of registered patients are receiving MDT and no drug resistance or significant relapses have been reported.

Chemotherapy of Leprosy

Chemotherapy differs according to the type of leprosy.

Treatment for Multibacillary Cases

Multibacillary cases (lepromatous and borderline lepromatous) are treated for a minimum of 1 year or up to smear negativity. The recommended treatment schedule is given below.

1. Rifampicin 600 mg, once monthly (supervised).
2. Dapsone 100 mg, daily (self-administered).
3. Clofazimine 300 mg, once monthly (supervised) or 50 mg, daily (self-administered).

Dapsone is given on body weight basis at 10 mg/kg of body weight to reduce toxicity. If intolerant to clofazimine, it may be substituted with 250–375 mg of ethionamide.

Treatment for Paucibacillary Cases

Paucibacillary cases (tuberculoid and borderline tuberculoid) are treated with rifampicin and dapsone. The recommended dose schedule is:

1. Rifampicin 600 mg, once a month for 6 months.
2. Dapsone 100 mg, daily for 6 months.

The duration of treatment should be extended till all signs of activity have subsided.

Other Drugs Used for Leprosy

Quinolones (ofloxacin), minocycline (a lipid-soluble tetracycline) and clarithromycin are the other bactericidal drugs available against *M. leprae.*

Advantages of Multidrug Regimen Therapy

1. Paucibacillary cases treated with MDT are cured within 6 months.
2. Multibacillary cases treated with MDT are cured within 12 months.
3. Patients become non-infectious to others after the first dose of MDT and so transmission of leprosy is interrupted.
4. No relapse is seen after the treatment is completed.
5. No resistance of the bacille to MDT has been detected.
6. It is cost-effective as a health intervention.

Since 1995, WHO has supplied MDT free of cost to leprosy patients in all endemic countries.

PARENTERALLY TRANSMITTED HEPATITIS B, C, D AND G

❑ HEPATITIS B

Hepatitis B is a serious public health problem throughout the world. Hepatitis B virus (HBV) induces acute hepatitis with a case fatality rate of about 1%. It becomes chronic in 5%–15% of infected individuals. About 25% of these chronic cases will die due to cirrhosis and hepatocellular carcinoma (HCC).

It is estimated that there are more than 200 million chronic HBV carriers in the world and 80% of them are from Asia and the Western Pacific. As of 2010, China has 120 million infected people, followed by India and Indonesia with 40 million and 12 million respectively. An estimated 600,000 people die every year related to HBV infection. In India this disease is a major public health problem. 30%–40% of viral hepatitis in India is likely to be due to HBV.

Causative Organism

A DNA virus originally known as Dane particle, causes hepatitis B. This virus has three antigens—a surface antigen known as 'Australia antigen' (HBsAg), a core antigen (HBcAg) and an e antigen

(HBeAg) (Delta agent is a defective virus, which requires hepatitis B as a helper virus in order to replicate. Therefore, infection occurs only in patients who are already infected with hepatitis B. It was identified in intravenous drug abusers in Italy. It causes increased severity of liver disease in hepatitis B carriers).

Reservoir and Source

Man is the only reservoir and carrier for this infection. Blood is the source of infection. Saliva, semen and vaginal secretion also have the virus and may transmit the infection.

Mode of Transmission

1. Hepatitis B virus is transmitted from the infected person to another person through blood and blood products. Procedures like blood transfusion, dialysis, dental procedures, immunization, tattooing, ear piercing and ritual circumcision, and fomites like contaminated syringes, needles, shared razor and tooth brushes have been found to transmit the disease. Intravenous drug users are at risk.
2. Perinatal transmission from mother to baby occurs in three ways:
   a. Transplacental transmission in utero (5%–15%) of newborns.
   b. Transmission during delivery, which is considered the main mode of perinatal transmission.
   c. Postnatal transmission from mother to newborn, which is not common. HBeAg is the main maternal factor that determines whether infection of newborns will occur or not. The expression of this antigen seems to be determined genetically.
3. Sexual transmission also takes place particularly among male homosexual partners and also among heterosexual partners during unprotected sex.

Transmission through blood sucking arthropods like mosquitoes and bed bugs is also suspected.

Incubation Period

The incubation period is 45–180 days.

Factors Facilitating Transmission

Promiscuity, male homosexual practices like anal intercourse, blood transfusion without screening for HBV and inadequate sterilization of syringes and surgical instruments all favor transmission of this disease.

Clinical Characteristics

Usually, it is an acute self-limiting infection. But in 5%–15% of cases, the disease becomes chronic and the affected persons become persistent carriers. Persistent infection may lead to progressive liver disease and carcinoma of liver.

Prevention and Control

Prevention of HBV infection is the best way for control. 3–4 doses of HBV vaccine in infancy and hepatitis B immunoglobulin (HBIG) within 24 hours of birth is the most effective way to prevent HBV infection. The vaccines are:

1. Plasma-derived vaccine: A formalin-inactivated subunit viral vaccine prepared from the surface antigen (HBsAg, obtained from carriers—plasma-derived vaccine) is available for prevention. Pre-exposure prophylaxis is indicated in places with high HBV prevalence; and postexposure prophylaxis is advised for newborn babies of carrier mothers and for individuals exposed to accidental transfusion of blood of HBV carriers. The usual dosage is 1 mL at 0, 1 and 6 months.
2. Recombinant DNA (RDNA) yeast-derived vaccine. A recombinant DNA vaccine, which is cheaper and safe, is also available.

Hepatitis B immunoglobulin can be given for immediate protection within 6 hours after exposure (but not later than 48 hours). Simultaneous administration of the vaccine and HBIG are more efficacious than HBIG alone.

The first universal HBV immunization program in the world was launched in Taiwan, after which HBV infection rates, chronicity rates, incidence of HCC and incidence of fulminant hepatitis in children have been effectively reduced.

Besides vaccination, measures like screening of blood for HBV before transfusion, proper sterilization of syringes, needles and surgical instruments, and health education about the mode of transmission will help to contain the spread of this disease.

❑ HEPATITIS C

Hepatitis C virus (HCV) is the major cause of parenterally transmitted non-A, non-B hepatitis. It eluded identification for many years. In 1989, the genome was cloned from the serum of an infected chimpanzee.

The infection is endemic worldwide; about 180 million people (3% of the world's population) are infected with HCV (WHO). Around 130–170 million of them are chronic HCV carriers who are at risk of developing liver cirrhosis and/or liver cancer. More than 350,000 people die from hepatitis C related liver disease each year. High rates of chronic infection are seen in Egypt (22%), Pakistan (4.8%) and China (3.2%). 3–4 million persons are newly infected each year.

In India, HCV infection accounts for one fourth of all cases of chronic liver disease. It is estimated that there are 12.5 million HCV carriers in the country. If screening for HCV among blood donors is not done efficiently, transfusion-induced chronic liver disease is likely to increase in the country.

Causative Organism

The HCV is an enveloped RNA virus in the flaviviridae family. It does not grow in cell culture.

Incubation Period

The incubation period is 6–8 weeks.

Reservoir and Source

Humans and chimpanzees are the only known species susceptible to infection. Blood and blood products and organs of infected individuals are the sources of infection.

Mode of Transmission

The HCV is transmitted through contaminated blood and blood products, and organ donation. Upto 50% of cases are related to intravenous drug users. Vertical transmission and sexual transmission are also suspected.

Factors Facilitating Transmission

Intravenous drug abuse, blood transfusion without screening for HCV and inadequate sterilization of syringes and surgical instruments all favor transmission of this disease.

Clinical Characteristics

Hepatitis C causes a milder form of acute hepatitis than caused by hepatitis B. But 50% of infected individuals develop chronic infection, as against 5%–15%, in the case of HBV.

Reliable serological tests have recently become available. HCV-specific IgG indicates exposure, but not infectivity. Polymerase chain reaction (PCR) assay detects viral genome in patient's serum.

Prevention and Control

Health education regarding the mode of transmission and the need to use sterilized needles and syringes to prevent its transmission and making cheap and affordable anti-HCV blood test kits available for screening are important preventive steps.

Currently no vaccine is available. But scientists have found monoclonal antibodies against HCV, which may make a successful vaccine a reality.

Treatment with interferon, INF-α, for at least 12 months has been approved as the standard treatment of hepatitis C. But in India, a 6 monthly treatment regimen is enough for eradication of HCV as the major type is the hepatitis C genotype 3. However, non-3 genotype requires a longer treatment.

Interferon and ribavirin can cause serious side effects. They are contraindicated in severe depression or in other psychiatric conditions, since drugs are dose dependent and reversible neuropsychiatric effect occurs in 30%–40% of patients during treatment.

Certain plant products like Picroliv, glycyrrhizin and *Phyllanthus amarus* have shown promising results with minimum side effects. They have antiviral properties through endogenous INF induction, as well as hepatocytoprotective effect. Glycyrrhizin has also been shown to inhibit RNA viruses through a hitherto unknown mechanism. The Indian Council of Medical Research is now conducting a multicentric, randomized, controlled clinical trial to evaluate the efficacy and safety of combined treatment regimens of INF and glycyrrhizin for the treatment of chronic hepatitis C. Several other herbal formulations have also shown promising results in hepatitis C treatment. However drug-induced interstitial pneumonitis has been caused by certain herbs.

❑ HEPATITIS G

A virus originally cloned from the serum of a surgeon with non-A, non-B, non-C hepatitis, has been called hepatitis G virus (HGV). It was implicated as a cause of parenterally transmitted hepatitis, but is no longer believed to be a major agent of liver disease. The virus has been classified as a flavivirus and is distantly related to HCV.

Acute hepatitis may also occur as part of the clinical course of a number of viral infections including human cytomegalovirus, Epstein-Barr virus, herpes simplex virus, yellow fever virus and rubella.

❑ SEXUALLY TRANSMITTED INFECTIONS

Sexually transmitted infections (STIs) [previously known as sexually transmitted diseases (STDs)] are showing an increasing trend throughout the world. Studies indicate that India also has a similar trend. Each year, 448 million new infections of curable STIs (syphilis, gonorrhea, chlamydia and trichomoniasis) occur according to 2005 estimates (WHO fact sheet 2011).

The STIs are caused by bacteria, viruses and parasites. Some of the most common infections are given below.

Causative Organism

Bacterial

1. *Neisseria gonorrhoeae.*
2. *Chlamydia trachomatis.*
3. *Treponema pallidum.*
4. *Haemophilus ducreyi.*
5. *Klebsiella granulomatis* (previously known as *Calymmatobacterium granulomatis*).

Viral

1. Human immunodeficiency virus.
2. Herpes simplex virus type 2.
3. Human papillomavirus.
4. Hepatitis B virus.
5. Cytomegalovirus.

Parasites

1. *Trichomonas vaginalis.*
2. *Candida albicans.*

Mode of Transmission

Transmission occurs mainly through direct sexual contact. Very rarely they are indirectly transmitted to doctors, nurses and laboratory workers. Besides sexual transmission, syphilis, hepatitis B and AIDS are transmitted also through contaminated blood and from infected mother to fetus.

Factors Facilitating Transmission

Media like TV and cinema showing pornographic scenes, which is a grave distraction from normal sexual behavior specially for the youth. Pornographic magazines also spread misinformation and spoil the youth.

Social factors such as prostitution, broken homes, sexual disharmony between husband and wife, urbanization and industrialization, population mobility, increased employment of women, homosexuality, social stigma associated with STIs, availability of contraceptives and liberalization of abortion laws, ignorance, local customs like polygamy, emotional immaturity, population explosion, economic affluence all favor transmission of STIs.

Clinical Characteristics and Incubation Period

Syphilis

Syphilis presents as indurated ulcer (chancre), usually single, in the genitals with enlargement of the regional lymph nodes as the initial feature. Smear from ulcer shows *Treponema pallidum.* If untreated secondary and tertiary syphilis will develop. Congenital syphilis results from mother-to-child transmission and is the second most common cause of stillbirth.

The incubation period is 10–90 days.

Gonorrhea

Gonorrhea manifests as purulent discharge from the genitals. If pregnant woman suffers from gonorrhea the baby may be born with ophthalmia neonatorum, an acute blinding eye disease. Smear from the discharge shows the gram-negative diplococci.

The incubation period is 2–10 days.

Chancroid

Chancroid is seen as ulcer, usually multiple, over the genitals and also extragenitally. Smear shows *Haemophilus ducreyi.*

The incubation period is 1–5 days.

Lymphogranuloma Venereum

Lymphogranuloma venereum (LGV) causes bubo in the groin as the earliest feature. Ulceration and elephantiasis of genitalia are late sequelae. Smear shows *Chlamydia trachomatis.*

The incubation period is 3–20 days.

Donovanosis

Donovanosis is seen as creeping exuberant ulcer over the skin and mucous membranes of external genitalia. Biopsy shows *Klebsiella granulomatis.*

The incubation period is 1–6 weeks.

Prevention and Control

Since STIs are the manifestations of social problems, special attention should be paid to remedy social ills. Removal of poverty and rehabilitation of prostitutes, marriage counseling and premarital examinations, health education, personal prophylaxis, teaching of moral values in schools and colleges, and control of cinema and other pornographic media are some of the measures that will help in the prevention of STIs.

Control is achieved through active case finding, case holding, establishment of separate STI clinics for males and females, effective chemotherapy and follow-up.

Syndromic Case Management of STDs

The traditional method of diagnosing STDs is by laboratory tests. However, such tests are very often unavailable or too expensive. For this reason, syndromic management of STDs has been recommended by WHO since 1990 for use in patients presenting with symptoms of STD. Its main features are:

1. Classification of the main causative pathogens by the clinical syndromes they produce.
2. Use of flowcharts derived from this classification to manage a particular syndrome.
3. Treatment for all important causes of the syndrome.
4. Notification and treatment of sex partners.
5. No expensive laboratory procedures required.

For example, a man presenting with urethral discharge would be treated for both gonorrhea and chlamydial infection. In a person with a genital ulcer, the treatment would most likely be for syphilis and chancroid. The syndromic approach permits STD treatment without costly laboratory tests. It offers accessibility and immediate treatment and is effective and efficient. Studies have shown that syndromic case management of STDs using flowcharts is more cost-effective than diagnosis based on either clinical examination or laboratory tests. Despite its shortcomings in women with vaginal discharge, this approach currently provides the best alternative guide to STD management, especially where resources for laboratory tests are limited. It performs well in the management of men with symptomatic urethral discharge and in the management of men and women with genital ulcer disease. A disadvantage of the syndromic approach is overtreatment in some patients. This is especially so in the case of vaginal discharge where cervicitis (due to gonorrhea and/or chlamydial infection) is not the predominant cause of the discharge.

The magnitude of the problem of STDs and the strong association with human immunodeficiency virus (HIV) transmission highlight the need to explore new and innovative approaches to prevent and control their spread. One such approach is the adoption of the 'public health package'. This package for STD control consists of the following components:

1. Promoting safer sex behavior.
2. Strengthening condom programming.
3. Promoting healthcare seeking behavior.
4. Integrating STD control in primary health care and other healthcare services.
5. Providing specific services for populations at increased risk.
6. Comprehensive case management.
7. The prevention and care of congenital syphilis and neonatal conjunctivitis.
8. Early detection of asymptomatic and symptomatic infections.

❑ ACQUIRED IMMUNODEFICIENCY SYNDROME (AIDS)

Acquired immunodeficiency syndrome (AIDS), first reported in early 1980s, is a sexually transmitted killer disease. It has now become a pandemic affecting all parts of the world, which has claimed more than 25 million lives over the past 3 decades.

There were approximately 34.2 million people living with HIV in 2011, while it was 32.9 in 2009. New HIV infections from 2008 till 2010 remains steady at 2.7 million. Number of deaths from AIDS related causes were 2, 1.9 and 1.8 million in 2008, 2009 and 2010 respectively.

In India, the total number of people living with HIV/AIDS in 2009 was estimated to be 2.4 million with a prevalence rate of 0.3%. There were 1.35 lakh new cases. About 1.72 lakh people died due to AIDS related causes. Andhra Pradesh (5 lakhs), Maharashtra (4.2 lakhs), Karnataka (2.5 lakhs) and Tamil Nadu (1.5 lakhs) are the high prevalent states.

Causative Agent

Causative agent of AIDS is a retrovirus named HIV, which infects actively dividing T lymphocytes (helper or CD4+ T cells). Two types are recognized—HIV-1 and HIV-2. HIV is easily killed by heat, ether, acetone, ethanol (20%) and β-propiolactone, but it is resistant to ionizing radiation and UV light.

Reservoir and Source

Cases and carriers form the reservoir pool. Symptomless carriers can infect others for years. The virus has been found in blood, semen and cerebrospinal fluid (CSF) abundantly. While in tears, saliva, breast milk, urine, and cervical and vaginal secretions, it is present in low level. But only blood and semen have been found to transmit the virus conclusively.

Mode of Transmission

1. Through sexual contact: The main mode of HIV transmission is through sexual contact—heterosexual, homosexual or anal intercourse. Presence of other STIs increases the chances of transmission of HIV.
2. Through blood: Transfusion of blood and blood products containing HIV, use of contaminated syringes, needles or any skin piercing instruments, needle sharing by drug users and procedures like ear piercing, tattooing, acupuncture all have

been found to transmit HIV. Shared razors and toothbrushes also can transmit HIV.

3. From mother to child: HIV transmission to the fetus takes place through placenta and to the infant during delivery and through breast milk. One-third of children of HIV-positive mothers contract the infection.

The most important mode of transmission in India is heterosexual transmission (87.4%). Injecting drug is the predominant route of transmission in north eastern states.

Mosquitoes, bugs or other insects, casual social contact, food or water have not been found to transmit HIV.

Factors Facilitating Transmission

Promiscuity, prostitution, multiple sex partnership, male homosexuality, intravenous drug abuse, sexually stimulating cinema, pornographic materials, ignorance, presence of STIs and carrier state in AIDS all favor transmission of HIV. It is paradoxical that the society, while not taking cognizance of the sexually stimulating media activities in TV, cinema, the internet, etc. preaches the youth to marry late. The materialistic society fails to recognize the negative impact of TV and cinema on children and the youth.

Clinical Characteristics

After contracting the infection, no symptom may be observed for the first 5 years or so in most people, but during this period they can transmit the virus to their sexual partners.

Antibody production against HIV in the infected individual takes place after a lapse of 2–12 weeks and this period is called 'window period'. Transmission can take place even during the window period. Though antibodies are produced against the virus they are not able to neutralize it.

After an unspecified asymptomatic carrier state period, AIDS-related complex ensues. Immune system of the individual is affected, but opportunistic infections and cancers related to AIDS are not seen in this stage. AIDS-related complex is characterized by unexplained diarrhea, fatigue, malaise, loss of more than 10% body weight, fever, night sweats and milder opportunistic infections like oral thrush and generalized lymphadenopathy or enlarged spleen. Count of T-helper lymphocytes in the blood is low.

Next the AIDS stage sets in. Many opportunistic infections occur in this stage. Active tuberculosis and Kaposi's sarcoma are seen. Serious fungal infections such as *Candida* esophagitis, cryptococcal meningitis, penicilliosis and parasitic infections like *Pneumocystis carinii* pneumonia and *Toxoplasma gondii* encephalitis occur as the T-helper lymphocytes (helper or CD4+ T cells), which are important in the immune reaction against pathogenic organisms are diminished to a very low level by the HIV, which infect and destroy them. Chronic diarrhea, severe weight loss, AIDS encephalopathy or AIDS dementia occur. Finally death is caused by uncontrolled or untreatable opportunistic infections.

Diagnosis of AIDS is made from clinical features and blood tests.

Enzyme-linked immunosorbent assay (ELISA) test is done to detect HIV antibodies and the Western Blot test to rule out false positive results. Tests using saliva or urine are also available. Rapid HIV tests can give results in 20 minutes. HIV can also be isolated from culture of lymphocytes from the patient.

Polymerase chain reaction (PCR) test finds either the RNA of the HIV virus or the HIV DNA in white blood cells infected with the virus. This test is very useful to find a very recent infection, to determine if an HIV infection is present when antibody test results were uncertain and to screen blood or organs for HIV before donation.

The CD4 cells are a type of white blood cell that are specifically targeted and destroyed by HIV. A healthy person's CD4 count can vary from 500 to more than 1,000. CD4 count less than 200 is seen in AIDS.

Prevention and Control

As there is no cure or vaccine against AIDS, the only option available for people is to change their unhealthy sexual behavior in order to prevent contracting HIV infection. Persistent health education through various media has increased the awareness of people about AIDS. But the society's reaction to AIDS patients is not favorable and many AIDS victims are stigmatized and neglected. It has to be understood that mere health education measures without concrete steps to remove the social causes that make the AIDS situation worse will not yield results.

Avoiding shared razors and toothbrushes, avoiding sharing of needles and syringes by drug abusers and avoiding pregnancy by HIV-positive women are important to prevent the spread of HIV.

Blood should not be transfused without screening for HIV. Needles, syringes and other surgical instruments should be thoroughly sterilized. Doctors and hospitals should use disposable syringes as far as possible. Antiretroviral therapy immediately after birth for infants born to HIV-positive mothers can prevent the development of AIDS in the infant.

Antiviral chemotherapy can prolong the life of AIDS patients. Nucleoside analogs [zidovudine (AZT), didanosine, zalcitabine, stavudine, lamivudine (3TC)], protease inhibitors (saquinavir, ritonavir, indinavir, nelfinavir) and nucleoside reverse transcriptase inhibitors (nevirapine, delavirdine) are the antiretroviral drugs employed in the treatment of AIDS.

Immediate postexposure prophylaxis (PEP) therapy with antiretroviral drugs within hours in accidental exposure to HIV is being practiced with some success in preventing AIDS. Healthcare workers accidentally exposed to HIV can be protected with combination treatment using AZT 300 mg 3 times daily plus 3TC 150 mg twice daily for 4 weeks. If an advanced AIDS case is the source, protease inhibitor nelfinavir 750 mg 3 times daily should be added to the above regimen. If the source is a resistant case (resistant to AZT and 3TC combination), stavudine plus didanosine should be used in the place of AZT plus 3TC.

Opportunistic infections also should be treated with appropriate drugs. When CD4 cell count is below 200 cells per microliter, primary prophylaxis with trimethoprim-sulfamethoxazole, aerosolized pentamidine and dapsone is indicated against *P. carinii* pneumonia. When a particular prophylactic regimen fails, alternate drugs should be thought. Rifabutin can be used to reduce the incidence of disseminated *Mycobacterium avium-intracellulare* after ruling out *Mycobacterium tuberculosis* in the patient. 300 mg of isoniazid (INH) daily for 9-12 months can be prescribed for prophylaxis against *M. tuberculosis.* Kaposi's sarcoma is treated with INF, chemotherapy or radiation. Ganciclovir for cytomegalovirus retinitis; fluconazole for cryptococcal meningitis, vaginal candidiasis and esophageal candidiasis; acyclovir or foscamet for herpes simplex and herpes zoster are also being prescribed.

❑ SCABIES

Scabies is an infestation of the skin by itch mite, an extremely small globular arthropod. The itch mite is known as *Sarcoptes scabiei* or *Acarus scabiei.* This disease is disseminated from an infected person by close contact. Acts while sleeping in the same bed, children playing with each other or nursing an affected individual can transmit the disease. Very often the entire family is affected. Transmission through contaminated clothes and bed linen can also take place.

Scabies is characterized by itchy lesions in the interdigital webs of hands, anterior aspect of the wrist and extensor aspect of elbows. Axillae, buttocks, lower abdomen, feet and ankles, and palms in infants are other common sites affected. Breasts in women and genitals in men are also affected. Secondary infection may complicate scabies.

In the control of scabies, treatment of all the members of the affected household or hostel or other institutions irrespective of whether all members have scabies or not, is important. Benzyl benzoate emulsion (25%) is applied all over the body from chin downwards and allowed to dry. Babies need the application on the head also. Bath is given after another application repeated after 12 hours of the first application. 0.5%–1% lindane also is an efficient sarcopticide. 2.5%–10% sulfur ointment is a cheaper remedy.

❑ PEDICULOSIS

Infestation, on the body surface, by lice is called pediculosis. Three kinds of lice infest man and they are *Pediculosis capitis* (head louse), *Pediculosis corporis* (body louse) and *Phthirus pubis* (pubic or crab louse). Lice infestation is a problem wherever hygiene standards are low.

Dissemination of louse is by close contact with infected persons. Overcrowding facilitates transmission. Children acquire the infestation easily in schools from other children.

Combs, bedding, clothing may also transmit lice form person to person.

Louse causes itching by their bites and it is the vector for epidemic typhus, trench fever and relapsing fever.

Head and pubic lice are controlled using 0.5% Malathion lotion application. The lotion is left, after application, for 12–24 hours after which the hair is washed. Malathion kills lice and the nymph-nits. Carbaryl dust is also effective against lice. Body louse is controlled by 1% Malathion powder or carbaryl powder which is blown down the neck of the shirt, up the sleeves and into the trousers from several angles. If necessary a second application may be advised after 7 days.

SECTION

3

Non-communicable Diseases

CHAPTER

8

Coronary Heart Disease

Consequent to the improvement in health care and standard of life, many live to old age. Lifestyle patterns pertaining to dietary intakes and behavior of modern man also have undergone significant changes, which cannot be considered as desirable changes. All these have resulted in an increase in the incidence of chronic diseases, especially in developed nations. In developing countries also, they are likely to increase in the future for the same reasons.

According to World Health Organization (WHO), non-communicable diseases (NCDs) kill more than 36 million people each year, out of which nearly 80% of NCD deaths (29 million) occur in low- and middle-income countries. Cardiovascular diseases account for most of these deaths.

Coronary heart disease (CHD), hypertension, stroke, diabetes mellitus (DM) and obesity are some of the chronic diseases, which have emerged as diseases of public health importance.

❑ CORONARY HEART DISEASE

Coronary heart disease (CHD), also known as ischemic heart disease (IHD), was observed in epidemic proportions in developed nations like USA and UK as early as 1920s and 1930s. But now it is seen to increase in developing countries, while there is a decline in its incidence in developed countries such as USA, Australia, Canada and New Zealand, attributed to lifestyle changes and the better control of hypertension in their population. But even in those countries showing a decline, CHD is still the leading killer. In 2008, an estimated 7.3 million people died due to CHD globally.

In India also, CHD has assumed epidemic proportions. In 2000, there were about 30 million patients; 14 million in urban areas and 16 million in rural areas and there were 1.6 million deaths due to CHD. The prevalence in rural adults was 3%–5% and in urban area it was 7%–10%. The WHO estimates that, by 2010, 60% of the world's cardiac patients will be in India. The CHD mortality is greater in South India, while stroke is more common in the eastern Indian states. Prevalence of CHD is higher in urban Indian populations, while stroke mortality is similar in urban and rural regions. Another important aspect is the fact that CHD appeared a decade earlier in India when compared to developed countries. Males are affected more than females. Hypertension, diabetes and heavy smoking are the important etiological factors in India.

Ischemia (reduction of blood supply) of the heart muscle, which is the basic etiology in CHD, occurs because of formation of block in coronary arteries that supply blood to the heart. When the occlusion is complete, sudden deaths may occur, while partial block causes pain in the chest called angina pectoris. Atherosclerosis and thromboembolism may be the basic pathology in the blocking of coronary arteries.

Risk Factors

Two kinds of risk factors have been identified for CHD—the non-modifiable risk factors and the modifiable risk factors.

Non-modifiable Risk Factors

1. Age: There is an increased risk after the age of 45 years in men and after 55 years in women.
2. Family history of early heart disease in parents and siblings: History of heart disease before 55 years in father and brother, and before 65 years in mother and sister.

Modifiable Risk Factors

1. High level of blood cholesterol.
2. High blood pressure (BP).
3. Overweight or obesity.

4. Sedentary lifestyles.
5. Stress.
6. Diabetes mellitus.
7. Cigarette smoking.

High blood level of C-reactive protein (CRP), which increases when there is inflammation, is also considered as a risk factor. Fibrinogen and homocysteine, an amino acid, are also linked to CHD.

Prevention

Prevention requires changes in lifestyle. Reduction in fat intake to less than 30% of total energy intake, restriction of saturated fat (egg, meat, milk) to less than 10% of total energy intake, reduction of dietary cholesterol to below 100 mg/1,000 kcal/day (one egg contains more than one day's requirement of cholesterol), increasing fiber content of diets by consuming vegetables, fruits and whole grain cereals and reduction of salt intake are advised for prevention of CHD. Effective control of high blood pressure, quitting cigarette smoking, regular physical activity and reduction of stress are also important in prevention.

CHAPTER

9

Hypertension and Stroke

❑ HYPERTENSION

Hypertension is the commonest cardiovascular disorder affecting about 20% of the adult population worldwide. The prevalence is rapidly increasing in developing countries also. The prevalence in India is ranging between 10% and 30.9%; 25% in urban and 10% in rural people. Hypertension is a major risk factor for stroke, myocardial infarction, cardiac failure, chronic kidney disease, peripheral vascular disease, cognitive decline and premature death.

World Health Organization defines hypertension as a systolic pressure equal to or greater than 160 mm Hg and/or a diastolic pressure equal to or greater than 95 mm Hg.

When the cause of high blood pressure (BP) is unknown, it is called primary or essential hypertension. In 90%–95% of hypertension cases, no identifiable causes can be found. If the high BP is due to some known causes like kidney disease, it is called secondary hypertension. Only in 5%–10%, some underlying causes can be incriminated.

In India, the prevalence is 10% in rural area and 25% in urban population. About 57% of all stroke deaths and 24% of all coronary heart disease (CHD) deaths are due to hypertension in India.

Risk Factors

Two kinds of risk factors for hypertension have been identified; the non-modifiable and the modifiable.

Old age and heredity constitute the non-modifiable risk factors.

Obesity, high salt intake, low-potassium intake, high saturated fat (animal fat) intake, stress, sedentary life, alcoholism and oral contraceptives are the modifiable risk factors.

Prevention

Primary prevention that involves reduction of modifiable risk factors enumerated above are discussed in Chapter 8, Coronary Heart Disease. Once identified, hypertension should be kept under check by proper and regular medication to prevent complications like CHD and stroke.

❑ STROKE

Stroke is a worldwide problem and it is one of the leading causes of death and disability throughout the world. Globally, 400–800/lakh strokes were reported in 2005 and stroke caused 5.7 million deaths in 2007. In developed countries, the incidence of stroke is declining largely due to efforts to lower BP and reduce smoking. However, the overall rate of stroke remains high due to the aging of the population.

The Global Burden of Diseases study estimated that the annual stroke incidence was 89/lakh population in 2005 and is likely to increase to 91/lakh in 2015.

World Health Organization defines stroke as rapidly developed clinical signs of focal or global disturbance of cerebral function lasting more than 24 hours or resulting in death. Stroke is caused by reduction or block in blood supply to parts of brain as a result of stenosis, clot or rupture of blood vessels supplying the area. In most cases, stroke may be considered as merely an incident in the progressive course of a generalized vascular disease. It may manifest as coma, hemiplegia, paraplegia, monoplegia, speech disturbances, nerve paresis, sensory impairment, etc. Hemiplegia is the most common manifestation.

The following syndromes are considered as stroke, according to WHO international classification of diseases:

1. Subarachnoid hemorrhage.
2. Cerebral hemorrhage.
3. Cerebral thrombosis or embolism.
4. Occlusion of precerebral arteries.
5. Transient cerebral ischemia or transient ischemic attack (TIA) of more than 24 hours.
6. Ill-defined cardiovascular disease (the underlying pathology in the brain is not determined).

Cerebral thrombosis is the most frequent form of stroke followed by cerebral hemorrhage.

Risk Factors

The risk factors for stroke are hypertension, cardiac abnormalities, diabetes, elevated blood lipids, obesity, smoking, glucose intolerance, blood clotting and contraceptives. Stroke is common in old age. But in India, it is found to occur in younger age groups (below 40 year of age) in one fifth of the total cases. Recurring TIAs caused by microemboli are a warning sign of stroke.

Prevention

Prevention of stroke involves control of hypertension and diabetes, avoiding smoking and identification and treatment of TIA.

CHAPTER

10

Diabetes Mellitus

❑ DIABETES MELLITUS

Over 180 million people have been diagnosed with diabetes mellitus (DM) worldwide. The incidence is expected to more than double by 2030. There is a rising trend in the incidence of DM in developing countries also. Almost 80% of diabetic deaths occur in low- and middle-income countries. The WHO projects that without urgent action, deaths from diabetes will increase by more than 50% in the next 10 years. Most notably, in upper-middle income countries, diabetic deaths are projected to increase by over 80% between 2006 and 2015.

Indian population is supposed to have an increased susceptibility to diabetes. According to Diabetes Atlas published by the International Diabetes Federation (IDF), there were an estimated 40 million persons with diabetes in India in 2007 and this number is predicted to rise to almost 70 million by 2025. The prevalence is 3.37% in 25 years and above (3.35% in male and 3.41% in female). The 40–49 age group has the highest prevalence. Impaired glucose tolerance (IGT) was also found to be very high.

Causes

Diabetes mellitus is caused as a result of defective production or action of the hormone, insulin—an endocrine secretion of pancreas. As insulin is essential for carbohydrate metabolism (besides its effect on fat and amino acid metabolism), blood glucose level rises (hyperglycemia) beyond normal levels in DM. The normal blood glucose level is 80–120 mg/100 mL.

The malnutrition-related diabetes mellitus (MRDM) is common in India and other developing countries. Mostly lean and young people between 15 and 35 years of age are affected with this diabetes. Though MRDM is often reported in Kerala and Orissa states, it is not at all unique to those two states and widely seen among underprivileged people all over the country. Two types of diabetes recognized are:

1. Non-insulin-dependent diabetes mellitus (NIDDM), the maturity onset type (type 2) occurring in the middle aged and the elderly.
2. Insulin-dependent diabetes mellitus (IDDM), the juvenile diabetes (type 1), occurring in young people below 30 years of age.

Gestational diabetes—hyperglycemia, first recognized during pregnancy. The IGT and impaired fasting glycemia (IFG) are intermediate conditions in the transition between normality and diabetes. The IGT can be detected by glucose tolerance test (GTT). People with IGT or IFG are at high risk of progressing to type 2 diabetes although this is not inevitable.

The etiological factors incriminated in causing DM are pancreatic disorders, destruction of β cells of pancreas by viral infections and toxins like cyanates/cyanides, defective insulin (less active) formation and decrease in insulin receptors resulting in less insulin sensitivity, genetic defects and autoimmunity. Obesity is also a risk factor for NIDDM, but not for IDDM. Prevalence of NIDDM increases with age.

Risk Factors

The risk factors identified are genetic predisposition, sedentary life, malnutrition during intrauterine period and infancy, viral infections like German measles, mumps and human coxsackievirus B4. Some chemicals like alloxan, streptozotocin and the rodenticide VALCOR—known toxins to β cells and stress in the form of surgery, trauma and stressful situations are also leading to β-cell destruction. Blood sugar estimation is done for the diagnosis of DM. Urine sugar test may be useful in monitoring the efficacy of treatment.

Screening for Diabetes Mellitus

Urine glucose, venous fasting plasma glucose, fasting capillary blood glucose, random blood glucose, glycated hemoglobin (HbA1c) are some of the tests performed to detect and monitor DM. Measurement of the 24-hour urinary excretion of C-peptide provides a useful monitor of average β-cell insulin secretion. Insulin concentrations are severely reduced in type 1 diabetes and some other conditions such as hypopituitarism. Insulin concentrations may be raised in type 2 diabetes, obesity, insulinoma and some endocrine dysfunctions such as Cushing's syndrome and acromegaly.

Complications

Long-standing diabetes can damage the heart, blood vessels, eyes, kidneys and nerves.

Diabetic retinopathy is an important cause of blindness. Approximately, 2% of people with diabetes for 15 years become blind and about 10% of them develop severe visual impairment. Diabetic neuropathy affects up to 50% of people with diabetes. Combined with reduced blood flow, neuropathy in the feet increases the chance of foot ulcers and eventual limb amputation. Diabetes is among the leading causes of kidney failure. About 10%–20% of people with diabetes die of kidney failure. Diabetes increases the risk of heart disease and stroke. About 50% of people with diabetes die of cardiovascular disease (primarily heart disease and stroke). The overall risk of dying among people with diabetes is at least double the risk of their peers without diabetes.

Diabetes and its complications impose significant economic consequences on individuals, families, health systems and countries.

Prevention and Control

Maintenance of normal body weight is an important preventive strategy. Avoidance of sweets, avoidance of excess calorie intake, intake of fiber-containing foods like whole grains, green leafy vegetables, fruits, etc. adequate protein intake, adequate physical exercise and elimination of food toxins like cyanates are considered important in the prevention of DM.

Once DM is detected, it must be treated properly in order to prevent serious complications. Routine monitoring of blood sugar, urine for albumin and ketones, blood pressure, visual acuity and weight are important in the control. In maturity onset type (NIDDM) diet alone or diet plus oral hypoglycemic drugs may be adequate for control. But in juvenile diabetes (IDDM) insulin use cannot be avoided.

Maturity Onset Diabetes of the Young

There are six known types of maturity onset diabetes of the young (MODY) caused by genetic mutations. Probably, there are other forms and causes still to be identified. Mutations in the *HNF4A* gene on chromosome 20 (MODY 1), the *GCK* gene on chromosome 7 (MODY 2), the *HNF1A* gene on chromosome 12 (MODY 3), the *IPF1* gene on chromosome 13 (MODY 4), the *HNF1β* gene on chromosome 17 (MODY 5) and the *IDDM7* gene on chromosome 2 (MODY 6) are the known entities.

These six types account for about 85%–90% of cases. One of the newest forms of monogenic diabetes is neonatal-onset diabetes due to KATP channel defects.

CHAPTER

11

Obesity

❑ OBESITY

Obesity is considered as a disease by WHO. It is the most common form of malnutrition in developed nations. About 20%–40% of adults and 10%–20% of children and adolescents are found to be obese in these countries. Obesity is found in developing countries also among the affluent. Obesity prevalence rises with age.

The highest obesity levels are in the WHO region of the America (26% of adults) and the lowest in the WHO Southeast Asia region (3% obese). In all parts of the world, women are more likely to be obese than men and thus at greater risk of diabetes, cardiovascular disease and some cancers.

Body weight more than '2' standard deviation, from the median weight for height is considered as obesity. Obesity has reached epidemic proportions globally with more than 1 billion adults overweight, at least 300 million of them clinically obese. An estimated 22 million children under five are estimated to be overweight worldwide. It is a major contributor to the global burden of chronic disease and disability. Obesity accounts for 2%–6% of total healthcare costs in several developed countries.

Etiological Factors

Economic growth, modernization, urbanization and globalization of food markets are just some of the forces thought to underlie the obesity epidemic.

Increased consumption of more energy-dense, nutrient-poor foods with high levels of sugar and saturated fats, combined with reduced physical activity, have led to obesity rates that have risen threefold or more since 1980 in some areas of North America, the United Kingdom, Eastern Europe, the Middle East, the Pacific Islands, Australia, Asia and China.

Body Mass Index

Body mass index (BMI) is a simple index of weight-for-height that is commonly used to classify underweight, overweight and obesity in adults (Table 11.1). It is defined as the weight in kilograms divided by square of the height in meters (kg/m^2), i.e.

$$\text{BMI} = \frac{\text{Weight (kg)}}{\text{Squre of the height (m}^2\text{)}}$$

For example, an adult with 70 kg weight and 1.75 m^2 height will have a BMI of 22.9 (70 kg/1.75 m^2 = 22.9).

TABLE 11.1: International classification according to BMI (adults)

Classification	Cutoff
Normal range	18.50–24.99
Underweight	< 18.50
Severe thinness	< 16.00
Moderate thinness	16.00–16.99
Mild thinness	17.00–18.49
Overweight	≥ 25.00
Preobese	25.00–29.99
Obese	≥ 30.00
Obese class I	30.00–34.99
Obese class II	35.00–39.99
Obese class III	≥ 40.00

Adapted from WHO website, http://www.who.int/bmi

A BMI of more than 25 kg/m^2 is defined as overweight. A BMI of more than 30 kg/m^2 in males and 28.6 kg/m^2 or more in females is considered as obesity.

The importance of obesity lies in the fact that it is the risk factor for diseases like hypertension, diabetes, gallbladder disease and CHD. It is also associated with lowered fertility, osteoarthritis of knee, hip and lumbar spine, and psychological stress.

Prevention and Treatment

The basic principle in the prevention and treatment of obesity is to limit the intake of energy, which should not exceed the energy expenditure. Promoting healthy behaviors will go a long way in this regard. Individuals should be encouraged and motivated to lose weight by the following:

1. Eating more fruits and vegetables as well as nuts and whole grains.
2. Engaging in the daily moderate physical activity for at least 30 minutes.
3. Cutting the amount of fatty, sugary foods in the diet.
4. Changing from saturated animal-based fats to unsaturated vegetable oil-based fats.

Obesity prevention and control strategies should focus on increasing the awareness of those factors that contribute to obesity among decision makers, health professionals and the general public, and lead them to plan/implement interventions that will create more favorable environment for healthier diet and lifestyle.

CHAPTER

12

Cancer

❑ CANCER

According to World Health Organization (WHO), cancer is a leading cause of death worldwide, accounting for 7.6 million deaths (around 13% of all deaths) in 2008. Lung, stomach, liver, colon and breast cancers cause the most of the cancer deaths each year; the most frequent types of cancer differ between men and women. About 70% of all cancer deaths in 2008 occurred in low- and middle-income countries, and cancer deaths worldwide are projected to rise to 13.1 million in 2030.

Tobacco use is the single most important risk factor for cancer causing 22% of global cancer deaths and 71% of global lung cancer deaths. In many low-income countries, up to 20% of cancer deaths are due to infection by hepatitis B virus (HBV) and human papillomavirus (HPV).

In India, 2–2.5 million cases of cancer are present at any given point of time. Over 7 lakh new cases and 3 lakh deaths (6% of total deaths) occur annually due to cancer and the leading sites of cancer are oral cavity, lungs, esophagus and stomach amongst men, and cervix, breast and oral cavity amongst women. The WHO has estimated that 91% of oral cancers in Southeast Asia are directly attributable to the use of tobacco and this is the leading cause of oral cavity cancer and lung cancer in India.

Types

Cancer is the abnormal growth of cells, which can invade adjacent tissues, get implanted in distant organs and cause death. Cancerous change can take place in all types of cells. Three types of cancers are recognized in general. These are cancers of epithelial cells (carcinomas) occurring in skin, mouth, esophagus, intestines and uterus, connective tissue cancers (sarcomas) occurring in fibrous tissue, fat and bone, and cancers affecting cells of bone marrow and immune systems (lymphomas, myelomas and leukemias).

The most frequent cancers seen worldwide are:

1. Among men (in order of number of global deaths): lung, stomach, liver, colorectal, esophagus and prostate.
2. Among women (in order of number of global deaths): breast, lung, stomach, colorectal and cervical (Table 12.1).

Etiological Factors

1. Physical carcinogens, such as ultraviolet rays and ionizing radiation.
2. Chemical carcinogens, such as asbestos, components of tobacco smoke, aflatoxin (a food contaminant) and arsenic (a drinking water contaminant).
3. Biological carcinogens, such as infections from certain viruses, bacteria or parasites.

TABLE 12.1: Main types of cancer and the mortality

Category	Mortality
Lung cancer	1.37 million deaths/year
Stomach cancer	736,000 deaths/year
Liver cancer	695,000 deaths/year
Colorectal cancer	608,000 deaths/year
Breast cancer	458,000 deaths/year
Cervical cancer	275,000 deaths/year

Aging is another fundamental factor for the development of cancer. The incidence of cancer rises dramatically with age, most likely due to a buildup of risks for specific cancers that increase with age. The overall risk accumulation is combined with the tendency for cellular repair mechanisms to be less effective as a person grows older.

Occupational exposure toward many chemical carcinogens like asbestos, benzene, polycyclic hydrocarbons, arsenic, etc. is linked to 1%–5% of all human cancers.

Risk Factors

Tobacco use, alcohol use, unhealthy diet and physical inactivity are the main cancer risk factors worldwide. Chronic infections from HBV, hepatitis C virus (HCV) and some types of HPV are leading risk factors for cancer in low- and middle-income countries. Cervical cancer, which is caused by HPV, is a leading cause of cancer death among women in low-income countries.

Primary Prevention Strategies

Modifying and Avoiding Risk Factors

More than 30% of cancer deaths could be prevented by modifying or avoiding key risk factors such as:

- Tobacco use
- Being overweight or obese
- Unhealthy diet with low fruit and vegetable intake
- Lack of physical activity
- Alcohol use
- Sexually transmitted HPV infection
- Urban air pollution
- Indoor smoke from household use of solid fuels.

Prevention

- Avoidance of the risk factors listed here
- Vaccination against HPV and HBV

- Control of occupational hazards
- Reducing exposure to sunlight.

Control

Early Detection and Treatment

Treatment is more effective when cancer is detected earlier. The aim is to detect the cancer when it is localized. There are two components of early detection programs for cancer:

1. Cancer education to promote early diagnosis by recognizing early signs of cancer such as lumps, sores, persistent indigestion, persistent coughing and bleeding from the body's orifices and the importance of seeking prompt medical attention for these symptoms.
2. Screening is the identification, by means of tests of people with early cancer or precancer before signs are detectable. Screening tests are available for breast cancer (mammography) and cervical cancer (cytology tests). Chest X-ray and sputum cytology are used to detect lung cancers.

Treatment of cancer is aimed at curing, prolonging life and improving the quality of life of patients with cancer. Some of the most common cancer types such as breast cancer, cervical cancer and colorectal cancer have a high cure rate when detected early and treated according to best evidence. The principal methods of treatment are surgery, radiotherapy and chemotherapy. Fundamental for adequate treatment is an accurate diagnosis by means of investigations.

Relief from pain and other problems can be achieved in over 90% of all cancer patients by means of palliative care. Effective strategies exist for the provision of palliative care services for cancer patients and their families, even in low resource settings.

World Health Organization has launched the non-communicable diseases action plan in 2008, which includes cancer-specific interventions.

CHAPTER

13

Rheumatic Heart Disease and Accidents

❑ RHEUMATIC HEART DISEASE

Rheumatic fever mostly affects children in developing countries, especially where poverty is widespread. Globally, almost 2% of deaths from cardiovascular diseases are related to rheumatic heart disease (RHD).

The incidence of RHD is much higher in India than the rest of the world. About 47%–59% of all cardiac admission to hospitals in major urban centers are said to be attributed to RHD.

A study by All India Institute of Medical Sciences (AIIMS) in and around Delhi found prevalence of 20.4/1,000 schoolchildren. It was twice as prevalent among children aged 11–15 years (prevalence of 26.5/1,000 children) compared to children aged 5–10 years (12.6/1,000 children). Girls had a higher prevalence of RHD (27.9/1,000 girls) compared to boys (13.3/1,000 boys).

Rheumatic heart disease occurs in 1%–3% of cases, as a sequelae of rheumatic fever caused by group A β-hemolytic streptococci. 'Rheumatic fever licks the joint, but bites the heart'. Valvular damage in the heart may cause heart failure and death.

Prevention

Prevention of rheumatic fever requires identification of streptococcal pharyngitis and its treatment with penicillin. This may be a difficult proposition.

Penicillin prophylaxis of rheumatic fever cases have to be continued for at least 5 years or till the child reaches 18 years of age in order to prevent the development of RHD. Improving living conditions is a long-term measure in the prevention and control of rheumatic fever and therefore of RHD.

❑ ACCIDENTS

An accident is defined as the unpremeditated event that produces unintended injury, death or property damage. Accidents just do not occur, but they are caused and therefore accidents are eminently preventable.

Accidents rank fourth among the leading causes of death. About 4 million people die due to injuries in the world every year. Three million deaths occur due to road accidents, domestic accidents, industrial accidents, fires, drowning, poisoning, falls and natural disasters every year. Road accidents alone claim about 885,000 lives. One million deaths occur due to intentional injuries or violence (homicides and suicides).

In India also, accidents are showing an upward trend. Fatality in road accidents in India is one of the highest in the world.

Proportional mortality rate [number of deaths due to accidents per 100 (or 1,000) total deaths] and death rate per 1,000 (or 1 lakh) registered vehicles per year are used to measure the problem of accidents.

Causes

Domestic accidents (drowning, burns, poisoning, falls, injuries from sharp or pointed instruments, and bites and other injuries from animals) cause death or disability frequently at extremes of life.

Industrial accidents also cause thousands of deaths and disabilities. But industrial accidents have been controlled more successfully because, they occur in stable environments where preventive action is relatively easy.

Railway accidents occur mainly because of human failure and claim many lives in India.

Road accidents may also be due to unfavorable and unphysiological conditions created by night driving and driving overtime besides the improper implementation of traffic guidelines.

The 10% of all accidental deaths and 7% of all suicides in India are due to fire accidents.

Human and environmental factors are responsible for accidents; 90% due to human failure.

Prevention

Prevention of accidents involves surveillance, safety education, promotion of safety measures, avoiding alcohol and drugs while driving, elimination of environmental factors that cause accidents, proper enforcement of laws pertaining to driving and industrial safety. Community-based interventions using relevant information on local patterns of injury and their causes have reduced the rates of injuries in many countries (especially the industrialized ones). Prevention of injuries is achieved through environmental modifications, changing the designs or structures (engineering), applying and/or reinforcing regulatory measures and overall changing of unsafe behaviors through education.

Regulatory measures, environmental changes and education play a crucial role in the prevention of injuries and accidents in children's environment.

Accident research (accidentology) is an important aspect in the control and prevention of accidents. The characteristics of accidents, the relationship between accidents and the personal attributes, finding out better methods of altering human behavior and safer environment are the important aspects for further research.

CHAPTER

14

Mental Health

❑ MENTAL HEALTH

Mental health is a state of well-being in which the individual realizes his/her own abilities, can cope with the normal stress of life, can work productively and fruitfully and is able to make a contribution to his/her community. A mentally healthy person will be able to satisfy his/her own conflicting instinctive drives without any serious conflict with social interest. A mentally healthy individual:

1. Feels comfortable about himself/herself; has the capacity to estimate own abilities and shortcomings, and has self-respect.
2. Feels right toward others, develops love, friendship and trust, and shows interest in the welfare of fellow men.
3. Is able to meet the demands of life and does not feel bowled over by own emotions of fear, anger, love or guilt.

Determinants of Mental Health

Determinants of mental health are broadly classified as:

1. Individual and family-related determinants.
2. Social, environmental and economic determinants.

Individual and Family-related Determinants

Proper nutrition and emotional satisfaction during pregnancy are important for normal mental development, besides physical growth of the fetus. The early formative years of the child is crucial in the making up of an individual and later as an adult. Warm and intimate relationship with both parents is essential for normal mental development of the child. Broken homes may cause behavioral disorders in children. Old age is affected by organic disease of the brain, economic insecurity, lack of a home, etc. Elderly people who are physically ill may suffer from chronic insomnia, alcohol problems, elder abuse, personal loss and bereavement.

Social, Environmental and Economic Determinants

Schools play an important role in shaping the character of children. Teacher-pupil relationship and the classroom environment will affect the mind of the young learner. Adolescent period is an important stage, which shapes the mental balance of an individual. It is the period of transition to adulthood. The basic needs of adolescents are:

- The need to be needed by others
- The need for increasing independence
- The need to achieve adequate adjustment with the opposite sex
- The need to rethink the cherished values of one's elders.

Poverty, war and inequity are the major socioeconomic and environmental determinants for mental health. Populations living in poor socioeconomic circumstances are at increased risk of poor mental health, depression and lower subjective well-being. Urbanization, war and displacement, racial discrimination and economic instability have been linked to increased levels of psychiatric symptomatology and psychiatric morbidity.

Global Mental Health Situation

More than 450 million people, the world over, suffer from mental disorders (WHO fact sheet, 2010). Mental and behavioral disorders are present at any point in time in about 10% of the adult population worldwide. One fifth of teenagers under the age of 18 years suffer from developmental, emotional or behavioral problems. One in eight has a mental disorder. Mental and neurological disorders account for 13% of the total disability-adjusted life years (DALYs) lost due to all diseases and injuries in the world. Five of the ten leading causes of disability worldwide are psychiatric conditions, including depression, alcohol use, schizophrenia and compulsive disorder. More than 150 million persons suffer from depression at any point in time. Nearly 1 million commit suicide every year. About 25 million suffer from schizophrenia. 38 million suffer from epilepsy and more than 90 million suffer from an alcohol or drug use disorder. Projections estimate that by the year 2020, neuropsychiatric conditions will account for 15% of disability worldwide, with unipolar depression alone accounting for 5.7% of DALYs.

The social and economic costs of poor mental health are high and the evidence suggests that they will continue to grow without community and government action.

Causes of Mental Illnesses

Mental illnesses are caused by a combination of biological, psychological and social factors.

Biological Causes

1. Deficiency or excess of chemical messengers (called neurotransmitters) in the brain and defects in or injury to certain areas of the brain have been linked to some mental conditions.
2. Heredity: Many mental illnesses run in families. Susceptibility is passed on in families through genes. Experts believe many mental illnesses are linked to abnormalities in many genes, not just one. This explains why a person inheriting susceptibility to mental illness does not necessarily develop the illness. Factors such as stress, abuse or a traumatic event can influence or trigger an illness in a person who has an inherited susceptibility to it.
3. Infections: Pediatric autoimmune neuropsychiatric disorders associated with the streptococcal infections (PANDAS) have been linked to the development of obsessive-compulsive disorder and other mental illnesses in children.
4. Prenatal damage: Loss of oxygen to the brain during childbirth may be a factor in the development of certain conditions such as autism.

5. Poor nutrition and exposure to toxins, such as lead, may play a role in the development of mental illnesses.

Psychological Factors

1. Severe psychological trauma suffered during childhood, such as emotional, physical or sexual abuse.
2. An important early loss, such as the loss of a parent.
3. Neglect.
4. Poor ability to relate to others.

Social Factors

1. Death or divorce.
2. A dysfunctional family life.
3. Feelings of inadequacy, low self-esteem, anxiety, anger or loneliness.
4. Changing jobs or schools.
5. Social or cultural expectations—a society that associates beauty with thinness can be a factor in the development of eating disorders.
6. Substance abuse by the person or the person's parents.

Classification

Mental illnesses are classified into two broad categories—major and minor illnesses. Schizophrenia, manic-depressive psychoses and paranoia are the major illnesses. Neurosis, personality and character disorders are the minor illnesses.

Promotion of mental health: Improvement in social, emotional and physical well-being of all people is necessary for primary prevention of mental illnesses.

Mental health promotion activities imply the creation of individual, social and environmental conditions that enable optimal psychological and psychophysiological development. It is an enabling process, done by, with and for the people.

Public health and social interventions for promotion of mental health should include the following:

1. Interventions during early childhood such as home visiting for pregnant women, psychosocial interventions during preschool period, and nutritional and psychosocial interventions among the disadvantaged populations.
2. Improving the accessibility of women to education, microcredit schemes, etc. and thereby empowering them economically and socially.
3. Social support to elderly population in the form of community and day centers for them.
4. Psychological and social intervention programs for the vulnerable groups such as minorities, indigenous people, migrants and people affected by conflicts and disasters.
5. Mental health promotion activities in schools.
6. Mental health interventions at workplaces such as stress prevention programs.
7. Improving the housing conditions through effective policies.
8. Violence prevention programs by involving the community.
9. Community development programs.

Prevention of Mental Disorders

Prevention of mental disorders is aimed at reducing the incidence, prevalence and recurrence of mental disorders, the time spent with symptoms or the risk condition for a mental illness, preventing or delaying recurrences and also decreasing the impact of illness in the affected person, their families and the society.

Well-established mental health services will go a long way in improving the mental health of the community. Routine screening programs will help to identity mental illnesses in their early stage and to initiate counseling and therapy.

SECTION 4

Demography and Family Welfare

CHAPTER

15

Demography

Demography as a scientific study of human population deals with three phenomena namely the size, composition and distribution of the population. These three characteristics get continually changed by five demographic processes namely fertility, mortality, marriage, migration and social mobility.

❑ WORLD POPULATION TREND

The population of the world was 1 billion in the year 1800. In 130 years (1930) a 2nd billion was added. The 3rd billion was added in only 30 years (1960). The 4th and 5th billions were added in just 15 (1974) and 12 (1987) years respectively. The 6 billion mark was reached in 12 years (1999). According to Population Reference Bureau (PRB) data sheet, the world population grew to 7.06 billion in mid-2012. More than half the world's 7 billion people now live in urban areas. Developing countries accounted for 97% of this growth because of the dual effects of continued high birth rates and young populations. Asia is the most populous continent with 4.3 billion people. China is the most populous nation accounting for 19.4% of the global population.

Europe's population is projected to decrease from the current 740 million to 732 million by 2050. Worldwide, the total fertility rate (TFR) is 2.4 and in the poorest countries it is 4.4. Highest TFR (7.1) is seen in Nigeria.

The growth rates of populations differ between different nations. In more developed countries, the growth rate is very low (0.1%), whereas it is high in less developed countries (around

1.4%) and very high in least developed countries (2.4%). In South Central Asia it is 1.6%, while in India it is 1.5%.

The 10 most populous countries in the world and their population are given in the Table 15.1.

Population Trend in India

Fertility (actual bearing of children) is high in India. It is the second most populous country in the world; several factors are held responsible for the high fertility. Universality of marriage, early marriage and the consequent long duration of married life, low level of literacy, poverty, lack of family planning practices, low status of women in society, preference for male child and polygamy are some of them.

However, now the fertility is showing a declining trend in India and the current TFR is 2.5 (2012). But it is still high when compared to the TFR in more developed countries (1.6) and higher than the TFR at world level (2.4).

Some Population Characteristics in India

India's population is 1,260 million (world's 17.5% population), the population has increased by more than 181 million during the decade 2001–2011 (Census report 2011). However, the growth is slower for the first time in 9 decades. The decadal growth has declined by 3.90%; from 21.54% in 2001 to 17.64% in 2011. The state of Bihar showed the highest decadal growth rate during this period (25.07%).

Uttar Pradesh is the most populous state with 199 million people and Lakshadweep the least populated at 64,429.

TABLE 15.1: Most populous countries and their population (2012)

Country	Population (million)
China	1,350 (19.4%)
India	1,260 (17.5%)
United States	314 (4.4%)
Indonesia	241 (3.37%)
Brazil	194
Pakistan	180
Bangladesh	153
Nigeria	170
Russia	143
Japan	128

Adapted from 2012 World Population Data Sheet

More than 50% of India's current population is below

the age of 25 and over 65% below the age of 35. About 72.2% of the population lives in some 638,000 villages and the rest 27.8% in about 5,480 towns and urban agglomerations.

The birth rate is 22.1 births/1,000 population (rural 23.7; urban 18; 2010 estimated), while death rate is 7.2 deaths/1,000 population (rural 7.7; urban 5.8; SRS 2011). Current fertility rate is 2.58 and infant mortality rate is 47 (rural 51; urban 31).

The literacy rate has gone up from 64.83% in 2001 to 74.04% in 2011 showing an increase of 9.21%. Kerala has the highest literacy rate at 90.86%; Mizoram (88.80%) is on the second position and Lakshadweep (86.66%) is on third. Bihar is at the bottom of the ladder with literacy rate of 63.82% followed by Arunachal Pradesh at 66.95%.

While India's land is only 2.4% of world's land area, it supports 17% of world's population.

Even as the overall sex ratio in India increased from 933 in 2001 to 940 in 2011, as per census figures, the child sex ratio dropped to 914 females in 2011 from 927 in 2001 – the lowest since, Independence. Highest sex ratio is reported in the states of Kerala (1,084) and Pondicherry (1,038).

Life expectancy or expectation of life at birth in India is increasing slowly since 1961. As of July 26, 2012, it is 67.14 years in the total population. But life expectancy in India is still very low, when compared to that in developed nations (above 75 years).

Population below poverty line is 29.8% (2010 estimated). As of 2011, India's per capita GDP was $ 3,700, while China had a per capita GDP (PPP) around $ 8,400/year.

Population Growth

Growth of population is measured by annual natural population growth rate, which is arrived at by subtracting death rate from birth rate and it is expressed in percentage.

Birth rate is a measure of fertility in populations. It is defined as the number of live births in 1 year in a specified population per 1,000 estimated midyear population.

It is calculated by the formula:

$$\frac{\text{Number of live births during the year}}{\text{Estimated midyear population}} \times 1{,}000$$

Birth rate as defined above is not a sensitive indicator of fertility as the whole population is not involved in reproduction. Therefore, other refined and sensitive indicators have been formed to measure the fertility. Some of them are:

1. General marital fertility rate (GMFR): It is the number of live births per 1,000 married women in the reproductive age group (15–44 or 49 years) in a given year.
2. Age-specific marital fertility rate: It is the number of live births in a year to 1,000 married women in any specific age group.
3. Total marital fertility rate is the average number of children that would be born to a married woman, if she experiences the current fertility pattern throughout her reproductive span.
4. General reproduction rate (GRR): It gives the average number of girls that would be born to a woman, if she experiences the current fertility pattern throughout her reproductive span assuming no mortality.
5. Net reproduction rate (NRR): It is the number of female children a woman will bear during her lifetime assuming fixed age-specific fertility and mortality rates. The NRR should be one to stabilize the population.

Adverse Effects of Overpopulation

Population growth is taking place in the world as a whole, but it has more significance or repercussions mainly in the developing countries. Overpopulation is said to exist when the population of a country is expanding faster than its economy at any point of time, thereby leading to a situation in which people cannot be adequately looked after. India with only 2.4% of world's land area, but supporting 16% of the world's population, is beset with lot of problems in improving the living conditions of its citizens. Overpopulation affects the environment very badly. Air, water, beaches and fishes are rendered less fit for breathing, drinking, swimming and eating respectively. Housing the ever-increasing population becomes a difficult proposition. Housing shortage in urban area was estimated at 11.9 million units by 1969 and the same in rural area was estimated at 60 million units by 1966. Clothes become scarce. Purchasing power of people is too low to buy adequate cloth. Production of cloth is also is not enough. The country is not able to provide electricity to all. In spite of massive investment in power sector, much remains to be done. Inadequacy in transport is acute in most areas of the country. Even the steady growth in transport has not been able to meet the transport requirement of the rapidly increasing population. Water supply and sanitation is far from adequate not only in rural areas but also in urban settlements. Education, employment and healthcare facilities fall short of the requirement, especially in rural areas. Many are found to suffer from undernutrition. Land holding becomes fragmented resulting in unremunerative returns.

Therefore, control of population is imperative, if the benefits of development in various fields are to reach all the people.

CHAPTER

16

Family Planning

Family planning refers to practices that help individuals or couples to attain the following objectives:

1. To avoid unwanted births.
2. To bring about wanted births.
3. To regulate the interval between pregnancies.
4. To control the time of births in relation to the age of the parent.
5. To determine the number of children in the family.

Family planning, which was discussed in only whispers in private quarters earlier, is being recognized as a basic human right now. Besides birth control it has many other scopes like advice on sterility, sex education, screening for pathological conditions related to reproductive system, marriage counseling and many others. As a collateral benefit, family planning helps to improve the health of the population, specifically women, fetus and children. By preventing unwanted pregnancies, spacing the pregnancy and limiting the number of births, many of the complications associated with pregnancy are averted and thereby health of the mother is improved. Similarly, by regulating pregnancy with reference to the age of mother, congenital anomalies like Down syndrome in the babies associated with advancing maternal age are prevented. Family planning also helps to reduce mortality, undernutrition, impaired growth, development and high incidence of infectious diseases in children by limiting the family size.

❑ ELIGIBLE COUPLES

Eligible couple is an important concept in family planning. Eligible couples are defined as currently married couples wherein the wife is in the reproductive age group of 15–45 years who need family planning services. In a population of 1,000, there will be 150–180 eligible couples. In 2001, the eligible couple rate per 1,000 population was 168.2 with 173 million eligible couples. The aim of all the family planning activities is to protect the eligible couples with one contraceptive method or other, so that unwanted births can be averted. The couple protection rate (CPR) has come down to 40.4 in 2011 from 45.6 in 2001. The long-term goal is to achieve a CPR of 60%. Only then the population of India can be stabilized at a particular level.

❑ CONTRACEPTIVE METHODS

Contraceptive methods are designed to prevent conception. There are temporary and permanent methods of contraception. It is not possible to create an ideal contraceptive method suitable for all. Therefore, the present strategy is to present various contraceptive devices and methods to the eligible couples, so as to enable them to choose any one of their choice (cafeteria approach), condoms, diaphragms, spermicides, etc. that are used at the time of coitus are termed as conventional contraceptives. Each contraceptive method has its own advantages and disadvantages. Broadly contraceptive methods are classified into:

1. Spacing methods:
   a. Barrier methods—physical, chemical and combined methods.
   b. Intrauterine devices.
   c. Hormonal contraceptives.
   d. Postconceptional methods.
   e. Miscellaneous methods.
2. Terminal methods:
   a. Vasectomy (male sterilization).
   b. Tubectomy (female sterilization).

❑ BARRIER METHODS

Physical Methods

Condom

Condom is the most widely used device by men all over the world. It is a simple device without any side effect. It also protects individuals from sexually transmitted diseases (STDs). It is for single use; worn on the erect penis before coitus. Occasional failures may be due to irregular and incorrect use. Condom for females is the latest.

Diaphragm

Diaphragm made of synthetic rubber is meant for women. It is a cup-like device with a rim strengthened by a metal or spring. Diaphragms are to be inserted deep into the vaginal canal before intercourse and kept inside for at least 6 hours after intercourse. This is not a popular device among Indian women.

Chemical Methods

Chemical methods comprise foam tablets, foam aerosols, creams, jellies, pastes and the like.

Combined Methods

In combined methods, a physical device like diaphragm is used smeared with a chemical spermicide like jellies.

Intrauterine Devices

Intrauterine devices (IUDs) are very popular in India. There are basically three types of IUDs. First-generation IUDs are made up of inert material—polyethylene or other polymers. Lippe's loop, a double S-shaped device is used in India. Two sizes (27.5 mm and 30 mm) are available. The lower ends of the loop will have attached threads useful for identification and removal. Second-generation IUDs are devices with metallic copper. Incorporation of copper has made it possible to make smaller devices, which can be fitted easily even in a nulliparous women. 'T' devices like

TCu220C, TCu380A or Ag and Nova T, and multiload devices like MLCu250 and MLCu375 are the different types of copper incorporated IUDs available now. Copper IUDs have the advantage of low expulsion rate, lower incidence of side effects besides its increased effectiveness in contraception. Third-generation IUDs are devices with progestogen. The incorporated hormone is released slowly into the uterine cavity.

Mechanism of Action of IUDs

The IUDs initiate a foreign body reaction causing cellular and biochemical changes in the endometrium and uterine fluids. These changes impair the viability of the gamete and thereby prevent fertilization. Copper seems to enhance the cellular response and affect the enzymes in the uterus. By altering the nature of mucus, copper ions may also affect sperm motility and their survival. Progestogen released from third-generation IUDs increases the viscosity of cervical mucus and thereby prevent the entry of sperm into the cervix. They also make the endometrium unfavorable for implantation. The overall effectiveness of IUDs is equal to that of hormonal contraceptives. Since, they have a longer continuation rates than hormonal contraceptives.

The IUD is preferably inserted during menstruation or within 10 days of beginning of menstruation because during this time insertion is easy. Immediate postpartum insertion of IUDs may have the risk of perforation and expulsion. Therefore, postpuerperal insertion (6–8 week after delivery) is preferable. The IUDs also can be inserted immediately after 1st trimester legal abortion, but are not advised after illegal and II trimester abortion.

Lippe's loop can be kept inside the uterine cavity as long as a woman desires provided there are no complications. But copper and hormonal devices have to be replaced periodically at 2–4 year intervals.

The ideal candidate for IUD insertion is a woman who has borne at least one child and who is in a monogamous relationship with no history of pelvic disease, with normal menstrual periods and with an access for follow-up.

Contraindications

Intrauterine devices are contraindicated absolutely in suspected pregnancy, pelvic inflammatory disease, undiagnosed vaginal bleeding, cancer of cervix, uterine or other pelvic tumors and in women with history of previous ectopic pregnancy. Anemia, purulent cervical discharge, distortions of uterine cavity and fibroids are relative contraindications.

Follow-up

Follow-up of IUD users should be done without fail in order to make sure that the IUD is in place and to treat any subsequent adverse effects. IUD users should also be advised to check the presence of threads regularly and to report to doctor if they miss their period.

Side Effects

Bleeding and pain are the major side effects associated with IUD use. If the pain and bleeding are severe, the device should be removed and some other family planning method advised. Pelvic inflammatory disease (PID), if it occurs, can cause sterility. Pregnancy sometimes occurs with the IUD in situ. Ectopic pregnancy is found to be more in IUD users. Expulsion of the device may also occur, especially during the 1st week after insertion or during menstruation. Uterine perforation may also be a rare complication.

Hormonal Contraceptives

Hormonal contraceptives are good spacing methods of contraception. They are available as oral pills or depot preparations.

Oral Pills

Combined pills: These contain both estrogen (30–35 μg) and progestogen (0.5–1 mg), e.g. Mala-N, Mala-D. They are available in packs containing 28 tablets (21 hormone tablets + 7 iron tablets). These pills are started on the 5th day of menstrual cycle and taken every day at a fixed time. If the user forgets to take the pill on any day, she should take it as soon as she remembers and the next day's tablet should be taken as usual. At the end of 21 days of ingestion of the pills, the woman gets withdrawal bleeding. If bleeding does not occur, the second pack of 28 tablets should be started 1 week after the preceding pack.

Combined pills can be used for postcoital contraception also. Two pills immediately after an unprotected intercourse and another two pills 12 hours later are advised for postcoital contraception. Insertion of copper IUD within 48 hours of intercourse also can prevent pregnancy.

Progestogen-only pill (mini pill): As the name implies, it contains only progestogen like norethisterone and levonorgestrel. High failure rate and poor cycle control preclude its widespread use. However, it may be indicated in older women for whom combined pills cannot be advised because of cardiovascular risks.

Hormonal contraceptives also include in its list once-a-month pill.

Mechanism of action: Hormonal contraceptives bring about their action by inhibiting ovulation. Progestogen-only preparations render the cervical mucus thick and thereby affect sperm movement, and also inhibit tubal motility.

Side effects: Common side effects are breast tenderness, weight gain, headache, migraine and bleeding disturbances. Cardiovascular complications like myocardial infarction, cerebral thrombosis and venous thrombosis are observed more in older women and it is due to estrogen content of the pill. Incidence of cervical cancer is found to be more in pill users. The progestogen component is known to lower high-density lipoproteins, elevate blood glucose and plasma insulin. Cholestatic jaundice, premature cessation of milk secretion and birth defects in the newborn when inadvertently taken during pregnancy and ectopic pregnancy are the other adverse effects.

Contraindications: Oral pills are intended primarily for spacing of pregnancies in young women. Continued use for long periods is to be avoided. Women above 35 years of age should not be advised oral pills.

Injectable Hormonal Preparations

Injectable depot hormonal preparations are also available for contraception. They contain progestogens. For example, depot medroxyprogesterone acetate (DMPA), norethisterone enanthate (NET-EN). They are administered as deep intramuscular injections in the buttock once in 3 or 4 months. Combined injectable contraceptives contain both progestogen and estrogen, and they act by inhibiting ovulation. They are administered at monthly intervals plus or minus 3 days. The side effects are similar to that of progestogen-only injectables and should not be prescribed to lactating women and those with risk factors for estrogen.

Others

Subdermal implants and vaginal rings containing progestogen are the other forms of hormonal contraceptives available.

Miscellaneous Methods

The methods enumerated here make use of the knowledge about menstrual cycle, fertilization and the changes that accompany ovulation to prevent conception. But these methods are mostly unreliable and they are meant for only committed and knowledgeable couples. Abstinence (abstaining from sex), coitus interruptus (withdrawal of penis from the vagina before ejaculation) and sex only during safe period (1 week before and 1 week after menstruation) can be practiced only by motivated couples. The other methods like basal body temperature method, cervical mucus method and symptothermal method advocate abstinence during the time of ovulation by noting down the rise in basal body temperature, which rises by 0.3°C–0.5°C and the changes in the consistency of cervical mucus, which becomes watery, raw egg white-like and profuse.

Postconceptional Methods

Menstrual regulation is a simple procedure requiring no legal sanction. It is aspiration of uterine contents 6–14 days after a missed period. Rarely uterine perforation can be caused during this procedure. Rh incompatibility also may be induced by this procedure.

Menstrual induction can be done by intrauterine application of prostaglandin F_2 (1–5 mg). The uterus contracts causing bleeding, which lasts 7–8 days.

The latest in postconceptional contraceptive methods is the use of antiprogestogen like mifepristone along with synthetic prostaglandin like misoprostol to induce abortion medically. An effective dosage regimen is 200 mg of mifepristone orally followed by 800 mg of misoprostol administered after 36–48 hours vaginally, under medical supervision. After the administration of misoprostol on the second day after mifepristone the woman is kept under observation for 4–6 hours during which time the expulsion of products of conception takes place. If no expulsion takes place, the woman is asked to report after 2 weeks for checkup. Abdominal cramps may be a problem after the administration of misoprostol needing medication.

Abortion

Abortion is termination of pregnancy before the fetus becomes viable (before 28 weeks). Abortions can be spontaneous or induced. Induced abortions can be legal or illegal performed by untrained quacks. Illegal abortions are dangerous and contribute to high maternal mortality. Mortality due to abortions is 7.8/1,000 random abortions in India, while it is low in developed countries.

The optimal time for abortion is 7th or 8th week of gestation. Second trimester abortion is dangerous even in experienced hands. After 12 weeks of pregnancy, opinion of two medical practitioners is necessary to perform abortion. In India, legal abortions can be performed only up to 20 weeks of gestation.

Medical Termination of Pregnancy Act (MTP Act) 1971: As the number of illegal abortions was high causing significant morbidity and mortality, Government of India legalized abortion by enacting the MTP Act in 1971, which came into force in April 1972. The MTP Act regulations were further liberalized in October 1975. But still illegal abortions continue to be high.

The MTP (amendment) Act, 2002: This Act stipulates three conditions:

1. The conditions for which abortion can be performed:
   a. Medical: Where continuation of pregnancy might endanger mother's life or cause grave injury to her physical or mental health.
   b. Eugenic: Where there is a substantial risk of the child being born with serious handicaps—physical or mental.
   c. Humanitarian: Where pregnancy is the result of rape.
   d. Socioeconomic: Where actual or reasonably foreseeable environments could lead to risk of injury to the health of the mother.
   e. Failure of contraceptives: Where the couple complain of failure of contraceptive method they adopted.
2. The person or persons who can perform abortion: Only doctors with requisite experience in obstetrics and gynecology are licensed to perform abortion.

   Note: Not withstanding anything contained in the Indian Penal Code, the termination of pregnancy by a person who is not a registered medical practitioner shall be an offence punishable with rigorous imprisonment for a term, which shall not be less than 2 years, but which may extend to 7 years under that Code and that Code shall, to this extent, stand modified. (3) Whoever terminates any pregnancy in a place other than that mentioned in section 4, (4) Any person being owner of a place, which is not approved under clause (b) of section 4 shall be punishable with rigorous imprisonment for a term, which shall not be less than 2 years, but may extend to 7 years.
3. The place where abortions can be conducted: No termination of pregnancy shall be made in accordance with this act at any place other than:
   a. A hospital established or maintained by government.
   b. A place for the time being approved for the purpose of this Act by Government or a District Level Committee constituted by that Government with the Chief Medical Officer or District Health Officer as the chairperson of the said Committee. Provided that the District Level Committee shall consist of not less than three and not more than five members, including the chairperson, as the government may specify from time to time.

The written consent of the guardian is necessary to perform abortion in a girl below 18 years of age and in mentally ill person.

❑ TERMINAL METHODS

Vasectomy and tubectomy are the terminal methods of contraception. These sterilization operations are provided free in government institutions. Female sterilization (tubectomy) accounts for 85% of all sterilizations and men do not come forward to get sterilized in sufficient numbers in spite of the fact that vasectomy is simpler and safer than tubectomy.

The following guidelines are to be followed before doing terminal methods of family planning:

1. The age of the husband should not be less than 25 years and more than 50 years.
2. The age of the wife should not be less than 20 years and more than 45 years.
3. The couple should have two living children at the time of the operation.
4. The age criteria can be relaxed, if the couple has three or more living children.
5. The acceptor should declare that he/she has the consent of the spouse and the spouse had not already undergone the sterilization operation.

Vasectomy

In vasectomy, the vas deferens is reached through an incision in the scrotum. It is cut and ligated after removing a piece of 1 cm length. It is important to warn the acceptor that he will not be sterile immediately after the operation and therefore, should use other methods of contraception at least for 30 ejaculations after the operation. Vasectomy, though a simple operation, is sometimes associated with some complications. Local pain, sepsis and hematoma and sperm granules due to accumulation of sperm may be distressing to the acceptor. Spontaneous recanalization may be a serious complication. Such a possibility should be informed to the acceptors. Some men also complain of diminution of sexual vigor and impotence, which are merely functional as the production of the male hormone is not affected by vasectomy.

Vasectomy, if properly done, is very effective, but sometimes failures (0.15 per 100 persons per year) may occur. It may be due to mistaken identification of vas by the surgeon, anatomical abnormality like two vases on one side and occasional spontaneous recanalization.

Vasectomized persons should be advised:

1. Not to lift heavy objects or ride bicycles for 15 days.
2. To use some contraceptive method until about 30 ejaculations to prevent failures.
3. To get the stitches removed on the 5th day after the operation.

No-scalpel Vasectomy

No-scalpel vasectomy has been introduced now and it is one of the most effective contraceptive methods available for males. It is more effective than the oral pill or the injectable contraceptive. It is an improvement on the conventional vasectomy with practically no side effects or complications. This new method is now being offered to men who have completed their families, as a special project, on a voluntary basis under the Family Welfare Program.

The no-scalpel vasectomy project is being implemented in the country to help men adopt male sterilization and thus promote male participation in the Family Welfare Program. Ensuring the availability of this new technique up to the peripheral level will help increase the acceptance of male sterilization in the country. The project is being funded by the United Nations Population Fund (UNFPA). The total contribution by UNFPA for the project is ₹ 9.15 crores. The contribution of the Government of India will be in kind such as providing centers for training and making available the necessary infrastructure at the training sites.

Tubectomy

Methods

Female sterilization is done by two methods namely minilap and laparoscopic.

Laparoscopic method: It has become very popular as it requires only a short stay in the hospital. An instrument called laparoscope is introduced into the abdominal cavity, the tubes are identified and the falope rings are applied to the tubes to occlude them. But this method is not advisable for postpartum women and it also requires experienced surgeons.

Minilap: In this operation a small incision (2.5–3 cm) is made on the abdominal wall and through the incision, the tubes are brought out and ligated. The procedure is suitable for postpartum women and useful as an elective procedure.

Complications

Complications in female sterilizations are uncommon. But occasionally serious complications like puncture of major blood vessels can occur in laparoscopic method.

Family Welfare Linked Health Insurance Scheme

Family Welfare Linked Health Insurance Scheme has been introduced since November 2005 to take care of the failure of sterilizations, medical complications for death resulting from sterilization and to provide indemnity cover to the doctor/heath facility (₹ 2 lakhs compensation for death during sterilization, ₹ 50,000 for death within 8–30 days after discharge and ₹ 30,000 for failure of sterilization).

Compensation for acceptors of sterilization is being provided since 1981 as a measure to encourage people to adopt permanent family planning methods.

CHAPTER

17

Maternal and Child Health

Mothers and children constitute a large group in any community. In India, women of childbearing age (15–44 year) and children below 15 years form about 22% and 35% respectively. Women and children are also a vulnerable group. The vulnerability is due to childbearing in the case of women, and growth and development in case of children. In developing countries infant, child and maternal mortality rates are high, when compared to that in developed nations. The causes responsible for high morbidity and mortality are mostly preventable.

❑ MATERNAL AND CHILD HEALTH PROBLEMS

The triad of problems that affect mothers and children are malnutrition, infection and the consequences of unregulated fertility. Besides these, poor socioeconomic conditions and lack of medical facilities are also important factors for their plight.

Malnutrition

Malnutrition in mothers leads to anemia, toxemia of pregnancy, maternal depletion and low birth weight of babies born to them. Many of the mothers are also short statured with inadequate pelvis due to chronic malnutrition since childhood. Inadequate food in the formative years of infants and children result in serious diseases like marasmus and kwashiorkor causing significant mortality. Such malnourished children are susceptible to infections easily.

Infections

Infections during antenatal period are also quite common. Cytomegalovirus, herpes simplex virus, etc. have been found to affect pregnant women. Such infections can lead to fetal growth retardation, low birth weight, embryopathy, abortion and puerperal sepsis. As far as children are concerned repeated attacks of diarrhea and acute respiratory infections are common causing significant mortality. Chronic infections like tuberculosis and malaria also may affect children in endemic areas.

Uncontrolled Reproduction

Uncontrolled reproduction affects women and children. Repeated pregnancy with less birth intervals can cause anemia and other complications associated with childbirth. Children of large families are found to suffer from under nutrition, repeated infectious episodes and low intelligence.

❑ MATERNAL HEALTH SITUATION IN INDIA

Maternal mortality ratio, an important indicator of maternal health in India is estimated to be 212/100,000 live births (SRS, 2007–2009). Kerala has the lowest MMR 81/100,000 live births (SRS 2007–2009). In Assam it is 390/100,000 live births. In Uttar Pradesh it is 359/100,000 live births.

Delay in accessing specialized maternal care is found to happen at all level leading to maternal mortality and severe morbidity.

Proportion of deliveries attended by a skilled birth attendant has to increase for reducing maternal mortality. Institutional deliveries have risen to 78.5% (2010–2011).

World Health Organization (WHO) defines a skilled birth attendant as "an accredited health professional such as a midwife, doctor or nurse, who has been educated and trained to proficiency in the skills needed to manage normal (uncomplicated) pregnancies, childbirth and the immediate postnatal period and in the identification, management and referral of complications in women and newborns."

It is also essential to build a continuum of care that increases access to and use of skilled care during pregnancy, birth and the postpartum period. Having a pool of skilled manpower for provision for this continuum of care is a major challenge for India towards improving its maternal health situation.

❑ REPRODUCTIVE AND CHILD HEALTH PROGRAM

Reproductive and Child Health (RCH) Program should focus not only on limiting births but also on healthy sexuality and childbearing. The reproductive health approach would enable women and men to achieve their personal reproductive goals without being subjected to additional burdens of disease and death associated with their reproduction.

Reproductive health implies that people are able to have a responsible, satisfying and safe sex life and that they have the capability to reproduce and the freedom to decide, if when and how often to do so. There is emphasis on the right of men and women to be informed of and to have access to safe, effective, affordable and acceptable methods of fertility regulation of their choice and the right to access to appropriate healthcare services, that will enable women to go safely through pregnancy and childbirth and provide couples with the best chance of having a healthy infant.

The major elements of RCH Program are given in Box 17.1.

Essential Components of RCH Program

1. Prevention and management of unwanted pregnancy.
2. Maternal care that includes antenatal, delivery and postpartum services.
3. Child survival services for newborns and infants.
4. Management of reproductive tract infections (RTIs) and sexually transmitted infections (STIs).

Maternal Health Program

The maternal health program, which is a component of the RCH Program aims, at reducing maternal mortality to less than 100 by 2010 through a number of interventions. They are:

1. Essential obstetric care, which intends to provide the basic maternity services to all pregnant women by ensuring early registration of pregnant women.
2. At least three antenatal checkups for taking preventive and promotive steps, and to detect complications early for prompt action.
3. At least three postnatal checkups to monitor the postnatal recovery. Emergency obstetric care is provided through first referral units established. Round-the-clock delivery services in primary health centers (PHCs)/composite healthcare system [community health centers (CHCs)] facilitate institutional delivery. The other interventions include provision of safe

BOX 17.1: Major elements of RCH Program

1. Reproductive health elements
   a. Responsible and healthy sexual behavior
   b. Interventions to promote safe motherhood
   c. Essential obstetric care for all
   d. Prevention of unwanted pregnancies: increase access to contraceptives
   e. Emergency contraceptives
   f. Safe abortion
   g. Pregnancy and delivery services
   h. First referral units (FRUs) for emergency obstetric care
   i. Management of RTIs/STIs
   j. Infertility and gynecological disorders
   k. Referral facilities by government/private sector for pregnant woman at risk
   l. Reproductive health services for adolescent health
   m. Global reproductive health strategy
2. Child survival elements
   a. Essential newborn care
   b. Prevention and management of vaccine preventable disease
   c. Urban measles campaign
   d. Elimination of neonatal tetanus
   e. Cold chain system
   f. Polio eradication—Pulse Polio Immunization Program
   g. Hepatitis b vaccine
   h. Measles, mumps, rubella vaccine
   i. Global Alliance for Vaccines and Immunization (GAVI)
   j. Diarrhea control program and ORS program
   k. Prevention and control of vitamin A deficiency among children

abortion services, prevention and management of RTIs/STIs, holding of RCH camps in remote areas and training of dais for clean and safe delivery.

Antenatal Care

Antenatal care is given to promote, protect and maintain the health of the mother during pregnancy. Detection of 'high-risk' cases (e.g. elderly and short statured primi, malpresentations, preeclampsia, anemia, previous cesarean, etc.) and their appropriate management forms an important strategy in antenatal care. Since, in India, a high percentage of mothers hail from rural and low socioeconomic background, regular number of checkups in antenatal clinics is difficult for them. Therefore a minimum of four checkups are advised—first before 3rd month, second during 6th month, third during 8th month and the fourth during the 9th month. One of these checkups should preferably be in the home of the mother (home visit).

During these antenatal checkups, the cases are registered. Physical examination and laboratory investigations (like hemoglobin estimation, VDRL test, urine analysis for albumin and sugar, blood grouping, etc.) are performed. Tetanus toxoid immunization of mothers to prevent neonatal tetanus is an important specific protection measure. Anemic women are supplied with iron and folic acid tablets containing iron (100 mg), and folic acid (500 μg) each. Prenatal advice regarding diet, personal hygiene, bowel habits, exercise, the importance of avoiding unnecessary drugs and the warning signs (like the swelling of feet, fits, headache, bleeding) is given. Vitamin A and D capsules, and milk are supplemented. Syphilis and gonorrhea, if found, are treated. Rh-negative women are given 200 or 300 μg of Rh immunoglobulin between 28 and 34 weeks. Sensitizing the mother for family planning is another important activity.

Intranatal Care

Intranatal care provides services to conduct the deliveries in thorough aseptic conditions with minimum injury to the baby and the mother. In urban areas, most deliveries are institutional.

But domiciliary midwifery is unavoidable in rural areas, even though most of the rural homes are unsuitable for it. Home deliveries may deprive the women of the necessary rest required for early restoration of her health and the services of trained nurses and the doctors. The peripheral level female health workers are trained to identify danger signals like prolapse of cord, excessive bleeding during labor, meconium-stained liquor, collapse during labor, etc. and refer such cases to PHCs.

Postnatal Care

The aim of postnatal care is to provide care for the rapid restoration of mother's health and prevent postnatal complications. Breastfeeding and family planning also are important aspects of postnatal care.

Development of postnatal complications like puerperal sepsis, thrombophlebitis, secondary hemorrhage, urinary infections and mastitis are looked for and treated. Physical examination in respect of pulse, respiration, involution of uterus and lochia are carried out and advice for perinatal toilet is given. Sufficient postnatal checkups during puerperal period and till 1 year after delivery are essential to detect early and late complications, and to treat them.

Postnatal care includes care of the newborn. It is carried out by both the obstetrician and the pediatrician. Resuscitation may be needed immediately after delivery, if the baby does not cry properly. The cut end of the cord is bandaged with acriflavin gauze and cleaned everyday till it drops off. Eyes are wiped with sterile cotton wool. The baby is also examined for any anatomical abnormality like imperforate anus and appropriate advice given. Advice on suitable family planning method for the needy mothers is given (Table 17.1).

❑ BIRTH WEIGHT

Birth weight is considered as a measure of maturity and fetal wellbeing. The WHO has fixed 2.5 kg as the cut off for normal birth weight for developing countries. Birth weight less than 2.5 kg is considered low birth weight.

TABLE 17.1: Vaccine use in pregnancy

Vaccine/Disease	Use in pregnancy	Comments
BCG*	No	
Cholera		Safety not determined
Hepatitis A	Yes	Administer, if indicated; safety not determined
Hepatitis B	Yes	Administer, if indicated
Influenza	Yes	Administer, if indicated; in some circumstances, consult a physician
Japanese encephalitis		Safety not determined
Measles	No	
Meningococcal disease	Yes	Administer, if indicated
Mumps	No	
Poliomyelitis (OPV†)	Yes	Administer, if indicated
Poliomyelitis (IPV‡)	Yes	Administer, if indicated; normally avoided
Rubella	No	
Tetanus/diphtheria	Yes	Administer, if indicated
Rabies	Yes	Administer, if indicated
Typhoid Ty 21		Safety not determined
Varicella	No	

*BCG, bacillus Calmette-Guerin; †OPV, oral polio vaccine; ‡IPV, inactivated polio vaccine.

Factors

Birth weight is dependent upon many factors. Some of the factors known to influence birth weight are maternal nutrition, genetic factors, height and age of mother, parity, duration of gestation, smoking in pregnancy, previous obstetric history, etc. Birth weight in affluent families is found to be higher (3.2 kg) than in poor families (2.9 kg).

Low birth weight is high in India when compared to developed nations; in India it is reported to be around 28% (UNICEF 2006–2010). But some workers are of the opinion that the high incidence of low birth weight is due to the high cut off fixed uniformly to all mothers ignoring the genetic characteristics and physical parameters of parents.

The cause of low birth weight is unknown in 30%–50% of cases. However, maternal malnutrition, anemia, infections during antenatal period and unregulated fertility are all known to cause low birth weight. The interplay of many other factors like hard physical labor, smoking, poor maternal weight gain, maternal height less than 145 cm, maternal weight below 40 kg and maternal age less than 20 years, is also incriminated in causing low birth weight.

Prevention of Low Birth Weight

Prevention of low birth weight is an important aspect of RCH care. Adequate food intake, correction of anemia, prevention and control of infections during pregnancy, early detection of disorders like toxemia, family planning and improvements in socioeconomic conditions of people are needed to prevent low birth weight. But increasing birth weight simply by giving more calories in the last trimester of pregnancy is not in tune with biological nature and such concepts can lead to nutritional imbalances in the mother seriously jeopardizing pregnancy outcome. Therefore, any program to improve birth weight should begin the intervention, when the future mothers are still children and not after they become pregnant.

❑ INFANT FEEDING

Feeding of infants properly is important to prevent protein-energy malnutrition (PEM). Faulty feeding practices are still prevalent. Breast milk, as a complete food, is adequate only up to 3rd month of extrauterine life. Supplementary feeds should be introduced to the baby after this period. Bottle feeding in Indian conditions is fraught with danger. Frequent diarrheal episodes are reported in bottle-fed infants. Presence of antimicrobial factors like macrophages, lymphocytes, secretory IgA, lysozyme and lactoferrin in breast milk give protection against diarrheas as well as acute respiratory infections. Breast milk prevents malnutrition and thereby reduces infant mortality. Therefore, breastfeeding is now advised as long as a woman can breastfeed her baby. The weaning foods advised are cow's milk, fruit juice and soft-cooked rice, dal and vegetables. By the time the child is 1 year, he/she should receive solid foods like his/her older siblings.

❑ GROWTH AND DEVELOPMENT

Increase in physical size of the body is growth, while increase in skill and function is development.

The factors that determine growth and development are genetic inheritance, nutrition and age besides many other socio-economic and biological factors. One of the methods of assessing growth is studying anthropometric indices like weight, height, midarm circumference, and head and chest circumferences.

Weight is an important indicator of physical growth. Normally growing baby doubles its birth weight at 5 months, trebles it at 1 year and quadruples it at 2 years of age. From then on 2.25–2.75 kg is added every year until adolescence.

Adolescent spurt occurs earlier for girls (10–11 year) and a little later for boys (12–13 year). During this period of growth spurt, boys put on some 20 kg and girls something like 16 kg.

About 50% increase in body length occurs in the 1st year from 50 to 75 cm and in the 2nd year some 12–13 cm is added. Afterwards, 5–6 cm is added every year until adolescence. During growth spurt, boys add up 20 cm and girls, 16 cm.

Reference standards for weight for age, height for age, weight for height, etc. for Indian children have been prepared by National Institute of Nutrition, which can be consulted to assess the growth pattern of children. To monitor the growth of preschool children a growth chart has been devised by WHO. It has two lines, an upper line for boys (50th percentile) and a lower line for girls (3rd percentile). Space between the two lines is described as 'road to health'. Children should be weighed ideally once every month in the 1st year, every 2 months in the 2nd year and every 3 months, thereafter up to 5–6 years. Weight is also recorded every time, the child is brought to the health center/hospital and all such weights recorded are plotted on the growth chart. If the growth curve of the child falls within the two lines in the chart and runs parallel to them, it indicates that the child is growing normally. If the curve falls below the lower line or if there are fluctuations even within the two lines, it indicates growth retardation.

In India, many modified growth charts are used, which have four reference curves (Fig. 17.1). The uppermost line corresponds to WHO reference standard. The lower lines in descending order represent 80%, 70% and 60% respectively of the standard weight.

As per Gomez classification, weight 90% is the standard and above is taken as normal. Weight between 89% and 75% is classified as first-degree (mild) malnutrition, between 74% and 60% as second-degree (moderate) malnutrition and that below 60% as third-degree (severe) malnutrition.

The growth charts (Fig. 17.2) are an important innovation in child growth monitoring. The chart creates a visual impression in the mother about her child's growth and thereby helping her to understand better the importance of good and adequate food for normal growth of her child.

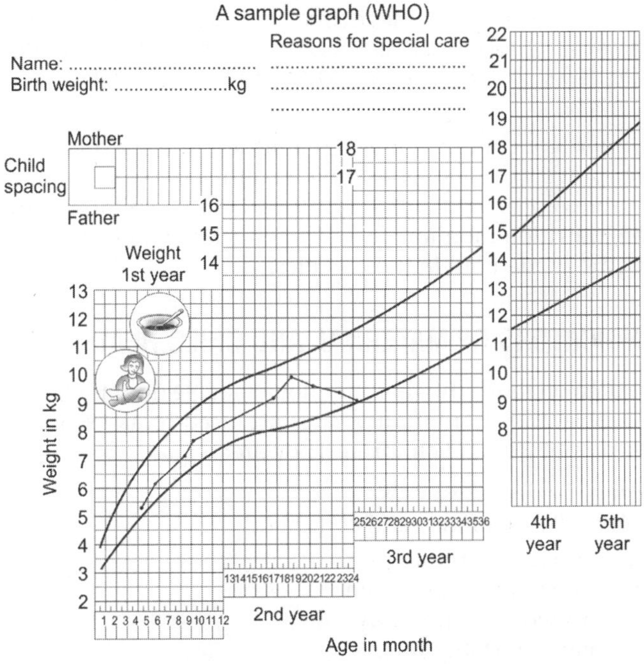

Figure 17.1: A sample growth chart (WHO)

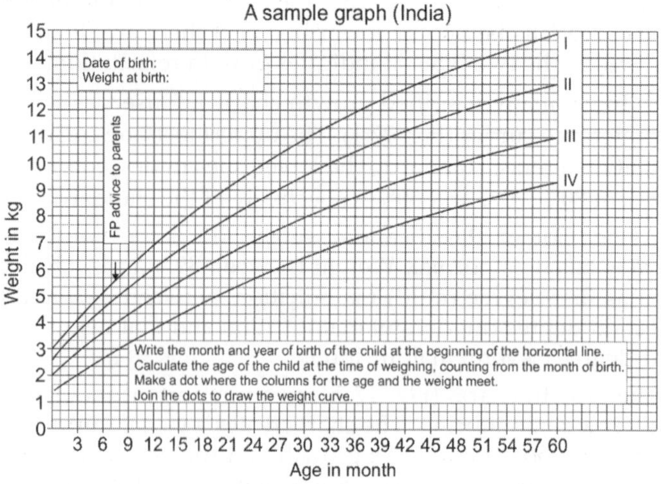

Figure 17.2: A sample growth chart (India). Weights of average well-fed healthy children should be above the upper most line I; children whose weights fall between lines I and III are undernourished and require supplementary feeding at home; children whose weights fall below line III are severely malnourished. Consult the doctor and follow his advice; children whose weights fall below line IV will have to be hospitalized (FP, family planning).

Under-five children clinics established in some areas give curative, preventive and promotive health services making use of non-professional auxiliaries. Treatment of sick children, immunization, nutrition monitoring, health education and growth monitoring are carried out in these clinics.

❑ INDICATORS OF MATERNAL AND CHILD HEALTH CARE

Since data on morbidity is either not available or not reliable even if available, mostly mortality rates are used to assess the health status of mothers and children. They are:

1. Maternal mortality rate.
2. Mortality in infancy and childhood:
   a. Perinatal mortality rate.
   b. Neonatal mortality rate.
   c. Postneonatal mortality rate.
   d. Infant mortality rate.
   e. Child (1–4 year) mortality rate.

f. Under-five mortality rate.
g. Child survival rate.

Maternal death is defined as death of a woman, while pregnant or within 42 days of termination of pregnancy, irrespective of the duration and site of pregnancy from any cause related to or aggravated by the pregnancy or its management, but not from accidental or incidental causes.

Maternal Mortality Rate

Maternal mortality rate (MMR) is expressed as number of maternal deaths per 1,000 live births. It is calculated by the formula:

$$\text{MMR} = \frac{\text{Total number of female deaths due to complications of pregnancy, childbirth or within 42 days of delivery from puerperal causes in an area during a given year}}{\text{Total number of live births in the same area and year}} \times 1{,}000$$

Causes

Major causes of maternal mortality in India remain hemorrhage (38%), sepsis (11%), abortions (8%), hypertensive disorders (5%) and obstructed labor (5%). Other conditions including anemia, medical disorders during pregnancy contribute to 34% of all maternal deaths (RGI-SRS, 2006). Delays in accessing specialized maternal care happen at all levels, which leads to maternal mortality and severe morbidity.

Globally, an estimated 287,000 women died in pregnancy and childbirth in 2010, a decline of 47% from levels in 1990.

India recorded around 57,000 maternal deaths in 2010. Maternal mortality is still high; 212/1 lakh live births (2007–2009). The country's Millenium Development Goals (MDG) in this respect is 109/1 lakh live births by 2015.

Causes of maternal mortality in India are:

1. Obstetric causes of maternal mortality are toxemias of pregnancy, hemorrhage during labor, infection, obstructed labor and induced abortion (Table 17.2).

TABLE 17.2: Causes of maternal deaths in different regions (2001–2003) in India

Regions	Hemor-rhage	Sepsis	Hypertensive disorders	Obstructed labor	Abor-tion	Other conditions
EAG* states and Assam	37%	11%	4%	5%	10%	33%
South	30%	17%	13%	9%	4%	26%
Others	40%	10%	6%	4%	3%	37%
India	38%	11%	5%	5%	8%	34%

*EAG, empowered action group

2. Non-obstetric causes are anemia, already existing diseases of the mother like heart disease, kidney disease, liver disease, malignancy and accidents.

Social factors like poverty, illiteracy, ignorance and prejudices, lack of maternity services delivery by untrained dais, and poor communication and transport facilities are also responsible for high MMR.

Maternal and child health (MCH) services are intended to reduce MMR through its various intervention methods.

Infant Mortality

Infant mortality (death of infants below 1 year of age) in India has come down to 47/1,000 in 2010 from 50/1,000 in 2009. But it is still high when compared to that in developed nations, where it is less than 10/1,000. Infant mortality rate (IMR) is expressed as the ratio of infant deaths to the total number of live births in a given year. It is calculated by the formula:

$$\text{IMR} = \frac{\text{Number of deaths of infants in a year}}{\text{Total number of live births in the same year}} \times 1{,}000$$

Causes

Causes of infant mortality in India are explained below.

During neonatal period: Immaturity, birth injury and difficult labor, congenital anomalies, hemolytic diseases of newborn, and placental and cord abnormalities are the main causes for infant mortality. Acute diarrheas and respiratory diseases (due to poor environment) also are rare causes for infant deaths in the neonatal period.

During postneonatal period: Difficulties due to bad environment are the common causes for infant deaths in postneonatal period. Acute diarrheal and respiratory diseases and other communicable diseases like whooping cough, influenza, pneumonia and malnutrition are the frequent causes. The less frequent causes are congenital anomalies and accidents.

Socioeconomic and cultural factors also contribute to infant mortality. Poverty, illiteracy, broken families, sex of the child (female infanticide), illegitimacy, unhygienic practices like application of cow dung to the cut end of umbilical cord, frequent purgation and faulty feeding practices, untrained indigenous dais practicing midwifery, lack of adequate medical care facilities and bad environment are some of the known contributing factors for high IMR.

The MCH services aim to reduce IMR through its various intervention measures.

Classification of Infant Mortality

Infant mortality can be subdivided into neonatal mortality and postneonatal mortality.

Neonatal mortality: As per SRS 2010 report of Registrar General of India, neonatal mortality rate (NMR) is 32 per 1,000 live births.

It is calculated by the formula:

$$\text{NMR} = \frac{\text{Number of deaths of newborn babies under 28 days of age in a year}}{\text{Total live births in the same year}} \times 1{,}000$$

Postneonatal mortality: The postneonatal mortality rate in India is 16 (2009) and it is calculated by the formula:

$$= \frac{\text{Number of deaths of infants aged between 28 days and 1 year in a given year}}{\text{Total number of live births in the same year}} \times 1{,}000$$

Perinatal Mortality

Perinatal mortality includes late fetal deaths (28 weeks gestation and more) and early neonatal deaths. There are 5.9 million perinatal deaths worldwide, almost all of which occur in developing countries. Perinatal mortality rate (PMR) is calculated by the formula:

$$\text{PMR} = \frac{\text{Late fetal deaths + deaths under 1 week of age in a year}}{\text{Total number of live births in the same year}} \times 1,000$$

Intrauterine and birth asphyxia, low birth weight, birth trauma and intrauterine or neonatal infections are the main causes for perinatal mortality. It is 35 (2009) in India.

Child Mortality Rate

Child mortality rate (1–4 year) is 14.1 (2009). Child mortality is considered a better indicator of the development of a country because it reflects the country's environmental, nutritional and economic levels. It is very high when compared to that in developed nations.

Under-five Mortality

The under-five mortality rate in India is 63 (UNICEF, 2010).

❑ INTEGRATED MANAGEMENT OF NEONATAL AND CHILDHOOD ILLNESS (IMNCI)

In India, there are nearly 17 lakhs child deaths each year and child mortality rates are one of the highest in the world. The Government of India constituted a core group comprising representatives from Indian Academy of Pediatrics (IAP), National Neonatology Forum of India (NNF), National Anti-malaria Program (NAMP), Department of Women and Child Development (DWCD), Child in Need Institute (CINI), WHO, UNICEF, eminent pediatricians and neonatologists and the representatives from the Ministry of Health and Family Welfare (MOHFW) and the Government of India.

Major Adaptations of IMNCI

The Integrated Management of Childhood Illness (IMCI) guidelines by WHO and UNICEF were adapted and the Integrated Management of Neonatal and Childhood Illness (IMNCI) was established. The major adaptations were as follows:

1. The entire age group of 0–59 months (as against 2 week to 59 month) in IMCI was included to address the neonatal mortality challenge.
2. The order of training was reversed, starting from the young infant (0–2 month) to the older child (2 month to 5 year).
3. The total duration of training was reduced from 11 to 8 days out of which, half of the training time was earmarked for the management of the young infants, 0–2 months, which contributes to a lot to the mortality rate.
4. Home-based care of newborns and young infants was included.

Components of IMNCI Strategy

The IMNCI strategy provides for home-based care for newborns and young infants. The home care component for newborns aims to promote exclusive breastfeeding, prevent hypothermia, improve recognition of illnesses by parents and reduce delays in seeking care. As per the IMNCI protocol, a health worker has to make at least three home visits for all newborns, the first visit should be within 24 hours of birth, second on day 3–4 and third at day 7–10. Three additional visits are scheduled for newborns with low birth weight at day 14, 21 and 28.

The strategy has the following three components:

1. Health worker component: Improvements in the case management skills of health staff through the provision of locally adapted guidelines.
2. Health service component: Improvements in the overall health system required for effective management of neonatal and childhood illness.
3. Community component: Improvements in family and community healthcare practices.

The IMNCI strategy promotes the accurate identification of childhood illnesses in outpatient setting and ensures appropriate combined treatment of all major illnesses, strengthens counseling of caretakers and speed up the referral of severely ill children. At a referral facility, the strategy aims to improve the quality of care provided to sick children. In the home setting, it promotes appropriate care seeking behaviors, improved nutrition and preventive care and the correct implementation of recommended care.

The IMNCI, a component of the World Bank-supported RCH II program, is being implemented through a joint effort of UNICEF, National Rural Health Mission (NRHM), Government and other child survival partners. The IMNCI was first piloted in six districts from end of 2002–2004.The program aims to reach out to 1 million people and provide a comprehensive newborn and child care package at all levels of care in 250 of the country's 602 districts by 2010. At the subcenter level, it shall be implemented through ANMs; at PHCs, through medical doctors, nurses and lady health visitors; at first referral units, through medical officers and nurses and at the village/household level through the AWWs. This approach could help the country in achieving the MDG of reducing the under-five mortality.

❑ FAMILY AND COMMUNITY HEALTH

The Family and Community Health (FCH) is a core program under WHO-India collaboration. It focuses on the health, development and well-being of individuals and their families and through them the community at large. The program has been envisaged to address key issues affecting life at various stages.

The FCH addresses the following:

1. Making pregnancy safe (MPS).
2. Child health and development (CHD).
3. Adolescent health and development (AHD).
4. Nutrition for health and development (NHD).
5. Reproductive health and research (RHR).
6. Nursing and midwifery.
7. Gender and women's health.

8. AYUSH.
9. Strengthening public health.
10. News and workshop.

Making Pregnancy Safer

The maternal health situation in India—each year in India, roughly 30 million women experience pregnancy and 27 million have a live birth (MOHFW, 2006). Maternal mortality ratio, an important indicator of maternal health in India, is estimated to be 212/100,000 live births.

Delay in accessing specialized maternal care happens at all levels leading to maternal mortality and severe morbidity. However, institutional deliveries have risen to 78.5% during 2010–2011.

The WHO defines a skilled birth attendant as "an accredited health professional—such as a midwife, doctor or nurse, who has been educated and trained to proficiency in the skills needed to manage normal (uncomplicated) pregnancies, childbirth and the immediate postnatal period and in the identification, management and referral of complications in women and newborns."

It is essential to build a continuum of care that increases access to and use of skilled care during pregnancy, birth and the postpartum period. The continuum of care need to extend from care in the household to the care provided by a skilled health professional at the primary care level to that provided at the referral facility for those women and newborns with complications.

Child Health and Development

Picture in India

Perinatal mortality in 2009 was 35. The IMR has declined from 114 in 1980 to 47 in 2009 (SRS Bulletin, Dec 2011).There are however, wide variations amongst and within the states in infant and child mortality. Kerala has recorded an IMR of 13; Madhya Pradesh 62. The other states with an IMR significantly above the national average are Orissa (61), UP (61), Rajasthan (55) and Assam (58) (SRS, 2011). Child mortality recorded in India in 2009 was 14.1.

Adolescent Health and Development

Situation in India

Adolescents (10–19 year) form a large section of population—about 22.5%, that is, about 225 million. They are living in diverse circumstances and have diverse health needs. The total population of young people (10–24 year) is approximately 331 million comprising nearly 30% of the total population of India (Census 2001).

The adolescents have a range of health problems that cause a lot of morbidity as well as definite mortality.

In spite of definite health problems they may have, it is a common observation that adolescents do not access the existing services. In India there have not been any designated services for this age group, so far leading to substantial unmet service needs. Absence of friendly staff, working hours that are inconvenient to adolescents and lack of privacy and confidentiality have been identified as important barriers in accessing health services by adolescents and young people. The health sector needs to respond by offering services to adolescents in a friendly manner and in a non-threatening environment.

WHO-India Collaboration

The WHO-India collaboration has worked closely with the Ministry of Health and Family Welfare for developing program for adolescent health and development. Technical assistance is provided for piloting adolescent friendly health services and adolescent reproductive and sexual health strategy under RCH-II.

SECTION 5

Nutrition

CHAPTER

18

Nutrients

Nutrition deals with the science of food and its role in body growth and development and in maintenance of normal health. The term 'nutrient' is applied to specific dietary constituents like protein, fats, carbohydrates, vitamins and minerals. Dietetics is the science, which deals with the practical application of the principles of nutrition.

❑ CLASSIFICATION OF FOODS

1. By chemical composition:
   a. Proteins.
   b. Fats.
   c. Carbohydrates.
   d. Vitamins.
   e. Minerals.
2. By predominant function:
   a. Body-building foods, e.g. milk, meat, poultry, fish, eggs, pulses, groundnuts, etc.
   b. Energy-giving foods, e.g. cereals, sugars, roots and tubers, fats and oils.
   c. Protective foods, e.g. vegetables, fruits, milk.
3. By nutritive value:
   a. Cereals and millets.
   b. Pulses (legumes).
   c. Vegetables.
   d. Nuts and oilseeds.
   e. Fruits.
   f. Animal foods.

g. Fats and oils.
h. Sugar and jaggery.
i. Condiments and spices.
j. Miscellaneous foods.

NUTRIENTS

Nutrients present in different foods are either organic or inorganic complexes. They are broadly divided into macro and micronutrients. Proteins, fats and carbohydrates are the macronutrients (also described as proximate principles) that are required by the body in larger amounts. Vitamins and minerals are the micronutrients needed in very small quantities.

❑ MACRONUTRIENTS

Proteins

Proteins are complex organic nitrogenous compounds composed of carbon, hydrogen, oxygen, nitrogen and sulfur. Phosphorous, iron and occasionally, other elements may also be present in some proteins. Element nitrogen is present only in proteins, while fats and carbohydrates do not contain nitrogen.

The basic units, which form larger protein molecules are called amino acids. Out of 22 amino acids only nine amino acids are needed by man, namely leucine, isoleucine, lysine, methionine, phenylalanine, threonine, valine, tryptophan and histidine. These are called essential amino acids (EAAs) because man cannot synthesize these amino acids. Man depends on dietary sources for these essential amino acids.

Animal proteins are said to be biologically complete because they contain all the EAAs needed for the human body. Egg proteins have amino acids most suitable for humans and therefore considered as reference proteins.

Sources

The sources of proteins are:

1. Animal sources, e.g. milk, meat, eggs, fish and fowl.

2. Vegetable sources, e.g. pulses, cereals, beans, nuts and oil seed cakes.

While animal proteins contain all the EAAs, vegetable proteins are deficient in one or the other EAA. The EAA, which is deficient in a vegetable food is called a 'limiting amino acid'. Cereal proteins are deficient in lysine and threonine, while pulse proteins are deficient in sulfur-containing amino acid, methionine. Consuming cereals and pulses as usual practice, in a cereal/pulse ratio of 5:1, can make good the deficiency of the limiting amino acids. This is what is called the supplementary action of proteins.

Digestibility of vegetable proteins is low due to the presence of trypsin inhibitors, but these antinutrient substances can be destroyed by adequate cooking.

Protein Nutritional Quality

The nutritional quality of dietary proteins is determined based on:

1. The content of essential amino acids.
2. The extent to which these amino acids are available for metabolism.

Functions

Proteins are vital to life processes. They are needed for the synthesis of plasma proteins, formation of muscle and other tissues, antibodies, enzymes and hormones, and for repair and maintenance of body tissues. Proteins yield 4 kcal, but they are not consumed for deriving energy.

Protein Digestibility

Protein digestibility, i.e. the proportion of food protein, which is absorbed is defined from measurements of the nitrogen content of foods and feces. True digestibility takes into account the extent to which fecal nitrogen is 'endogenous', which in turn is measured as fecal nitrogen loss on a protein-free diet.

$$\text{Apparent protein (N) digestibility (\%)} = \frac{I - F \times 100}{I}$$

$$\text{True protein (N) digestibility (\%)} = \frac{I - (F - Fk) \times 100}{I}$$

(I, nitrogen intake; F, fecal nitrogen loss on the test diet; Fk, fecal nitrogen loss on a protein-free diet).

Biological Value

The amino acid profile is assumed to determine the effectiveness with which absorbed dietary nitrogen can be utilized, which is usually defined in terms of biological value.

$$\text{Apparent protein (N) biological value (\%)} = \frac{(I - F - U) \times 100}{I - F}$$

True protein (N) biological value (%)

$$= \frac{I\,(F - Fk) - (U - Uk) \times 100}{I - (F - Fk)}$$

(U, urinary nitrogen loss on the test diet and Uk, urinary nitrogen loss on a protein-free diet).

Amino Acid Score

The amino acid score determines the effectiveness with which absorbed dietary nitrogen can meet the essential amino acid requirement at the safe level of protein intake. This is found out by comparing the content of the limiting amino acid in the protein or diet with the requirement pattern.

Factors Other than Diet Affecting Protein Requirements

The daily requirement of protein varies with age and physiological conditions like pregnancy. Infants and children require more protein than adults. The requirement during pregnancy and lactation is also more (Table 18.1). Intracellular infection leads to increased loss of N_2, K, Mg, P and vitamin C and therefore increases the need of these nutrients.

Fats

Fats (lipids) are concentrated sources of energy yielding per unit weight twice the energy furnished by either proteins or carbohydrates. Fats yield 9 kcal/g.

Fats are made up of smaller units called fatty acids. Most of the body fat (99%) is stored in the form of triglycerides in the adipose tissue. Fatty acids and glycerol combine to form triglycerides. Fatty acids are of two kinds, saturated (e.g. lauric, stearic and palmitic acids) and unsaturated with double bonds (e.g. linoleic and linolenic acids). Among the unsaturated fatty acids, monounsaturated fatty acids (e.g. oleic acid) and polyunsaturated fatty acids (PUFAs) (e.g. linoleic acid) are found to be important in human nutrition.

Sources

Vegetable oils, butter and ghee are called visible fats. Cereals, pulses, oilseeds, milk, egg, meat, etc. also contain fats, which are invisible. Most people derive their fat requirements mainly from invisible fat sources. Monounsaturated fats are found in nuts and avocados. Animal fats except fish oils (e.g. ghee, butter, milk, cheese, eggs) are mostly saturated fats and so deficient in essential fatty acids (EFAs), while vegetable fats except coconut oil (e.g. groundnut, sesame, mustard, safflower and sunflower oils) are rich sources of EFAs.

Functions

Monounsaturated fats lower low-density lipoprotein (LDL)

TABLE 18.1: The requirement of protein for different categories

Category	Requirement
Infants	
Age	**Daily requirement (g/kg)**
0–3 month	2.3
3–6 month	1.85
6–9 month	1.65
9–12 month	1.50
Adults	
Pregnant woman	**Additional requirement (g/day) WHO**
I trimester	0.5
II trimester	9.6
III trimester	24.9
Lactating women	**Additional requirement (g/day) WHO**
0–6 month	25
6–12 month	18

cholesterol, while possibly raising high-density lipoprotein (HDL) cholesterol. PUFA cannot be synthesized by body and therefore, are to be supplied through diets. Because of this fact, these fatty acids are called EFAs. They are essential for physical as well as mental growth of infants and children and for the integrity of epithelial tissues in all. EFAs are also known to reduce low-density lipoproteins like LDL cholesterol in blood thereby reducing the incidence of atherosclerosis, hypertension and heart attacks. PUFAs are the precursors of prostaglandins, which are known to play an important role in many physiological functions. Cholesterol is the precursor for the synthesis of steroid hormones and bile acids and is an essential part of membranes and nervous tissue. Fats are needed for the absorption of fat-soluble vitamins. They also improve the palatability of foods in cooking.

Deficiency Feature

Deficient intake of EFA causes the disease phrynoderma, which is characterized by thorny projections in the skin over the elbow, knee and buttock.

Requirement

The intake of fat is based on the EFA requirement (Table 18.2). Invisible fats supply 50% of the EFA needs. To meet the balance, visible fat has to be consumed preferably in the form of vegetable oils.

However, intake of visible fats should be kept below 50 g per day to prevent complications like atherosclerosis and heart attack associated with high fat intake.

TABLE 18.2: Recommended intake fats for different categories

Categories	g/day
Adults	
Sedentary	25
Heavy work	30–40
Young children and adolescents	30–50
Pregnant women and lactating women	30

Adapted from NIN Dietary guidelines for Indians, 2nd edition; 2011

Carbohydrates

Carbohydrates form the bulk of food in India and therefore

the main source of energy; contributing 60%–80% of the total energy consumed. They are classified as monosaccharides (e.g. glucose), disaccharides (e.g. sucrose) and polysaccharides (e.g. starch, cellulose).

Many molecules of monosaccharides join to form bigger carbohydrate molecules. Starch is the polysaccharide present in rice, potato, etc. Glucose is stored in the liver and muscles as glycogen. Some carbohydrates (e.g. cellulose) cannot be digested by man's digestive system due to lack of the enzyme necessary for their digestion. But, such non-digestible carbohydrates form what is called the fiber content of the diets. These fiber compounds prevent constipation as they increase the bulk of feces. They are also known to reduce cholesterol in blood by interfering with its absorption from the gut. However, excessive intake of fiber (more than 40 g/day) may interfere with the absorption of important minerals like calcium, iron and zinc.

❑ MICRONUTRIENTS

Vitamins

Vitamins are micronutrients required by the body in very small amounts. Since the body cannot synthesize most of the vitamins, they have to be supplied through diet. Vitamins do not yield any energy, but are essential for the body for utilizing other nutrients like carbohydrates, fats and proteins. They are classified into water-soluble (e.g. B-group vitamins and vitamin C) and fat-soluble (e.g. A, D, E and K) vitamins.

Fat-soluble Vitamins

Vitamin A

Retinol and β-carotene have vitamin A activity. β-carotene is converted to retinol in the intestine and absorbed. In some individuals, β-carotene conversion to retinol may not be efficient.

Sources: Retinol is present only in animal foods. Liver, eggs, butter, cheese, whole milk and fish are rich in retinol. β-carotene, which is provitamin A, is present in plant foods. Green leafy vegetables like amaranth and spinach, yellow fruits and vegetables like papaya, mango, pumpkin and carrot are rich in β-carotene. Some foods are also fortified with vitamin A (e.g. vanaspathi, margarine).

Functions: Vitamin A is essential for normal as well as dim-light vision. It is also necessary for the integrity of epithelial tissues and growth of children. As an antioxidant it is considered cancer preventive.

Deficiency features: Deficiency of vitamin A is common in preschool children. Night blindness (nyctalopia) is the earliest symptom. The affected child is unable to see objects clearly in dim light. Conjunctival xerosis is the earliest sign, which can be detected by trained doctors and paramedical workers. Bitot's spots are pearly white or yellowish raised spots over the bulbar conjunctiva on either side of cornea and they indicate current vitamin A deficiency only in small children. But, in older children and adults, it may be just a remnant of past deficiency. Corneal xerosis is fairly a serious condition. The cornea appears dull and does not have the moist appearance. In severe deficiency cornea may ulcerate, which on healing may leave a white scar (leukoma). Keratomalacia, a serious emergency condition, is an important cause for blindness in India. In this condition, cornea becomes soft and may burst open. If the eye collapses, vision is lost.

Dry skin, follicular hyperkeratosis and growth retardation are the non-ocular deficiency features.

Subclinical deficiency: Serum retinol values below 0.70 mmol/L is a generally accepted population cut-off for preschool children to indicate risk of inadequate vitamin A status. Above 1.05 mmol/L indicates an adequate status.

Requirement: The recommended dietary allowance (RDA) of vitamin A for different categories is enlisted in Table 18.3.

Excessive intake of vitamin A (without medical advice) can cause toxic symptoms. High intake during pregnancy is suspected to cause teratogenicity in the newborn.

Vitamin D

Cholecalciferol is the naturally occurring vitamin D. It is first converted into 25-hydroxycholecalciferol in the liver and then into 1,25-dihydroxycholecalciferol in the kidney, which is the active form of vitamin D. Vitamin D is now considered as a hormone.

TABLE 18.3: Recommended dietary (daily) allowance (RDA) of Vitamin A for different categories

Category	Retinol (μg/day)	β-carotene (μg/day)
Adults (both sexes)	600	4,800
Pregnancy	800	6,400
Lactating women (0–12 month)	950	7,600
Infants		
0–6 month	350	350
6–12 month	350	2,800
Children		
1–6 year	400	3,200
7–9 year	600	4,800
Boys and girls 10–17 year	600	4,800

Sources: Dehydrocholesterol in the skin is converted into vitamin D by the action of UV rays of the sunlight. This is the way the vitamin D requirement of Indians is met. Our diets do not supply even 1/10th of the recommended vitamin D allowance. Only foods of animal origin contain vitamin D. Liver, egg yolk, butter, cheese and some fish are good sources of vitamin D. Fish liver oils are the richest source of vitamin D.

Functions: Vitamin D is essential for the absorption of dietary calcium in the intestine and for the deposition of the same in bone and teeth.

Deficiency features: Vitamin D deficiency is rare in India. Deficiency in growing children results in rickets. Gross deformities of bone such as pigeon chest, bowlegs, rickety rosary, enlarged lower end of radius and ulna and frontal bossing are the skeletal deformities characteristic of rickets. In girls, deformities of pelvic bone may become apparent at the time of childbirth later in their lives.

In adults, deficiency causes osteomalacia, which manifests as pain in bones. This usually starts during pregnancy and may become severe during subsequent pregnancies.

Requirement: Indian Council of Medical Research (ICMR) has not recommended any dietary intake of vitamin D because of the availability of abundant sunlight in India. Vitamin D requirement is usually met from the synthesis by the skin. However, 400 IU (10.0 mg) may be recommended during pregnancy and lactation. Excessive intake of vitamin D will cause toxic manifestations.

Vitamin E

Tocopherols and tocotrienols are found to have vitamin E activity. Tocopherols are widely distributed in foods. Alpha-tocopherol is the form that is preferentially absorbed and accumulated in humans.

Sources: Richest sources are the vegetable oils, egg yolk and butter. Palm oil is a rich source of tocotrienols, etc.

Function: Vitamin E is an antioxidant and so cancer preventive.

Deficiency feature: There is no clear indication of dietary deficiency.

Requirement: The suggested intake of vitamin E is 0.8 mg/g of essential fatty acids.

Vitamin K

It is found in two forms, namely vitamin K_1 and vitamin K_2.

Sources: Vitamin K_1 (phylloquinone) is present in green leafy vegetables and some fruits. Vitamin K_2 (menaquinone) is normally produced by bacteria in the intestines. Cow's milk is a better source than breast milk.

Function: Vitamin K is essential for the formation of prothrombin needed for blood clotting.

Deficiency feature: Deficiency of vitamin K is not seen except sometimes in newborn babies, manifested as bleeding tendency. Such cases may need 0.5–1.0 mg of vitamin K intramuscularly once.

RDA: 55 microgram per day is needed in adults including pregnancy and lactation, 1 mg/kg is considered adequate.

Water-soluble Vitamins

Thiamine (B_1)

This vitamin as coenzyme, is essential for the metabolism of carbohydrates.

Sources: Whole grain cereals, wheat germ, yeast, pulses, oil seeds and nuts (particularly groundnuts) are the important sources of thiamine. Vegetables, fruits, meat, fish and eggs contain small amounts.

Processing: During milling and washing before cooking, significant amount of vitamin B_1 is lost from rice. Excessive cooking and storage of foods also are deleterious to this vitamin. But, par-boiling helps to retain the vitamin.

Deficiency features: Deficiency of this vitamin causes beriberi, which may be wet, dry or infantile type. Wet beriberi is characterized by edema and cardiac failure and the dry beriberi is manifested as peripheral neuritis. 2–4 months old infants develop infantile beriberi when the mothers have B_1 deficiency. Wernicke's encephalopathy and Korsakoff's syndrome are seen in alcoholics, which respond to large doses of thiamine.

Requirement: The requirement of thiamine is based on calorie intake. The RDA is 0.5 mg/1,000 kcal.

Riboflavin (B_2)

This, as part of a coenzyme, is essential for several oxidative processes and is concerned with energy and protein metabolism.

Sources: Milk, eggs, liver, kidney and green leafy vegetables are rich sources of vitamin B_2. Cereals and pulses are poor sources, but on germination riboflavin content increases. Colonic bacteria also synthesize this vitamin.

Deficiency features: Deficiency of vitamin B_2 is quite common in India. Angular stomatitis is the commonest manifestation. Cheilosis, glossitis, nasolabial dyssebacia, scrotal dermatitis, vascularization of cornea are the other manifestations.

Requirement: The requirement of riboflavin is also based on calorie intake. The RDA is 0.6 mg/1,000 kcal.

Nicotinic Acid (Niacin)

This, as a coenzyme, is necessary for the metabolism of carbohydrate, fats and proteins. Body can synthesize this vitamin from the essential amino acid tryptophan.

Sources: Whole cereals, pulses, nuts, particularly groundnuts and meat are good sources. Milk is pellagra preventive because of its high tryptophan content.

Deficiency features: Deficiency of niacin causes pellagra, which is characterized by diarrhea (involvement of alimentary canal), dermatitis (affection of the skin) and dementia (involvement of the nervous system). These are the three Ds. Deficiency features are seen in people whose staple diet is maize because niacin in maize is in bound form and therefore not absorbed. Jowar (*Sorghum vulgare*) eaters in India also manifest pellagra. The protein of jowar contains excess of leucine, which causes an imbalance between leucine and isoleucine. Such imbalance interferes with the conversion of tryptophan into nicotinic acid.

Requirement: RDA is 6.6 mg/1,000 kcal.

Vitamin B_6 (Pyridoxine)

As a coenzyme, it is essential for the metabolism of proteins and fats.

Sources: Meat, pulses and wheat are rich sources. Liver, vegetables and other whole grains are good sources of B_6.

Deficiency features: Deficiency disorders of vitamin B_6 are not been clearly established. Certain type of anemia, peripheral neuritis and some types of angular stomatitis are been cured by the administration of B_6. The drug isonicotinylhydrazine (INH) can induce B_6 deficiency in TB patients.

Requirement: RDA is between 0.6 mg and 2 mg/day. Pregnant women require 2.5 mg/day.

Folic acid

This vitamin is required for the maturation of RBCs and for the synthesis of nucleic acids (DNA). This is a heat-sensitive vitamin, easily destroyed by heating.

Sources: Fresh green vegetables, liver and pulses are good sources of folic acid. Excessive heating during cooking destroys this vitamin and it is considered an important cause for the deficiency of this vitamin in India.

Deficiency features: Deficiency is common in pregnant and lactating women and children. Deficiency causes megaloblastic anemia. Deficiency during pregnancy is associated with neural tube defects such as spina bifida.

Requirement: The Table 18.4 illustrates the daily requirement of folic acid.

TABLE 18.4: Requirement (RDA) of folic acid

Category	μg/day
Adults and adolescents	100
Pregnant women	400
Lactating women	150
Infants	25
Preschool children	50
School children	70

Cyanocobalamin (B_{12})

This vitamin, like folic acid, is required for the synthesis of DNA. It is also required for the metabolism of folic acid and the synthesis of fatty acids in myelin in the nervous system. Unlike folic acid, this vitamin is heat stable.

Sources: The sources of vitamin B_{12} are only non-vegetarian foods such as liver, kidney, meat, fish, eggs and milk. However, it is presumed that vegetarians get their B_{12} from contaminated foods. Bacteria in human colon also can synthesize this vitamin.

Deficiency features: Deficiency of B_{12} causes megaloblastic anemia in which the RBCs are oversized (macrocytic). B_{12} forms a complex with intrinsic factor secreted in the stomach and this union is needed for its absorption in the ileum. When absorption of B_{12} is affected due to deficiency of intrinsic factor in the stomach, the resultant anemia is called pernicious anemia. B_{12} deficiency causes demyelination of peripheral nerves and spinal cord giving rise to the clinical condition called subacute combined degeneration.

Requirement: RDA for adults and children is 1 μg/day. Lactating women need 1.5 μg/day.

Vitamin C (Ascorbic acid)

Vitamin C is needed for the formation of collagen and calcification of bone and teeth. It also facilitates the absorption of iron from plant foods. Heating and exposure to air can easily destroy this vitamin.

Sources: Fresh fruits, especially citrus fruits and green leafy vegetables are the good sources. Gooseberry is a cheap and rich source of this vitamin. Germination of pulses increases the vitamin C content in them.

Deficiency features: Deficiency of vitamin C causes scurvy. It is characterized by bleeding tendency, which is due to defective collagen present in the capillary walls. Bleeding gums, bleeding into the skin and other parts like muscles and brain may be seen. Healing of wounds is also delayed in deficiency.

Requirement: RDA for adults, children and pregnant women is 40 mg/day. Infants require 25 mg/day. Lactating women need 80 mg/day.

Minerals

Physiological functions are carried out by means of exchange of ions. The proximate principles supply energy to carry out these ionic exchanges. Therefore, minerals play a very vital role in the physiological processes of the body.

Some minerals are required in large quantity—major minerals, while some others are needed in only very small amounts—trace elements. Some minerals may also find their way into the physiological systems as contaminants.

Major minerals needed by the body are calcium, phosphorus, sodium, potassium and magnesium and the trace elements required are iron, iodine, flourine, zinc, copper, cobalt, chromium, manganese, molybdenum, selenium, nickel, tin, silicon and vanadium.

Major Minerals

Calcium

It is essential for the formation of bone and teeth. 98% of body calcium is present in bones. Blood calcium (10–11mg/100 mL) is required for vital body functions like cardiac contraction, contraction of muscles, transmission of impulses to the interior of cells, blood coagulation, etc.

Sources: Milk and milk products are the best sources of calcium. Cheap source of this mineral is green leafy vegetables. While rice is deficient in calcium, millet ragi is a good source of this mineral. Drinking water may also be an important source of calcium.

Deficiency features: Deficiency of calcium is not known to cause any disorder, if vitamin D intake is adequate. Blood level of calcium is a very well-maintained parameter in all species indicating its vital role in physiological processes. Blood calcium level is maintained by mobilizing calcium from the bones, if the dietary intake is not adequate.

Requirement: The RDA of calcium for various categories is given in Table 18.5.

Phosphorus

This is another major element in the body. Calcium is deposited in bones and teeth as calcium phosphate. Phosphorus is a component of nucleic acids and plays an important role in cellular metabolism of carbohydrate, fats, etc. Cereals, pulses, nuts and oilseeds are rich sources of phosphorus. Since our habitual diets meet the physiological requirement, phosphorus deficiency is rarely seen.

RDA of phosphorus is similar to that of calcium for all except in infants in whom the requirement is slightly high.

Magnesium

This is essential for cellular metabolism. It is also found in bones along with calcium. Magnesium occurs widely in foods and plant foods are rich in it. Therefore, deficiency of magnesium is unlikely in population.

Sodium and potassium

These two are important constituents of cellular and tissue fluids, and blood. Compounds of these elements dissociate in the plasma to form electrolytes, which are essential for the maintenance of osmotic pressure.

Sodium and potassium are present in all foods particularly in fruits and vegetables. Plants contain high level of potassium.

Deficiency of these electrolytes does not occur except in disease conditions like vomiting and diarrhea. Sodium depletion can occur in manual laborers working in hot sun in summer months.

TABLE 18.5: Requirement (RDA) of calcium

Category	g/day
Adults	0.4
Pregnancy and lactation	1
Infants	0.5
Children	
1–9 year	0.4
10–15 year	0.6
16–18 year	0.5

Trace elements

These elements are required for body in minute quantities for important functions. Trace elements known to be required by man are iron, zinc, copper, chromium, cobalt, iodine, manganese, molybdenum, fluorine and selenium. Iron and iodine deficiency are widespread. Deficiency of other elements may be encountered rarely.

Iron

This element is essential for the formation of hemoglobin, which transports oxygen to all cells. Cells require iron for various oxidation-reduction reactions.

Sources: Non-vegetarian foods like liver, meat, poultry and vegetables, especially green leafy vegetables, are rich sources of iron. Milk is a poor source. Millets like bajra and ragi, cereals and pulses, dates and dried fruits are the other iron sources. Iron vessels used for cooking also contribute iron significantly.

Absorption of iron (only 2%–5%) is an important constraint in habitual mixed vegetarian diets. Therefore, diets should supply 10–25 fold of required iron daily. Absorption from non-vegetarian diets is better (10%–20%).

Deficiency features: Deficiency of iron causes iron-deficiency anemia (IDA) in which the RBCs are small in size (microcytic hypochromic anemia). It is quite common in India; two thirds of pregnant and half of non-pregnant women suffer from anemia. Anemia is common in preschool children also. Iron deficiency has an adverse effect on psychomotor and mental development in children. Mortality and morbidity of mother and infant during pregnancy is increased.

Cut-off levels (WHO) for the diagnosis of anemia in different groups is given in Table 18.6.

Requirement: RDA of iron for various categories are enlisted in Table 18.7.

TABLE 18.6: Cut-off levels for the diagnosis of anemia

Category	g/100 mL
Adult males	13
Non-pregnant females	12
Pregnant females	11
Children 6 month to 6 year	11
6–14 year	12

Iodine

This element is essential for the synthesis of thyroid hormones—thyroxine and triiodothyronine.

Sources: Seafoods like sea fish, sea salt and cod liver oil are good sources of iodine. Other food articles also contain smaller amounts. The human requirement is met mainly from food articles (90%) and to some extent from water.

Deficiency features: Iodine deficiency has been identified all over the world. It is a significant health problem in 130 countries and affects 740 million people. One third of the world population is exposed to the risk of iodine deficiency disorders (IDDs).

Iodine deficiency disorders are seen in vast areas of and is not restricted to only sub-Himalayan areas as was thought earlier. Deficiency of iodine in the soil in hills is responsible for the high prevalence of goiter in sub-Himalayan areas.

Deficiency of iodine may cause:

1. Goiter.
2. Subnormal intelligence.
3. Neuromuscular weakness.
4. Endemic cretinism.
5. Stillbirth.
6. Hypothyroidism.
7. Defect in vision, hearing and speech.
8. Spasticity.
9. Intrauterine death.
10. Mental retardation.

Requirement: RDA is 150 μg/day for adults.

TABLE 18.7: Requirement (RDA) in different categories

Category	mg/day
Adults	
Male	17
Female	21
Pregnancy	35
Lactation	25
Infants 6–12 month	46 μg/kg/day
Children	
1–3 year	9
4–6 year	13
7–9 year	16
Boys	
10–12 year	21
13–15 year	32
16–17 year	28
Girls	
10–12 year	27
13–15 year	27
16–17 year	26

Adapted from ICMR guidelines 2010

Fluorine

It is essential for normal mineralization of bones and teeth enamel. 96% of body fluorine is present in bones and teeth. *Sources:* Drinking water is the main source of fluorine and other food articles also may contain traces of it. Excess fluorides in water, causing dental and skeletal fluorosis, is the problem in India and not lack of it.

Deficiency feature: Lack of fluorides is associated with dental caries.

Requirements: The recommended level in drinking water in India is 0.5–0.8 mg/L. In temperate countries, it is 1–2 mg/L.

Zinc

This element is a cofactor for a number of enzymes and it is a constituent of insulin molecule.

Sources: Non-vegetarian foods are rich in zinc. Liver is the richest source. Pulses are good sources. Leafy and other vegetables contain less.

Deficiency features: Deficiency results in dwarfism and hypogonadism. Zinc deficiency is not reported in India even in poor income groups.

Requirement: The daily requirement is in the range of 4–7 mg. In pregnancy and lactation, the requirement is slightly more.

Copper

This is an essential constituent of oxidative enzymes like cytochrome oxidase. It plays an important role in iron absorption. It is also involved in cross-linking of connective tissues, neurotransmission and lipid metabolism.

Sources: Sea food (shell fish), liver, whole grains and legumes, nuts including peanuts, dart green leafy vegetables, apples and papaya are reasonable source. Rice is a poor source, human milk has the highest concentration.

Deficiency features: Copper deficiency causes poor iron absorption, normocytic hypochromic anemia, abnormal GTT, hypercholesterolemia, etc. Copper deficiency is not seen in India.

Requirement: RDA is 2–3 mg/day, which is usually met by well-balanced diets.

Selenium

Selenocysteine functions as a redox center for the selenium-dependent glutathione peroxidases, iodothyronine deiodinases type I, II and III and thioredoxin reductases.

Sources: Fish, shellfish and offal (liver, kidney) are rich sources of selenium. Meat and egg are good sources, while cereals are poor sources. Wheat may be a major contributor because many consume it as staple food.

Table 18.8: Requirement (RDA) of selenium for various categories

Category	µg /day
Infants and children	6–21
Adolescents	26–32
Pregnancy	28–30
Lactation	35–42
Children (6–14 year)	12

Deficiency: Suboptimal selenium states may be widespread in human populations. Keshan disease, manifested as cardiomyopathy in children and women of child-bearing age is seen in the selenium-deficient regions of China. Harmless viruses become virulent in selenium-deficient status.

Requirement: The RDA of selenium for various categories are given in Table 18.8.

Molybdenum

Molybdenum acts as a cofactor for the iron-and flavin-containing enzymes that catalyze hydroxylation of various substrates.

Sources: Milk, beans, bread and cereals are good dietary sources.

Deficiency features: Deficiency symptoms cannot be induced in humans.

Requirement: Requirement is in microgram quantities.

Chromium

Trivalent form (chromium III), the most stable one in biological systems is essential for both humans and animals. It is essential for carbohydrate, lipid and nucleic acid metabolism.

Sources: Whole grains, black pepper, brewer's yeast, mushrooms, prunes, raisins, nuts, asparagus, beer, wine, meat and liver are the good dietary sources. Refining cereals and sugar removes chromium. Stainless steel vessels in contact with acidic foods can contribute to the intake.

Deficiency features: Marginal deficiency causes impaired glucose tolerance.

Requirement: Requirement is in microgram quantities.

Manganese

Bivalent (+2) form is predominant in biological systems. Manganese is a catalytic cofactor for mitochondrial superoxide dismutase, arginase and pyruvic carboxylase.

Sources: Cereals contain high concentration of manganese. Non-vegetarian foods (egg, milk, fish, poultry and red meat) contain low amounts.

Deficiency has never been observed in people on usual diets.

Requirements: 2–5.5 mg/day.

❑ ENERGY

Energy is needed by the body for all the metabolic functions and growth. Inadequate supply of energy results in growth failure in children and weight loss in adults.

Energy is measured as kilocalories or kilojoules. Energy needs are driven from the three proximate principles namely carbohydrates, fats and proteins. Carbohydrates and proteins yield 4 kcal/g, while fats yield 9 kcal/g. Proteins are not utilized by the body for yielding energy when fat and carbohydrate are consumed in adequate amounts (Table 18.9).

For calculation of energy requirements, concepts like Indian reference man and Indian reference woman are being used. Indian reference man is 18–29 years of age, free from disease and physically fit, weighing 60 kg. Indian reference woman is 18–29 years of age, free from disease and physically fit, weighing 55 kg (Table 18.10).

TABLE 18.9: Energy requirements of infants, children and adolescents (computed for reference children)

Category	kcal/day	kcal/kg/day
Infants		
0–6 month	500	92
6–12 month	670	80
Children		
1–3 year	1,060	82

Contd...

Contd...

Category	kcal/day	kcal/kg/day
4–6 year	1,350	75
7–9 year	1,690	67
Boys		
10–12 year	2,190	64
13–15 year	2,750	58
16–15 year	3,020	55
Girls		
10–12 year	2,010	57
13–15 year	2,330	50
16–15 year	2,440	47

Adapted from Nutrient requirement and recommended dietary allowances for Indians-A report of the expert croup of ICMR-2009

TABLE 18.10: Energy requirement of adults

Adults	Body weight	Activity		
		Sedentary (kcal/day)	Moderate (kcal/day)	Heavy (kcal/day)
Reference man (18–29 year)	60 kg	2,320	2,730	3,490
Reference woman (18–29 year)	55 kg	1,900	2,230	2,850

The cut-off point for determining the extent of poverty and energy inadequacy in India is fixed at 2,200 kcal per caput per day and the survival ration during famines is placed at 1,800 kcal per caput. The additional energy requirement during pregnancy and lactation is given in Table 18.11.

TABLE 18.11: Additional energy requirement during pregnancy and lactation additional requirement—kcals/day

Category	Additional requirement (kcal/day)
Pregnancy	350
Lactation	
1–6 month	600
7–12 month	520

Adapted from Recommended dietary allowances for Indians (macronutrients and minerals). Dietary guidelines for Indians, 2nd edition; 2011

CHAPTER

19

Balanced Diet and Nutritional Contents of Foods

❑ BALANCED DIET

A balanced diet should meet the daily body requirements in respect of energy and all the essential nutrients necessary for maintaining health, vitality and general well-being. It should also provide a small amount of extra nutrients to withstand short periods of deficient intake.

The Tables 19.1 and 19.2 gives the balanced diets for different categories of people.

The Table 19.3 illustrates additional allowances during pregnancy and lactation.

TABLE 19.1: Balanced diet for adults

Food items	g/portion	Sedentary		Moderate		Heavy	
		Man	Woman	Man	Woman	Man	Woman
		Number of portions					
Cereals and millets	30	12.5	9	15	11	20	16
Pulses	30	2.5	2	3	2.5	4	3
Milk (mL) and milk products	100 mL	3	3	3	3	3	3
Roots and tubers	100	2	2	2	2	2	2
Green leafy vegetables	100	1	1	1	1	1	1

Contd...

Contd...

Food items	g/portion	Sedentary		Moderate		Heavy	
		Man	Woman	Man	Woman	Man	Woman
		Number of portions					
Other vegetables	100	2	2	2	2	2	2
Fruits	100	1	1	1	1	1	1
Sugar	5	4	4	6	6	11	9
Fat	5	5	4	6	5	8	6

To calculate the days requirement of above mentioned food groups for an individual, multiply grams per portion with number of portions.

❑ NUTRIENT CONTENT OF COMMON FOODS

Cereals and Millets

Rice, wheat (cereals), jowar, bajra and ragi (millets) are the major grains consumed in India contributing 70%–80% of energy requirement of majority of our people. Cereals contain 6–12 g of protein per 100 g and meet more than 50% of protein requirements as they are consumed in bulk quantities. They also provide minerals like calcium, iron and vitamin B. But, most of them do not have β-carotene or vitamin C. Their fat content is low, but because they are the staple diet, their contribution of essential fatty acid (EFA) may be up to 50% of recommended dietary allowance.

Pulses

Pulses contain 17–25 g of protein per 100 g and therefore, are rich source of protein. They are also rich in B-group vitamins, but lack in vitamin A and vitamin C. Germinated pulses contain more vitamin C. Fat content of pulses also contribute fair amount of EFA.

TABLE 19.2: Balanced diet for infants, children and adolescents (number of portions)

Food items	g/ portion	Infants 6–12 month	1–3 year	4–6 year	7–9 year	10–12 year		13–15 year		16–18 year	
						Girls	Boys	Girls	Boys	Girls	Boys
Cereals and millets	30	0.5	2	4	6	8	10	11	14	11	15
Pulses	30	0.25	1	1.0	2	2	2	2	2.5	2.5	3
Milk (mL) and milk products	100	4*	5	5	5	5	5	5	5	5	5
Roots and tubers	100	0.5	0.5	1	1	1	1	1	1.5	2	2
Green leafy vegetables	100	0.25	0.5	0.5	1	1	1	1	1	1	1
Other vegetables	100	0.25	0.5	1	1	2	2	2	2	2	2
Fruits	100	1	1	1	1	1	1	1	1	1	1
Sugar	5	2	3	4	4	6	6	5	4	5	6
Fat/oil (visible)	5	4	5	5	6	7	7	8	9	7	10

*Quantity indicates top milk. For breastfeed infants, 200 mL top milk is required.
One portion of pulse may be exchanged with one portion (50 g) of egg/meat/chicken/fish.
For infants introduce egg/meat/chicken/fish around 9 month.

Nuts and Oilseeds

Oilseeds and nuts are rich in protein and fat, but they do not contain appreciable amount of carbohydrate. Nuts contain monounsaturated fatty acid; oleic acid that is known to reduce LDL cholesterol and raise HDL cholesterol. They also contain high level of B-group vitamins. Groundnuts are particularly rich in thiamine and niacin.

TABLE 19.3: Additional allowances during pregnancy and lactation

	During pregnancy		During lactation	
Food items	Quantity (g)	Calories (kcal)	Quantity (g)	Calories (kcal)
Cereals	35	118	60	203
Pulses	15	52	30	105
Milk	100	83	100	83
Fat	–	–	10	90
Sugar	10	40	10	40
Total		293		521

Fats and Oils

Fats and oils (visible fats) are the concentrated sources of energy yielding 9 kcal/g. Vegetable oils like groundnut oil, safflower oil, gingelly oil, etc. contain good amount of EFA and vitamin E. But butter and ghee are poor sources of EFA and vitamin E, while they are rich in saturated fats.

Fruits and Vegetables

Fruits are good sources of vitamin C. Yellow fruits contain β-carotene, the precursor of vitamin A. Banana is a good source of energy. Dates contain good amount of iron. Green leafy vegetables are rich sources of minerals like calcium and iron and vitamins like β-carotene, riboflavin, vitamin C and folic acid.

Roots and tubers (potato, carrots, yam, colocasia, tapioca, etc.) are rich sources of carbohydrate. Carrots are rich in β-carotene. Tapioca and yam are rich in calcium. Vegetables like brinjal, ladies finger, beans, gourds, tomatoes, etc. provide vitamins and minerals. Because they are rich in fiber, they add bulk to the diet and prevent constipation.

Milk and Milk Products

Milk is a good source of high-quality protein, riboflavin and calcium. Milk is pellagra preventive as it is rich in the essential amino acid tryptophan. However, it is deficient in iron and vitamin C. Skimmed milk powder has no fat, but its protein and carbohydrate contents are higher. Curd is rich in probiotic lactic acid. As milk is a nutritious food, it should be made available to vulnerable groups like infants, preschool children, and pregnant and lactating women.

Eggs

Eggs are good sources of high-quality proteins and fats. They also contain all the fat-soluble and water-soluble vitamins except vitamin C. Minerals like calcium, phosphorus, iron, zinc and other trace elements are also present in egg. As egg yolk contains large amount of cholesterol (one egg contains 250 mg), middle-aged and old people with history of coronary heart disease (CHD) may restrict egg consumption. Consumption of raw egg should be avoided as it contains an antinutrient compound avidin, which will interfere with the absorption of vitamin biotin.

Fish

Fish are rich in proteins (15–25 g/100 g). As fish fats are rich in EFAs (omega-3 fatty acids), their consumption is considered beneficial in preventing cardiovascular diseases. Sea fish are also sources of iodine.

Flesh Foods

Meat and poultry are rich in good-quality proteins and also provide B-group vitamins. Flesh foods contain vitamin B_{12}, which is absent in vegetarian foods. Offals like liver are rich in vitamin A,

B_{12} and iron. Iron present in non-vegetarian foods is much better absorbed than that in vegetarian foods.

Condiments and Spices

The nutritive value of spices and condiments is limited. Minerals like iron, other trace elements and potassium may be present in some spices. Chillies and coriander contain β-carotene and green chillies provide beta carotene and vitamin C. One disadvantageous aspect of spices is their high content of tannins, which interfere with the absorption of iron. Asafetida and garlic have antibacterial property and inhibit putrefying bacteria.

CHAPTER

20

Nutritional Problems in India

❑ NUTRITIONAL PROFILE OF INDIA

Malnutrition is a leading contributor to infant, child and maternal mortality. The infant mortality rate, though on the decline, is still high when compared to developed nations.

Chronic malnutrition among preschool children is reflected as stunting and wasting. Preschool children are found to be underweight. Chronic energy deficiency, as assessed by body mass index (BMI), is also prevalent among adults.

The prevalence of Bitot's spots (vitamin A deficiency) among the preschool children in rural West Bengal was 0.6% (NIN, Hyderabad), which is more than public health significance. Subclinical deficiency was seen in 61% of preschool children, especially from the low socioeconomic groups.

Studies on prevalence of nutritional anemia in India show that 65% of infant and toddlers, 60% of 1–6 years of age, 88% of adolescent girls and 85% pregnant women have anemia. The prevalence of anemia was marginally higher in lactating women as compared to pregnancy. 3.3% of adolescent girls (with hemoglobin < 7 g/dL) and 9.9% of pregnant women are found to have severe anemia.

Surveys have clearly demonstrated that not even a single state/union territory (UT) is free from the problem of iodine deficiency disorders (IDDs). Sample surveys in 28 states and 7 UTs have revealed that out of 324 districts surveyed so far, 263 districts are IDD endemic, i.e. the prevalence of IDD is above 10%.

Nearly one third of all children born have low birth weight, i.e. weight < 2.5 kg at birth.

Common Nutritional Problems

Protein energy malnutrition (PEM), vitamin A deficiency (VAD), IDA and IDDs and B complex deficiencies are the common nutritional problems in India.

Protein Energy Malnutrition

Protein energy malnutrition (PEM) is an important nutritional problem affecting infants and children. Save the children data (2012) shows that almost half of Indian children (47% – UNICEF; 2012) are underweight besides being stunted. India has the second highest percentage of underweight children below the age of 5 years. Severe PEM affects not only physical growth but also mental development.

The most important characteristic of PEM is underweight for age. In third degree PEM, the body weight is less than 60% of the expected weight. Two distinct clinical, severe forms are described namely kwashiorkor and marasmus. The primary cause of PEM is inadequate intake of food due to poverty. Infectious diseases like diarrhea, respiratory disease, measles and worm infestations often precipitate PEM. Integrated Child Development Services (ICDS) scheme of Government of India and Tamil Nadu Integrated Nutrition Project (TINP) are being implemented with the aim of controlling PEM.

Vitamin A Deficiency

Vitamin A deficiency (VAD) is one of the highest in the world especially among preschool children; 31%–57% of preschool children have subclinical deficiency and 1%–2% have clinical VAD. In pregnant women, the incidence of subclinical VAD was 5% (NPCB Newsletter April–June 2012). Out of 6 million blindness cases in India, 1% is due to VAD.

Clinically this may manifest as the earliest conjunctival xerosis to the most severe form keratomalacia.

The cause of VAD is inadequate intake of vitamin A – containing foods such as milk, eggs and vegetables containing β-carotene. Ignorance, infections (measles) and worm infestations also contribute to this problem. VAD is often seen in PEM cases. Under Vitamin A Prophylaxis Program, massive doses of vitamin A (2 lakhs IU) are administered to preschool children once in 6 months.

Nutritional Anemia

Anemia can arise due to deficiency of different kinds of nutrients. But, the commonest nutrient deficiency for anemia in India is iron deficiency. Studies on prevalence of nutritional anemia in India show that 65% of infant and toddlers, 60% of 1–6 years of age, 88% of adolescent girls and 85% of pregnant women have anemia. The prevalence of anemia was marginally higher in lactating women as compared to pregnancy. 3.3% of adolescent girls (with hemoglobin < 7 g/dL) and 9.9% of pregnant women are found to have severe anemia. Rural people are found to suffer from anemia more than the urban.

Anemia results mainly because of inadequate intake of iron containing foods in our habitual diets. Absorption (bioavailability) of iron from the mixed vegetarian diet is also poor, less than 5%. Loss of iron from monthly menstruation and repeated and close pregnancies are also responsible for anemia in women. Hookworm infestation and malaria also contribute to the problem of anemia in India.

Destruction of folic acid, a heat-sensitive vitamin commonly present in foods, by excessive heating during cooking is an important cause for folic acid deficiency among the people.

Anemia impairs cellular immunity, causes significant morbidity and mortality in pregnancy and also affects the working capacity. In children, anemia is found to affect their scholastic performance. Anemia prophylaxis program supplies iron and folic acid tablets to girls, women and children with a view to reduce anemia prevalence.

Iodine Deficiency Disorders

Surveys have found iodine deficiency disorders (IDDs) not only in the goiter belt of sub-Himalayan regions but also in other parts of India as well. Sample surveys conducted in 325 districts covering all the states/UTs have revealed that 263 districts are endemic where the prevalence of IDDs is more than 10%. It is estimated that more than 71 million persons are suffering from goiter and other IDDs.

Iodine deficiency in neonatal period seriously affects physical growth as well as mental development. IDDs control program is being implemented with the aim of supplying iodized salt throughout the country.

Deficiency of B-group Vitamins

Rice and wheat are the staples for many populations of the world. Processes such as excessive refining and polishing of cereals removes considerable proportions of B-group vitamins from these cereals. Though overt clinical manifestations of Thiamine, Niacin and riboflavin deficiency are not seen now there is evidence that subclinical deficiency of these vitamins (especially of riboflavin and pyridoxine) is widespread. These subclinical deficiencies exert deleterious metabolic effects. There are periodic reports of outbreaks of B-complex deficiencies in populations under various distress conditions (refugee and displaced population groups-20 million people by current united nations estimates). Cereal foods used under emergency situations are not fortified with micronutrients. An economic blockade in cuba resulted in the outbreak of peripheral neuropathy and visual loss in the adult population due to low B-complex content of diets. Pregnant and lactating women, infants and children are at high risk of developing deficiency.

CHAPTER

21

Community Nutrition Programs in India

❑ COMMUNITY NUTRITION PROGRAMS

Balwadi Nutrition Program

Balwadi Nutrition Program was started in 1970–71. Under this program, food supplement providing 300 kcal of energy and 10 g of protein per child is being supplied to children in the age group of 3–5 years through balwadies established in rural areas for 270 days in a year. Department of Social Welfare is responsible for the implementation of the program. Children also get preprimary education in the balwadies.

Mid-day Meal Program for School Children

National Program of Nutritional Support to Primary Education, popularly known as the Mid-Day Meal Scheme (MDM) was started in 1995 in an attempt to enhance enrolment, retention and attendance, while simultaneously improving nutritional levels among children in school. It currently covers nearly 12 crore children. The main objectives of the scheme (as per the 2006 revision) are to:

1. Improve the nutritional status of children in classes one through five in government schools and government-aided schools.
2. To encourage children from disadvantaged backgrounds to attend school regularly and help them to concentrate in school activities.

3. To provide nutritional support to students in drought-ridden areas throughout summer vacation as well.

In October 2007, the scheme was revised to cover children in the upper primary section as well, i.e. classes 6–7. The scheme provides a cooked mid-day meal with a minimum of 300 calories and 8–12 g of protein to all children studying in classes 1–5 and 700 calories and 20 g of protein to upper primary students.

Tamil Nadu Integrated Nutrition Project

The Tamil Nadu Integrated Nutrition Project was started in 1980 targeting 6–36 months old children, and pregnant and lactating women.

Objective

1. To reduce malnutrition up to 50% among children under 4 years of age.
2. To reduce infant mortality by 25%.
3. To reduce VAD in the under 5-year-old children from about 27% to 5%.
4. To reduce anemia in pregnant and nursing women from about 55% to 20%.

Components

1. Nutrition services.
2. Health services.
3. Communication.
4. Monitoring and evaluation.

Under this scheme, children are weighed periodically and the 'failing to gain weight' children are given supplementary feeding. Pregnant and nursing mothers also receive supplements. Health services are also provided to antenatal women and children in collaboration with primary health cares (PHCs) and subcenters.

This project is assisted by World Bank. With the goal of universalization of ICDS, all the TINP blocks will be converted to ICDS blocks.

Note: In courtesy of National Institute of Health and Family Welfare.

Integrated Child Development Services Scheme

Integrated Child Development Services (ICDS) Scheme was launched on 2nd October, 1975, during 5th five year plan, in pursuance of the national policy for children, in 33 experimental blocks. The program has now been made universal. As of 31-12-2010, 1,241,749 anganwadi centers are functioning under the scheme. The primary responsibility for the implementation of the program is with the Department of Women and Child Development, Ministry of Human Resources Development at the center and the nodal departments at the state, which may be Social Welfare, Rural Development, Tribal Welfare, Health and Family Welfare or Women and Child Development.

Beneficiaries

Children below 6 years, pregnant and lactating women, women in the age group of 15–44 years and adolescent girls in selected blocks are the beneficiaries.

Objectives

1. Improving the nutrition and health status of children in the age group of 0–6 years.
2. Laying the foundation for proper psychological, physical and social development of the child.
3. Effective coordination and implementation of policy among the various departments.
4. Enhancing the capability of the mother to look after the normal health and nutrition needs through proper nutrition and health education.

The package of services provided:

- Supplementary nutrition, vitamin A, iron and folic acid
- Immunization
- Health checkups
- Referral services
- Treatment of minor illnesses

- Nutrition and health education to women
- Providing non-formal preschool education to children in the age group of 3–6 years
- Convergence of other supportive services like water supply, sanitation, etc.

Anganwadi is the peripheral level unit, which implements this program. Anganwadi worker is the key person responsible for all the activities of the center. Each center caters to a population of 1,000.

Scheme for Adolescent Girls

A scheme for adolescent girls in ICDS was launched by the Department of Women and Child Development, Ministry of Human Resource Development in 1991. All adolescent girls in the age group of 11–18 years receive the following common services:

- Watch over menarche
- Immunization
- General health checkups once in 6 months
- Training for minor ailments
- Deworming
- Prophylactic measures against anemia, goiter, vitamin deficiency, etc.
- Referral to PHC, district hospital, in case of acute need.

Vitamin A Prophylaxis Program

As part of the national program for control of blindness, vitamin A prophylaxis is being given to preschool children since 1970 by the Ministry of Health and Family Welfare. Under the scheme, 2 lakhs IU (110 mg) of retinyl palmitate in oil solution is administered orally to all preschool children once in 6 months. After the introduction of this scheme, vitamin A deficiency has been reduced, it is claimed. But skepticism about this program is also being voiced in some quarters as such massive dose of vitamin A may not be physiological and may cause adverse effects.

Prophylaxis Against Nutritional Anemia

Anemia due to deficient intake of iron and folic acid is very common among women and preschool children. Government of India launched the anemia prophylaxis program during the 4th and 5th year plan to prevent nutritional anemia among the vulnerable sections of society. Under this program, iron and folic acid tablets are being supplied to women and children (1–12 years of age) through MCH centers (in urban areas), PHCs (in rural areas) and ICDS centers.

IDDs Control Program

Iodine deficiency disorders are found not only in the goiter belt of Himalayan region but also in many other parts of the country. It is estimated that nearly 145 million people are living in goiter endemic zones. In order to control this problem, Government of India launched the IDDs control program in 1986. Under this program, it is proposed to supply iodized salt to all areas of the country. Sale of uniodized salt is being banned.

Short-term programs like the ICDS scheme, Vitamin A Prophylaxis Program and anemia prophylaxis program are only palliative. Only long-term socioeconomic development can prevent the nutritional deficiency diseases permanently.

Family and Community Health

The family and community health (FCH) is a core program under WHO-India collaboration. It focuses on the health, development and well-being of individuals and their families and through them the community at large. The program has been envisaged to address key issues affecting life at various stages. FCH endeavors for the improvement of nutrition under the program nutrition for health and development.

Nutrition is an input to and foundation for health and development. Better nutrition is a prime entry point to ending poverty and a milestone to achieving better quality of life. Freedom from hunger and malnutrition is a basic human right and their alleviation is a fundamental prerequisite for human and national development.

Under the WHO-India ongoing Technical support and Collaborative programs, the focus of activities of the WHO vis-à-vis nutrition is not only limited to the vast magnitude of various forms of nutritional deficiency but also to obesity and long-term implications of unbalanced dietary and lifestyle practices that result in chronic diseases such as cardiovascular disease, cancer and diabetes.

❑ ASSESSMENT OF NUTRITIONAL STATUS

Assessment of the nutritional status of populations requires examination of different aspects pertaining to human nutrition. Nutritional status assessment comprises the following:

1. Clinical examination.
2. Anthropometric examination.
3. Study of biochemical profile.
4. Diet survey.
5. Vital and health statistics.
6. Ecological studies.

Clinical Examination

Clinical examination is a simple and practical method of assessing nutritional status of groups of individuals. Clinical signs associated with specific nutrient deficiency such as angular stomatitis in riboflavin deficiency, conjunctival xerosis in VAD, etc. are looked for and assessed. Head to foot is examined for deficiency features in clinical examination.

Anthropometry

Height, weight, skin fold thickness and midarm circumference of people in general and children in particular indicate their nutritional status. Serial measurements can indicate the pattern of growth in children.

Laboratory and Biochemical Assessment

Tests like hemoglobin estimation, serum levels of albumin and vitamins are useful to detect subclinical deficiency early, much before they become clinical. But, they are expensive and cannot be applied to a whole community.

Diet Survey

Diet surveys throw light on the actual nutritional intake of populations. There are three methods by which diet consumption pattern can be assessed:

1. Weighment of raw foods: This is the most practical method and also widely employed. The raw foods that are to be cooked in a day in the sample household is weighed and the average per capita consumption unit is calculated by dividing the total quantity of foods cooked by the total number of members in the family including the guests, if any. Ideally, the survey should be conducted for 21 days in the households, but it is usually restricted to 7 days. National Institute of Nutrition (NIN), Hyderabad conducts diet surveys for only 3 consecutive days for ordinary purposes.
2. Weighment of cooked foods: This method, though better and more accurate is not practicable as people object to the weighment of cooked foods.
3. Oral questionnaire method: This method is suitable to conduct diet survey on a large scale. People are asked to give the details of the foods consumed during the previous 24 hours. If conducted properly, this method can give reliable results.

   Diet surveys will throw light on whether people consume diets adequately or not and also on the dietary habits and deficiency diseases of populations.

Vital Statistics

Morbidity and mortality statistics may also indirectly indicate the nutritional status of populations.

Assessment of Ecological Factors

Information on food production, per capita food availability, family size, occupation, customs and cultural practices related to nutrition, healthcare services available in the area and the prevalence of infections and worm infestations among the people are all important to assess the nutritional status of populations.

CHAPTER

22

Food Adulteration

❑ FOOD TOXICANTS

Toxic substances present in some foods can cause ill health in man. They may get into foods accidentally or by deliberate adulteration. Some of them are discussed below.

Lathyrism

Lathyrus sativus (khesari dal) is a wildly growing dal having a toxin called beta-oxalyl-amino-alanine (BOAA). When consumed over a period of 2–6 months, this dal causes a spastic paralytic disease called neurolathyrism. This disease is prevalent in Madhya Pradesh, Uttar Pradesh, Bihar and Orissa where this dal is being given as wages for workers. Traders also may adulterate toor dal with khesari dal. Banning the crop or processing the dal to remove the water-soluble toxin, before consumption will help in the prevention of neurolathyrism. Traders who adulterate can be dealt with under Prevention of Food Adulteration (PFA) Act.

Aflatoxicosis

When food materials such as groundnut, maize, parboiled rice, wheat, rice, etc. are stored under moist conditions (moisture more than 16%), the storage fungi *Aspergillus flavus* and *A. parasiticus* infest them and elaborate aflatoxins (e.g. B1, G1). Consumption of such fungus-infested grains results in aflatoxicosis. Milk and eggs can also cause aflatoxicosis, if the cattle and poultry are fed with fungus-infested feeds. The toxins are dangerous to liver (hepatotoxic) and may also cause cancer of liver.

Proper storage after drying (moisture below 10%) and discarding of fungus-infested grains will prevent this disease.

Epidemic Dropsy

Traders adulterate mustard oil with argemone oil. Argemone seeds, which resemble mustard seeds may also be mixed with mustard seeds. Argemone oil contains a toxic alkaloid sanguinarine. Consumption of adulterated mustard oil causes epidemic dropsy, which is manifested as bilateral swelling of legs and diarrhea. Cardiac failure and death may follow. Prevention requires health education and punitive action against the traders under PFA Act.

Ergotism due to consumption of field fungi (*Claviceps fusiformis*) infested bajra, rye, sorghum and wheat and endemic ascites due to consumption of millet *Panicum miliare* contaminated with seeds of crotalaria are also seen in some parts.

❑ PREVENTION OF FOOD ADULTERATION

Prevention of Food Adulteration Act

Unscrupulous traders indulging in adulteration of food articles with cheap and harmful substances to make huge profits is well known. Government of India, therefore, enacted an act in parliament in 1954 to deal with food adulteration.

Mixing, substitution, abstraction, concealing the quality, putting up decomposed foods for sale, misbranding or giving false labels and addition of toxicants constitute adulteration. The PFA Act has been amended in 1964, 1976 and in 1986 to make it more stringent. All food items sold in India should conform to PFA standards. Any deviation from PFA standard is considered as adulteration.

Under PFA Act food inspectors from public health department takes samples of suspected foods and send to laboratories for analysis. If found adulterated, the trader is prosecuted as per

PFA Act. Minimum fine of ₹ 1,000 and minimum imprisonment for 6 months can be imposed on the guilty. Life imprisonment and fine of ₹ 5,000 also can be awarded in serious cases. The 1986 amendment empowers consumer and voluntary organizations also to take samples of suspected food items.

While the PFA Act prescribes stringent punishments, implementation of the act is far from satisfactory.

Food Safety and Standards Act, 2006

The Indian Parliament has enacted a new Act called the Food Safety and Standards Act, 2006 (FSSA) in August 2006. With the coming into effect of the new Act, the PFA Act 1954 will stand repealed from the date on which the new Act comes into force.

The Food Safety and Standards Authority of India (FSSAI) has been established under the Act as a statutory body for laying down science-based standards for articles of food and regulating manufacturing, processing, distribution, sale and import of food so as to ensure safe and wholesome food for human consumption.

The FSSAI consists of a chairperson and 22 members, of which one third shall be women. In their endeavor to carry out provisions of the Act, the FSSAI shall be assisted by Central Advisory Committee (CAC), Scientific Panels (SPs) and Scientific Committee (SC) each with specific responsibilities.

In order to strengthen the food safety infrastructure in the country, a 5-year World Bank-aided capacity building project for food safety and quality control of drugs has been launched by the central government.

Other Standards

There are also other standards like the Agmark standards and the ISI standards, which vouch for the good quality of the products. But, they are not mandatory.

CHAPTER

23

Role of Nutrition

❑ NUTRITION, HEALTH AND EUGENICS

Nutrients broadly classified as carbohydrates, fats, proteins, vitamins and minerals are essential for body growth, development, maintenance and repair. Nutrition is the most important determinant of health. This is amply illustrated by the saying 'Man is what he eats'. Nutrition, it appears, decides the very quality of people. Physical characteristics like height and weight, health and well-being, ability to resist infections, improving longevity and freedom from chronic degenerative diseases including cancers are all linked to nutrition.

Nutrition and Intrauterine Life

A good pregnancy outcome (a healthy mother and a healthy baby at the end of pregnancy) requires adequate nutrition besides freedom from other harmful influences.

Effects of Undernutrition During Pregnancy

Undernutrition during pregnancy results in intrauterine growth retardation (IUGR) and low birth weight in babies besides complications such as anemia and toxemia in the mother. Growth spurt in human brain takes place between last 8 weeks of gestation and several months in postnatal life. As cell division and myelination take place at certain predetermined chronological times, deprivation of nutrients during this critical period may result in restricted brain development. Number of brain cells may become less and the deficit will persist into adult life.

Balanced Pregnancy Diet

It is important that obstetrics (the medical science of pregnancy and childbirth) sees beyond just bringing forth a baby with adequate birth weight. Obstetricians, obsessed with birth weight as an important criterion of good pregnancy outcome, are responsible for the alarming increase in the incidence of cesarean sections, which cause significant morbidity and even mortality in the mother. Therefore, increasing calorie intake to increase birth weight at the last stages of pregnancy is not a sound concept. A balanced diet throughout pregnancy and in postnatal life should be ensured to create a healthy and better generation in future.

Prepregnancy Nutrition

In fact, prepregnancy nutrition of the mother is also decisive in this regard. Events prior to conception influence the long-term physiological process of fat storage and the nature of the fat store. This is the fat, which is available during the critical period of cell commitment and division during embryonic and placental development in the I trimester. Poor maternal nutrition or metabolic status prior to pregnancy represents a significant risk of compromizing embryonic development, cell commitment and the rate of DNA replication in a manner, which cannot be compensated later.

Nutrition and Physical Stature

Nutrition also decides the physical stature of man. Human beings in the developed nations are taller and heavy when compared to people in developing countries. This is attributed to good nutrition, which has enabled the former to grow to their predetermined maximum genetic potential. Even in India, Punjabis are much taller and well built than the rest of the population, which is is again due to better quality food consumed by them.

Malnutrition and Diseases

Impact of Malnutrition

Besides the overall impact of undernutrition on the physical growth and mental development, deficiency of specific nutrients also causes significant morbidity and even mortality. PEM in infants and children is an important deficiency disease, which inflicts heavy casualties besides its impact on the physical and mental development of the surviving children. Osteoporosis (weak bones) is common in women who have given birth to many children. Deficiency of vitamin A, if severe, can cause blindness. Iron and folic acid deficiency causes anemia, which contributes to poor pregnancy outcome and impairment of scholastic performance of children. Niacin deficiency causes abnormal mental behavior. Riboflavin deficiency has been incriminated in cataract formation and delayed wound healing.

Effects of Excess Nutrients

While, at one extreme, deficiency diseases are common in developing countries like India, at the other extreme, excess intake of food and its harmful effects are also observed in developed nations. High calorie intake can lead to obesity with its attendant adverse effects. Hypertension, diabetes mellitus and atherosclerosis are all linked to the dietary habits of people. Excessive intake of fat-soluble vitamins A and D can cause toxicity. Excess fluoride in water causes crippling fluorosis.

Antinutrient Compounds and Health

Another aspect that should receive due consideration in nutrition is the fact that some antinutrient compounds present in common foods can interfere with the utilization of some nutrients by the body. Trypsin inhibitors in soy and egg white can cause protein indigestion, which can be prevented by cooking them well. Phytates, tannins and oxalates present in vegetable diets can affect the absorption of minerals like iron, calcium, zinc and magnesium. Consumption of raw eggs affects the absorption of vitamin biotin due to a substance called avidin present in them. Though adequate fiber content in diets is beneficial, too much of it (more than 40 g/day) in the diet can affect absorption of some minerals. This may be especially important in diabetes mellitus for which lot of green leafy vegetables (rich in fiber) are advised.

Toxic Substances and Health

Besides the antinutrient compounds, there are some naturally occurring toxic substances, which cause nutritional diseases in man. Lathyrism, a crippling disease can occur as a result of consumption of khesari dal, which contains a toxic alkaloid, BOAA. Epidemic dropsy reported in Delhi as recently as a few years ago is caused by a toxic substance in argemone seeds, which are used to adulterate mustard seeds and oil. Consumption of fungus-infested groundnuts and other grains cause aflatoxicosis (a condition, which affects liver). This fungus grows on food articles when they are stored with high moisture content. Aflatoxicosis in man can also result from consumption of eggs and milk if the poultry and cattle had been fed with fungus-infested feeds. Food poisoning can occur due to consumption of food contaminated by bacteria or their toxins as a result of improper handling or storage. Personal hygiene and refrigeration can avert food poisoning.

Nutrition and Food Processing

Faulty food processing techniques also can result in loss of nutrients and therefore, contribute to nutritional deficiency diseases. Washing rice with plenty of water before cooking and removal of excess water from cooked rice can cause loss of thiamine as it is a water-soluble vitamin. Other water-soluble vitamins also may be lost in the same way. Raw rice also will be deficient in thiamine. Vitamin C, a heat-sensitive compound can be very easily destroyed during cooking. Even exposing vegetables for long after cutting will result in vitamin C loss. Browning results in loss of lysine, an essential aminoacid. At the same time, technique like germination of pulses and cereals increases riboflavin and vitamin C content.

Nutrition and Immunity

It is nutrition, which decides the immune status of an individual. Lymphoid tissues, which play a dominant role in immunity are highly vulnerable to undernutrition. Thymus derived-lymphocytes (T cell), bone marrow-derived lymphocytes (B cell) and macrophages involved in immune responses are affected in undernutrition. Protein, lipids, vitamins A, B_6 and trace minerals zinc, iron and copper are known to affect immune responses. Vitamin C and zinc deficiency impair phagocytosis, a process involved in engulfing pathogens and destroying them. Opportunistic infections may setin in undernutrition. Immunization in children evokes only suboptimal response in undernutrition. Undernutrition leads to frequent infection, which in turn leads to further malnutrition, forming a vicious cycle.

Bioactive Phytochemicals in Nutrition

Foods like cabbages, carrots, cauliflower, onions, pepper, cloves, garlic, green leafy vegetables, chillies, ginger, citrus fruits, amla, guava, turmeric, sesame oil and sunflower oil contain what are called bioactive phytochemicals, which are found to play a dual metabolic role in prevention of diseases and retardation of pathological processes. Flavonoids, coumarins, lignins, indoles, diterpenes are some of those phytochemicals, which bring about their beneficial effects by acting as antioxidants (carotenoids), detoxifying agents (indole derivatives) or as blocking or suppressing agents (allelic sulfides in garlic).

Nutrition and Aging

Specific nutrients are known to retard aging process:

1. By minimizing reduction of functional enzymes (e.g. tocopherols, carotenoids, vitamin C).
2. By overcoming suboptimal immunocompetence, thereby reducing vulnerability to infections in old age (e.g. iron, zinc, vitamin C).
3. By improving mental functions. Vitamins B_1, B_6 and vitamin C, and mineral copper are needed in the pathways of

neurotransmitter synthesis. Vitamins niacin, folate, cyanocobalamin (B_{12}), riboflavin (B_2) and minerals zinc, potassium and magnesium are important in brain metabolism. Low cholesterol is associated with depression and impaired cognitive functions in the elderly.

Nutrition and Coronary Heart Disease

Diet modifications are found to be beneficial in either preventing or reducing the severity of coronary heart disease (CHD) (heart attacks). A calorie intake appropriate to body weight, fat intake between 15% and 30% of the total energy requirement, saturated fat (animal fat) less than 10%, polyunsaturated fat below 8%, cholesterol less than 300 mg/day (an egg contains more than a day's cholesterol requirement), sugar less than 10%–15% of the calorie intake, salt not more than 5–7 g/day, dietary fiber at 40 g/day are the recommendations to prevent CHDs.

Nutrition and Cancer

High intake of saturated fat, animal protein, red meat, salt, nitrate, nitrosamine and aflatoxins in food (fungal-infested food) are all incriminated in carcinogenesis in man. Cooking practices such as grilling, broiling or smoking can initiate formation of carcinogenic compounds in foods. At the same time, β-carotene, vitamin A, vitamin B_{12}, vitamin C and trace minerals like zinc and selenium are known to prevent certain types of cancers. Vegetables and fruits rich in micronutrients are protective against cancers of epithelial origin. Bioactive phytochemicals such as isothiocyanate, indoles, flavones, phenols, protease inhibitors and allium compounds have been found to protect against carcinogenesis. Chinese green tea, phytoestrogens in soy, curcumin in turmeric have also been found to be beneficial in cancer prevention.

Undernutrition in Fetal Life and Chronic Adulthood Disease

Recent studies have indicated a possible link between undernutrition in intrauterine life and the development of chronic degenerative diseases in adulthood. It appears that the kind of adult one is going to make is decided in the womb itself. When essential nutrients are not made available to a growing fetus through maternal nutrition, it leads to different types of organ or tissue damages in the fetus, the deleterious consequences of which may be manifested in adult life. Those individuals who had deficiencies during their intrauterine period with consequent organ or tissue damage, when exposed to a life of affluence later when they become adults are likely to develop chronic degenerative diseases.

Therefore, it is understood that a good nutrition in pregnancy is crucial for producing a healthy population and many diseases seen now have nutritional connections, which can be prevented by paying attention to nutritional intake of the population through poverty alleviation programs and nutrition education.

SECTION

6

Health Education and School Health Service

CHAPTER

24

Principles of Health Education

❑ SOME TERMS AND CONCEPTS

Values

Values are affectively charged sets of beliefs culturally determined and acquired through the process of socialization and they influence human behavior. For example, religious and moral values are seen to influence gender and sexual behavior in social groups. Socially created values may influence choice of food and breastfeeding.

Attitudes

An attitude can be defined as a tendency to respond positively or negatively to other people, to decisions, to institutions and to organizations.

It has cognitive, affective and conative components. Positive attitude towards somebody will recognize some good aspects in him/her; the person will be liked and interacted with as often as possible. Cognition is knowledge, opinions, beliefs and thoughts about people or institutions and organizations. Feeling pity on poor people is an affective element. Doing something to mitigate their suffering is the conative (action) component.

Attitudes are more or less permanent ways of behaving. Attitudes are not learnt from textbooks, but acquired by social interaction. Prevailing social norms decide the development of attitudes. As attitudes once developed are difficult to change, people should develop healthy attitudes. Parents, teachers, religious leaders and elders play a vital role in the development of attitudes. An individual's behavior is also decided by the basic instinctive motivational factors, such as hunger, sex and pain. For example, a teenager's values and attitudes may succumb to sexual passion.

Traits

Traits are more general and also more stable. While attitude has both subject and object, trait has only subject. Traits vary in degrees (trait of sociability).

Habits

Habits are an accustomed way of doing things. When an act is done repeatedly it becomes a habit. Habits, when followed through generations, become customs. Habits influence human behavior and build personality. Good habits should be cultivated in the young. Washing hands (ablution) with soap after defecation should be taught to children from early childhood to make it a routine habit.

Customs

Customs control the behavior and conduct of individuals, and they are needed to enforce discipline among the varied types of individuals of a society. Laws are generally custom based.

Health Behavior

Health behavior refers to all activities that apparently healthy individuals might undertake in order to minimize the likelihood of developing a disease in future. Health behavior will lead to primary prevention.

Illness Behavior

Illness behavior refers to those activities undertaken by individuals in response to some symptom experience. Symptomatic persons may indulge in mental debate about the significance and the seriousness of the symptoms, consult layman in this field, think of other activities including self-medication and consulting doctors. Appropriate illness behavior results in secondary prevention.

Sickness Role

In sickness role, patients diagnosed to suffer from some disease will expect to be exempted from normal activities and seek help from others. They will also obediently comply with the medical advice in order to recover from the illness.

Motivation

Motivation is an inner force, which drives an individual to a certain action. It also determines the individual's behavior. It may be positive or negative. Without motivation, behavior changes cannot be expected to take place. It is not manipulation. Motivated person acts willingly and knowingly.

Man has biologic needs (food, water), social needs (need for company, love and affection), economic needs and ego-integrative needs (desire for prestige, power, self-respect). It is induced by human examples and this finding is used in community health work like promotion of latrine use. A household using sanitary latrine will motivate its neighbor to construct one in his/her home. In the same way, eligible couples can be motivated for adoption of family planning. Incentives stimulate motivation and energize specific behaviors.

Socialization

Socialization is the process by means of which an individual acquires the beliefs, customs, traditions and prejudices that prevail in a society and gradually becomes a member of the social group. Since socialization is an important matter for society, it is desirable that the children's socialization should not be left to mere accident, but should be controlled through institutional channels. School is an important place for children to get socialized.

Culture

Culture is defined as learned behavior, which has been socially acquired. Culture stands for customs, beliefs, laws, religion and moral precepts, arts, and other capabilities and skills acquired by man as a member of the society. Prevailing culture conditions the behavior and conduct of individuals. Culture is not static, but dynamic, keeps on changing.

Acculturation

When two people from different cultural backgrounds come into contract, there is diffusion of culture both ways and it is called 'acculturation'. The British brought their culture into India. Trade and commerce, industrialization, propagation of religion, education and conquest of nations all facilitate acculturation.

Society

Society is not a group of people; it is the system of social relationship that exists between individuals of the group. The society controls and regulates the behavior of individuals by both customs and law. Society can exert pressure on individuals to conform to norms. Scientific concepts can be translated into practice only with the help of societies.

Community

World Health Organization (WHO) expert committee describes community as a social group determined by geographic boundaries and/or common values and interests. Another definition says that community is a cluster of people living within a contiguous small area who share a common way of life. Community sentiment that is a feeling of belonging together is an important feature of a community. Social capital depends on community life. In countries like India, community life is seriously eroded by the caste structure and community sentiment is observed only within the members of a caste group. In such a scenario, programs that depend upon community participation are likely to fail. Creation of a broader community feeling beyond caste confinement is an important necessity for success of all programs. Programs are based on scientific concepts. But when the society is unscientific due to the influence of castes, religions and the like, the programs mostly fail.

Social Institutions

Social institutions are social structures and machinery through which human society organizes, directs and executes the multifarious activities required for human need. The family, school, caste, religion, church, club, the hospital, political parties, professional associations and the panchayats are all social institutions.

❑ HEALTH PROMOTION

Health is determined by four factors namely:

1. Genetic predisposition.
2. Health services.
3. Individual behavior and lifestyles.
4. The environment.

Health promotion involves the last three spheres.

Environment is considered to have a major influence on health. Health promotion concerns not only with physical environment but also the cultural and socioeconomic circumstances.

The principles that should form the basis in health promotion activities are:

1. Health is a positive state; it is an essential commodity, which people need in order to achieve socially and economically productive life.
2. Substantial progress in health promotion depends on rectifying inequalities in health within and between nations.
3. Health promotion depends on the existence of an active empowered community. Medical services should be reoriented and the focus should be on empowerment, cooperation and quality of life.
4. Health is not just an individual responsibility. Ignoring the social and environmental circumstances, which conspire to make people ill, is fundamentally a defective strategy and unethical. Healthy public policy is a must.

   Health promotion = Health education + healthy social policy.

Successful health promotion leads to health gain, which is conceptualized as adding years to life, adding health to life (reducing disease and disability) and adding life to years (enhancing quality of life).

❑ HEALTH EDUCATION

Health education is any intentional activity that is designed to achieve health- or illness-related learning. It influences human decision-making and behavior. Effective health education may produce changes in knowledge and understanding, or ways of thinking; influence or clarify values; bring about some shift in belief and attitude; facilitate acquiring skills and even affect changes in behavior or lifestyle. Health education deals with how health might be promoted and disease prevented by the judicious application of educational strategies. To prevent disease at the primary, secondary and tertiary levels and to promote the proper use of medical services are the twin goals of health education. In the process, cajoling and coercing people to adopt lifestyles that would prevent the onset of any given disease and persuading them to use appropriate screening services to detect precursor manifestations and asymptomatic disease are needed. Health education emphasizes the need to consult a doctor for treatable conditions at an early stage and the need to comply with the medication regimes in order to prevent relapse and teaches how to readjust to normal life after having suffered from some disabling conditions.

Health education should enhance self-confidence and provide a variety of skills in individuals and the community, so that policy-making process is influenced. Health education should not merely bring health issues to the attention of the public, but rather should generate the kind of indignant concern critical consciousness raising. Concerted force of public pressure is needed to bring about substantial policy changes needed. Changes in beliefs, attitudes and competences are necessary to bring about desired community action.

Health education plays an important role in improving the health of the community. It is given to encourage people:

1. To adopt and sustain health promoting lifestyle and practices.
2. To promote proper use of health services available.

3. To arouse interest, provide new knowledge, improve skills and change attitudes for making rational decisions, which will help people in solving their own problems.
4. To stimulate individual and community self-reliance and participation to achieve health development through individual and community participation. Health education should become part of medical health and general educational disciplines for better impact.

Health education to be effective must use the knowledge derived from different branches of social sciences like sociology, psychology and social anthropology.

Principles

In the delivery of health education, certain principles have to be adopted for effective communication. They are as follows.

Credibility

People accept new information only from sources with credibility.

Interest

Health education should create interest in the audience. To accomplish this it should first start from the felt needs of the target group and then go on to talk about the new programs to be implemented there.

Participation

People should be made to actively participate in the planning and implementation of healthcare programs. Then only the programs will be successful. Programs imposed on people without their involvement will be rejected.

Motivation

Awakening the fundamental desire to learn is motivation. Motivation is of two types. Primary motivation arises in respect of sex, hunger and survival. Praise, love, rivalry, rewards and punishments evoke secondary motivation. People can be motivated to change for better lifestyles by explaining the benefit. A motivated person becomes the motivational force for others in the group.

Comprehension

Comprehending capacity of the people should be borne in mind, while giving health education. Communicating message in the language people understand is necessary for the message to reach them.

Reinforcement

Health education will be effective only when given repeatedly. When repeated in different ways, it is much more effective.

Learning by Doing

If people are involved in the program to be implemented for them, they learn the importance of the program better. This is amply illustrated by the Chinese proverb, which runs as follows. "If I hear I forget; if I see I remember; if I do I know."

Known to Unknown

While imparting health education, we must first begin from what is known to the people already about the topic and then gradually build up new knowledge.

Setting an Example

Health educator should set an example for the message he/she delivers. When advising people to adopt small family norm, the educator also should have a small family.

Good Human Relation

Health educator should develop good human relationship with the people for whom he/she works. Then the message he/she gives will be well accepted.

Feedback

Opinions expressed by the participants should be considered and desirable change in the current strategy in the delivery of health education should be adopted.

Leaders

Using community leaders like the village headman, teachers and political leaders in health education process will be very effective in driving home the health message.

If the above health education principles are used in the delivery of health education, it will go a long way in the effective communication of the health education message.

Strategies in Health Education

Influencing Health Beliefs

A belief is a subjective probability judgment about a particular circumstance or relationship. Influencing health beliefs is a main concern of health education. Convincing people of medically received wisdom as true is necessary. For example, health education message may try to make people believe that smoking is associated with many diseases and that immunization will prevent childhood diseases. Beliefs should be built at community level and population should be persuaded to accept what is considered true. Only when people are convinced that:

1. They are susceptible to a given disease.
2. The disease is serious.
3. The recommended preventive measure will benefit.
4. It will not incur excessive costs or disadvantages, they will accept the advice. Beliefs about the cause of a disease, the risks associated with it and the effect will decide whether behavior change strategy will work or not.

Motivating People

Values are affectively charged sets of beliefs culturally determined and acquired through the process of socialization and they influence behavior. For example, religious and moral values are seen to influence gender and sexual behavior in social groups. Socially created values may influence choice of food and breastfeeding.

Attitudes are more or less permanent ways of behaving. Prevailing social norms decide the development of attitudes. It makes an individual respond in some preferential manner. Parents, teachers, religious leaders and elders play a vital role in the development of attitudes.

Normative Pressure

Despite one's own beliefs and personal preferences, other people also may influence intentions. Individuals may follow general social norms. They may be influenced by spouse, family or peer group also. Such, normative pressures might influence utilization or non-utilization of specific health services.

Effective health education strategies should result in:

1. Implementation of healthy public policy, which will reduce inequalities in the distribution of disease and its socioeconomic determinants.
2. Creation of reoriented (i.e. demystified, accessible and responsive) services.

❑ HEALTH COMMUNICATION

Health education methods adopt three types of approaches for communicating health information. They are:

1. The individual approach (personal contact, home visits and personal letters).
2. Group approach (lectures, demonstrations and discussion methods).
3. Mass approach (television, radio, newspapers, printed material, direct mailing, posters, health museums and exhibitions, folk methods and the internet).

Individual Approach

While dealing with individuals, the health educator must first create an atmosphere of friendship and allow individuals to talk as much as possible. Health education on various aspects such as diet, causation and nature of illness and its prevention, personal hygiene, environmental hygiene, etc. can be given to individuals. Doctors can play an effective role in providing health education as they enjoy people's confidence. Public health nurses, health visitors and health inspectors who frequently meet people in connection with their professional work also can deliver health information.

Group Approach

While giving health education to a group, the interest of the group should form the primary aspect. For example, schoolchildren should be taught about personal hygiene, oral hygiene, etc. and antenatal women about childbirth and baby care. Appropriate method should be selected to provide health education to a group to achieve success of health education.

Methods

Methods in the health education of groups are described as given below.

Lectures: Target group should not have more than 30 members and the lecture should not exceed 15–20 minutes. Audiovisual aids, such as flipcharts, flannelgraph, exhibits, and film and charts can be used for communication in lectures.

Limitations: The limitations of lectures are that they do not stimulate thinking or problem-solving capacity in the group. Comprehension of the subject lectured may also vary with the individuals. Hence, health behavior is not necessarily affected.

Demonstration: Principles of 'seeing is believing' and 'learning by doing' are used in demonstration. A procedure is demonstrated step-by-step before a target group. Demonstration arouses interest and persuades the onlookers to adopt recommended practices. It has a high motivational value and can bring about desirable changes in the behavior pertaining to the use of a new practice. Installation of hand pumps, chlorination of water, construction of a sanitary latrine and preparation of oral rehydration therapy (ORT) solution, all can be demonstrated with good impact.

Group discussion: A group is an aggregation of people who interact with each other unlike a group of students in a classroom who simply passively listen to a teacher. Group discussion is a very effective method of health communication as it allows people to exchange ideas and opinions freely and learn. For effective communication the group should not be less than 6 members and more than 12. A group leader initiates and facilitates the discussion by encouraging everyone to participate in the discussion. Members should be asked to express clearly, listen to what others say, not to interrupt when others speak, make only relevant remarks, accept criticisms gracefully and help to reach some conclusions. A person may be asked to record the proceedings and prepare a report. Decision taken in group discussions is likely to be adopted by group members easily. Although, unequal participation may be a limitation in group discussions, a well-conducted one may be useful in helping learners to come to a group decision needed to solve their common problem. Group decision is better than individual decision.

Panel discussion: In this method, 4–8 experts discuss a specific topic in front of a large group or audience. The chairman of the panel welcomes, introduces the panel members and initiates the discussion. The panel members are requested to give their viewpoints on the topic. Once the discussion by the panelists is over, the audience is invited to take part in the discussion. This can be an effective way of driving home the message, if properly planned and conducted.

Symposium: In symposia, experts give a series of speeches on a selected topic before an audience. At the end, the audience is allowed to raise questions. Finally a summary is presented by the chairman.

Workshop: In workshops, the participants divide themselves into smaller groups of 4 or more and hold discussions on some aspect of the issue under discussion. Each group discusses in a friendly atmosphere under expert guidance and come out with a plan of action on the issue. Workshops provide the participants an opportunity to improve their effectiveness as professional workers.

Role play: This method is particularly useful for schoolchildren and is used to impart value education, which cannot be expressed adequately in words. The situation is enacted as a drama by a group of about 25. The spectators do not remain passive, but actively participate by demonstrating how they feel that a particular role should be handled in their opinion. Human relationships can be portrayed properly in such sociodramas.

Conferences and seminars discuss a single topic in depth for a period ranging from half a day to 1 week. Many formats can be used to aid the learning process.

Mass Approach: Education of the Public

To educate the whole community mass media is used. Newspapers, radio and television are the important media that reach large number of the public quickly. Television has now become an indispensable item of the households in the world.

Unfortunately, the focus given to cinema and commercial advertisements in television belittle the importance of other useful messages. This trend should be checked to make it really beneficial to the masses.

As mass media alone is not adequate in changing human behavior, they should be used in combination with other methods. It should be ensured that the programs are culturally appropriate in order to achieve effective communication. Mass media can be used to create political will in favor of health and healthy social policy, to raise health consciousness of the people and to foster community involvement.

Internet has great potential as a medium to spread health messages very quickly. Printed materials such as magazines, pamphlets, booklets and handouts are useful tools to reach many with health educational information. Folders, newsletters and booklets on topics like family planning, immunization, nutrition, etc. can be used to educate people in remote areas. Eye-catching posters, billboards and signs can be used advantageously to spread health messages. Motives like humor or fear can be effectively used to transmit messages in posters. Posters should be periodically replaced with new ones for the desirable impact as their life is short. Health museums and exhibitions attract large number of people and help to increase the knowledge and awareness. As people explain the various specimens kept in museums and exhibitions, it gives a personal touch to the communication. Folk media like keerthan, katha, folk songs, dances, dramas and puppet shows are quite useful in creating health consciousness among the rural masses.

Some Agencies Involved in Health Education

The WHO has a new division of health education and health promotion. International Union for Health Education is functioning with headquarters in Paris. It started the South-east Asia Regional Bureau (SEARB) at Bengaluru in 1983.

Government of India has established the Central Health Education Bureau in the Ministry of Health. State Government also has established health education bureaus in their health directorates. Directorate of Advertising and Visual Publicity (DAVP), Press Information Bureau, Doordarshan (Indian official television channel) and All India Radio are also actively involved in health education.

❑ SCHOOL HEALTH SERVICE

School health service, if provided properly, can be an effective way of improving community health and it is much more relevant in developing countries like India as most of the students hail from poor families. The Government of India constituted a school health committee (Renuka Ray) in 1960 to assess the standards of health and nutrition of schoolchildren. Subsequently, many state governments allocated funds for school health and feeding programs. But it can be said that the school health service provided now in our country is far from satisfactory.

Health problems of schoolchildren may vary from place to place, but in general schoolchildren are found to suffer mainly from malnutrition, infectious diseases, intestinal parasites, diseases of the skin, eye and ear, and dental caries.

School health service can be an effective way to take care of millions of schoolchildren by providing promotive, preventive and curative services, which include health education and provision of a healthful school environment.

School Health Program

School Health Program is a program for school health service under National Rural Health Mission (NRHM). It intends to cover 1,288,750 government- and private-aided schools covering around 22 crore students all over India.

The School Health Program, the only public sector program specifically focused on school-age children, addresses the health needs of children, both physical and mental and in addition, it provides for nutrition interventions, yoga facilities and counseling. All the services are provided in a cost-effective manner.

The program at the national level has been developed to provide uniformity/guidance to states who are already implementing or plan to implement their own versions of program and to give guidance in proposing a coherent strategy for school health program in next year's NRHM Program Implementation Plan (PIP) to those states that have not yet started their program.

It is proposed that an auxiliary nurse midwife (ANM) may be spared once a week for school health only, if she has either multipurpose worker (MPW) (male) or second ANM to support her at the health subcenter. The MPW (male) will be more appropriate for exclusive boys' senior basic schools. Training of trainers (ToTs) will take place at state and district levels, and teachers will be oriented on the program, so that they internalize the core values and strategies of the program. Apart from the teachers screening the children, area ANMs/MPWs will visit one school every week on an average for detailed screening and treatment of minor ailment and required referral. In addition, a medical officer will also visit one school per week for additional screening, treatment and referral. The program may be taken up in a phased manner covering 20% schools in the 1st year and 40% schools each in 2nd and 3rd year.

Various school health promotion committees have been recommended at state, district, block and school levels.

Components of School Health Program

Screening, Health Care and Referral

1. Screening of general health, assessment of anemia/nutritional status, visual acuity, hearing problems, dental checkup,

common skin conditions, heart defects, physical disabilities, learning disorders, behavior problems, etc.

2. Basic medicine kit will be provided to take care of common ailments prevalent among young school going children.
3. Referral cards for priority services at the district/subdistrict hospitals.

Immunization

- As per national schedule
- Fixed day activity
- Coupled with education about the issue.

Micronutrient (Vitamin A, Iron and Folic Acid) Management

- Weekly supervised distribution of iron-folate tablets coupled with education about the issue
- Administration of vitamin A in needy cases.

Deworming

- As per national guidelines
- Biannually supervised schedule
- Prior information, education and communication (IEC)
- Siblings of students also to be covered.

Health Promoting Schools

- Counseling services
- Regular practice of yoga, physical education, health education
- Peer leaders as health educators
- Adolescent health education; existing in few places
- Linkages with the out-of-school children
- Health clubs, health cabinets
- First aid room/corners or clinics.

Capacity Building

Development of knowledge, skills and attitudes in individuals and groups.

Monitoring and Evaluation

To assess the quality and impact of one's work against the strategic plan needed for reorientation and fine tuning.

Midday Meal

Noon meal provided to schoolchildren at school premises.

Health Appraisal

Appraisal of the health of the students is the first activity to be undertaken. The initial examination at school entry should be thorough, which should include a careful history, physical examination, tests for vision, hearing and speech, stool examination for parasites, routine blood and urine examination, and examination for nutritional deficiency diseases. Screening for tuberculosis should also be done. The parents should be advised to be present during the periodic medical examination of their children and the class teachers should play an active role in conducting the medical examination. Subsequent examinations should be done once in 4 years or more frequently, if facilities are available. Health appraisal should cover school personnel also as they form part of the school environment. In addition to periodical medical examination, daily morning inspection by the teachers for any change in the appearance and behavior of students will help to diagnose any illness or growth failure. Teachers should be adequately trained in this respect during their teacher training courses.

Remedial Measures and Follow-up

After each periodic medical examination, children should be followed up and appropriate treatment given. Special clinics should be conducted at primary health centers in the rural areas and in one of the selected schools in urban areas after giving due advance information. As dental, eye, ear, nose and throat defects are common among schoolchildren, specialists should be invited to examine them. Separate beds should be earmarked in referral hospitals for schoolchildren for admission, investigation and treatment.

First Aid

Establishing first aid posts in schools is essential to attend to emergencies like accident and acute medical conditions like gastroenteritis, epileptic fits, etc. Teachers should be equipped with the knowledge on first aid.

Health Education

Health education in schools should deal with three important aspects. Knowledge on personal hygiene practices like bathing, brushing of teeth and use of clean clothes should be imparted. Attention should be paid to healthy postures, while sitting in the classroom. Ergonomically designed chairs and tables should be provided. Students should be weaned away from bad habits like cigarette smoking. Involving students in environmental sanitation programs such as construction of sanitary latrines and wells, and fly control activities will help them in understanding the importance of clean environment for prevention of diseases. Family life education imparted through health education will go a long way in creating healthy attitudes in adolescents toward reproduction.

Services

Dental health services for prevention and treatment of dental caries and promotion of oral hygiene, and eye health services for early detection and treatment of refractive errors and vitamin A deficiency, etc. are provided. A positive school environment (for example, an inclusive social climate with supportive peers) and good school adjustment (as shown by academic achievement and low levels of school-related stress) can increase the sense of success and competence. This in turn leads to greater well-being and life satisfaction and fewer subjective health complaints. In contrast, lack of academic achievement and poor peer acceptance can result in a decrease in positive health outcomes and an increase in risk behavior. Accordingly, the school context seems to be both a risk factor and a resource for physical, emotional and social well-being. Mental health services for detection and prevention of juvenile delinquency, maladjustment and drug addiction should become an important aspect of school health service, so that the students become mature, responsible and well-adjusted adults in future.

Midday meal program, providing at least one third of calories and half of protein requirement of children, can help to prevent malnutrition besides improving school attendance.

Healthful School Environment

Creation of healthful school environment is very important. Location of school building in an elevated centrally located place away from busy places and roads, cinema theaters, factories, railway tracks and markets should be ensured. Site is selected in high lands to prevent water logging. School health committee (1961) recommended 10 acres of land for higher elementary schools and 5 acres for primary schools with an additional one acre of land per 100 students. Playground facilities should be provided. Nursery schools should be preferably single storied and the external walls should have a minimum thickness of 10 inches to prevent heat radiation. Classrooms should not accommodate more than 40 students and the per capita space for students in a class room should not be less than 10 square feet. It is desirable to provide single desks and chairs, ergonomically designed. Combined doors and windows area should be at least 25% of floor space and the windows should be placed in such a way that they ensure cross ventilation. Ventilators should be at least 2% of the floor area. The walls are painted white. Sufficient natural lights should light the classrooms and the lights should come from behind and not from front. Adequate water supply and eating facilities should be provided. One urinal for 60 students and one latrine for 100 students, and separate privies for boys and girls must be provided.

Implementation of School Health Program

School Health Committee

School health committee is an essential part of the school organization and administration. Principal/Headmistress/Headmaster will be responsible for the formation of health committee in the school.

Members: The health committee may consist of up to four teachers from the school and a student from each class/grade/standard or as appropriate for the school size. Selected parents and community members should also be invited to become members of the committee. Members of the parent/teacher association may wish to elect two members to serve on the committee.

School health coordinator: Every school should be required to appoint a suitably trained teacher who has the designated responsibility for coordination and promoting the total health program.

School health club as a cocurricular activity: School health coordinator may be the sponsor of the club with the nominated teachers as cosponsors. All the children studying in the school would be eligible for membership of the club. Two health leaders from each class may be selected. They will form the committee to organize the club activities

The school health committee is responsible for the maintenance of the healthy school environment, the development of school grounds that are sound for the development of children, for provision and cleanliness of healthy classrooms, premises and toilets. More than the healthy physical environment, the committee should be conscious of the need to create an emotional environment of care and respect. It will take strong measures to involve parents and the community in a practical way.

Committees at national, state, district and village level are established to monitor the implementation of the program. Primary health centers assist through their medical team in conducting periodic medical examination of schoolchildren.

❑ HEALTH CULTURE

Health culture can be defined as the healthy way of life that people adopt to prevent diseases and promote health.

Promotion of health culture demands continuous education on simple personal hygiene practices to be followed in day-to-day life and persuasion to discontinue lifestyles that are inimical to healthful living.

Personal hygiene can be defined as the way of life that an individual should adopt in his or her everyday life necessary to prevent diseases and promote health culture.

Maintenance of high standard of hygiene and sanitation is a long-term proposition, and it cannot be affected in the near future in developing countries like India because of the kind of social situation that exists. Therefore, there is a need for enlightening people on hygiene practices, so that they will adopt healthy lifestyles and protect themselves from diseases. Concerted efforts are needed to educate people on healthy lifestyles.

With that in mind some undesirable habits and practices commonly observed and the desirable changes needed for healthful living are discussed below. Here, it is beyond the scope to attempt an exhaustive analysis of various aspects of human lifestyles.

Practices Associated with Food and Water

Preventing contamination is an important aspect to be kept in mind in respect of food and water. Selling eatables uncovered and exposed to flies on the roadside, in busy bus stands and in front of schools by petty vendors is a very common scene. Foods exposed to dust and flies can cause diseases. House flies carry disease causing organisms, deposit them on exposed foods and thereby transmit diseases like typhoid, jaundice, diarrhea, dysentery and intestinal worms. Dusts also carry eggs of intestinal worms, deposit on eatables and transmit worm infestations like thread worm disease. Therefore, the practice of eating fruits and vegetables like grapes, tomatoes, carrot, etc. exposed to dirt and flies directly without washing them well should be avoided. This is essential not only to prevent infectious diseases like diarrhea but also to avoid poisoning by insecticides.

Infant feeding is another important area, which demands a high standard of hygiene. Feeding bottle in the hands of ignorant mothers is a dangerous tool. While traveling in the bus or train, mothers are found to carry the feeding bottles exposing them to flies and dusts, and the bottle as such is used to feed the baby. This is an unhygienic practice and it often leads to frequent diarrhea in the infant and even death due to dehydration, if not treated properly. Feeding bottle should be either kept covered or avoided. For the same reason washing feeding bottles with sand should be avoided and the need to boil the feeding bottles for at least 10–15 minutes should be emphasized.

As food articles also act as vehicle for transmission of diseases like diarrhea, food poisoning, typhoid, jaundice, etc. it is desirable to be choosy in selecting the food items in hotels and even the eatery. It is better to dine only in standard hotels. Preparations like chutney often mixed with raw water before serving can be avoided. Only food items, which are likely to be freshly prepared, may be chosen rather than fancy and tasty items.

Another aspect to be considered in this respect is the nutritional aspects of foods. Common cooking practices often result in loss of nutrients leading to deficiency features in the consumers.

As rice is the staple diet of majority, people mainly depend on it for vitamin thiamine intake. Since thiamine is a water-soluble vitamin, it can be lost very easily during the process of washing. So, minimal washing with little water can reduce thiamine loss. Discarding the cooked water also contributes to this vitamin loss. So, pressure cooking is desirable. In this regard, parboiled rice is preferable to raw rice as thiamine is retained in parboiled rice even after washing, but not in raw rice. Thiamine intake can be ensured, if people consumed products made of whole wheat.

Another very sensitive vitamin, which gets easily destroyed during cooking, is the vitamin C. Even exposure of cut vegetables to air, for a while, can result in vitamin C loss. Boiling significantly destroys vitamin C. Therefore, tomatoes should be added in curries just before removing the vessel from the stove in order to retain at least some amount of vitamin C. Regular intake of fruits containing vitamin C like lemon, gooseberry, orange, grapes, tomatoes, guava, etc. can manage the requirement of vitamin C. Germinated pulses (e.g. Bengal gram) also provide vitamin C.

Yet another vitamin sensitive to heating is folic acid. Its deficiency is common in women and preschool children, resulting in anemia. Deficiency of this vitamin is common, especially in pregnancy. As cooking in high temperatures results in loss of this vitamin, foods containing folic acid namely green leafy vegetables, meat, milk, dairy products, eggs, etc. should be cooked in low heat to reduce the vitamin loss. Iodized salt should be added in the last stages of cooking in order to retain the mineral iodine. If added much early in the cooking, it gets removed.

Drinking water, without any discrimination, from all available sources is a very common habit. But it is not a healthy one as water is often a vehicle for carrying many disease causing germs. People should be especially careful about drinking water from hotels, cinema theaters, bus stands, railway stations and in melas, festivals and marriage feasts. Water in these places is invariably contaminated with some germ or the other and is likely to transmit waterborne diseases mentioned earlier. Drinking boiled water in such situations is desirable. But mixing boiled water with raw water before drinking, as is the common practice, defeats the very purpose of boiling, which is done to kill the disease causing germs. Alternately, aerated water can be consumed when the quality of drinking water available is suspected. Even at homes, where water is stored in pots or drums without tap collection of water for drinking by means of a tumbler dipping fingers in the water is not a healthy practice. Water gets contaminated by fingers and so can transmit waterborne diseases. Such pots or drums can be tilted to pour water into the collecting vessel like tumbler. It is also a common scene that people tend to collect water for drinking from a drum or can kept in public places directly through the mouth of the vessel by opening the lid even though the vessel is fitted with a tap. Therefore, besides emphasizing storing of water in vessels fitted with a tap, people also should be educated to collect water only through the tap and not through the mouth of the vessel.

Practices Associated with Excretory Functions

Many of the waterborne and food-borne diseases are due to contamination of water and food by human excreta. The most important cause for fecal contamination of food and water is the age-old practice of open-air defecation. From feces in the open fields, disease-causing germs are transferred to food and water through insects like houseflies. Wind also plays a role in such transfer of germs to food articles like vegetables and fruits, and exposed food-items sold on the roadside. So, if this obnoxious practice of open-air defecation is avoided, most of the waterborne and food-borne diseases can be prevented.

Lack of personal hygiene is found to be very common. Water taps, door handles and latches in public lavatories may get soiled with feces from the user's improperly washed fingers. So, washing one's hands well after using such public conveniences with soap becomes essential to protect oneself from fecal-borne diseases. Immediately after using latrines, especially public latrines or after handling a busy watertap in public places, fingers should not be used to rub the eyes, blow nose or meddle with the mouth in order to prevent the transfer of disease germs from taps or door handles soiled by the previous user. Washing hands after urination is also necessary as hands may get soiled by organisms present in the urine. Typhoid germs can get transferred through urine-soiled hands to food and water. Therefore, it is essential that any user of conveniences should take care to wash the taps in latrines and wash basins after using them to prevent the spread of diseases to the subsequent user. This is absolutely necessary when the user suffers from diarrhea, dysentery, common cold or eye diseases like trachoma.

Ablution after defecation is here performed using water unlike in the West where tissue paper is used for the purpose. In this process, hands get soiled with feces containing disease-causing germs. If soiled hands are not washed thoroughly with soap after defecation, there are ample chances for transfer of germs from soiled hands to food and water. If the person happens to be a food handler like housewife, cook or hotel servant who handles food items, there are plenty of chances for transmission of disease germs to the susceptible consumers through contaminated food and water. So, washing hands with soap after defecation is an absolute necessity. This practice should be inculcated very early in childhood.

Indiscriminate spitting is a common unhealthy practice and it facilitates the spread of diseases like tuberculosis. People suffering from common cold, sore throat and chest infection should not spit everywhere indiscriminately for fear of spread of those diseases to others through air. People, while coughing or sneezing, should cover their face and nose with a handkerchief to prevent airborne transmission of diseases to neighbors. In the absence of a kerchief or towel, turning the face away from neighbors, while coughing or sneezing should be practiced. During pandemic H1N1 outbreaks, people exposed to the infected individuals or large crowds should wash their hands frequently and should not touch their nose or mouth without washing their hands in order to protect themselves from contracting the infection.

Practices Associated with Some Miscellaneous Activities

Sharing of other's articles is an unhealthy practice. Garments, especially undergarments like vests and underwears, when shared, can spread fungal diseases like tinea versicolor and ringworm disease from person to person. Similarly, pillows, towels, soaps and khajals, when shared, can transmit eye diseases like trachoma, a blinding eye disease. Shared razors and toothbrushes can spread killer disease AIDS and another serious liver disease, serum jaundice. Similarly, shared combs can transmit louse infestation.

Sycosis barbae, which is contracted from barber shop, can be prevented by washing the shaven area with soap immediately after shaving and by applying antiseptic lotions. Similarly, using home-washed undergarments as against laundry-washed ones can save us from the distressing tinea cruris (dhobi's itch) in the groin.

Picking one's ear by whatever stick one can lay his or her hand on is a dangerous practice. It can result in chronic ear discharge leading to even deafness. This practice also can transfer the spores of tetanus bacilli from the ground to the ear and cause the killer disease tetanus. Likewise, picking the teeth with dirty sticks, pins and safety pins can cause infection of gums.

During outbreak of communicable eye diseases like trachoma or Madras eye, people may contract them from sufferers, while traveling in a bus or train or from cinema theater. The habit of cleaning one's eyes with fingers in such situations should be avoided and only the back of one's hand or fingers should be used to relieve any itching sensation in the eyes, if needed. Immediately after reaching home or office, hands should be washed with soap to prevent contracting such diseases.

Unhealthy practices result in not only infectious diseases but also poisoning sometimes. For example, taking out children frequently for a walk along busy roads may result in lead poisoning from the automobile exhausts. Since children are short, they inhale more exhaust containing lead than the adults.

It is hoped that the above tips, if highlighted regularly, will help to promote healthy lifestyles in society.

SECTION

7

Environment and Health

CHAPTER

25

Physical Environment and Health

Environment in which man lives can be divided into three components namely physical (water, air, soil, housing, radiation, etc.) biological (plants and animal life including microorganisms) and social (customs, culture, habits, occupation, religion, etc.) environments. Physical and biological environments are amenable for modification, but the social environment is a complex one. Environmental sanitation deals with the physical environment and to some extent biological environment. The aim of environmental sanitation is to create and maintain environmental conditions that will promote health and prevent diseases. Providing safe water and improving sanitary conditions are the two important health promotional activities of public health.

❑ PHYSICAL ENVIRONMENT

Air

Air contains primarily nitrogen (78%), oxygen (21%) and carbondioxide (0.03%). It also contains argon, neon, krypton, xenon and helium in traces. Water vapor, traces of ammonia and suspended matter such as dust, bacteria, spores and vegetable debris are also present in the air.

Air Pollution

Air is considered as polluted when harmful substances are present in it. Gases, mixtures of gases and particulate matter generated by man's activities get into the atmosphere in concentrations that affect the health of human beings and the entire ecosystem.

Indoor Air Pollution

Indoor air pollution also contributes significantly to ill health, especially in rural homes affecting mainly women and children. About 5% of deaths and diseases are due to indoor pollution caused by burning of solid fuels for cooking in 21 of the most heavily impacted countries according to WHO. Tobacco smoke, nitrogen oxide (NO_2), carbon dioxide (CO_2) from cooking and non-ventilation type heating, allergens such as mites and moulds in airtight rooms cause air pollution of the interior environments where people spend most of their time (nearly 90%). More than half of the world's population (over 3 billion) relies on dung, wood, crop waste or coal to meet their most basic energy needs. Cooking and heating with such solid fuels on open fires or stoves without chimneys lead to indoor air pollution. This indoor smoke contains a range of health-damaging pollutants including small soot or dust particles that are able to penetrate deep into the lungs. In poorly ventilated dwellings, indoor smoke can exceed acceptable levels for small particles than outdoor air by 100-fold. Indoor air pollution is responsible for the death of 1.5 million people mostly children and women annually, i.e. one death every 20 seconds.

Adverse effects: Exposure to indoor air pollution increases the risk of pneumonia among children under 5 years, and chronic respiratory disease and lung cancer (in relation to coal use) among adults over 30 years old. Exposure to biomass smoke has been linked to lung cancer, asthma, cataracts and tuberculosis. There is tentative evidence for an association between indoor air pollution and adverse pregnancy outcomes, in particular low birth weight or ischemic heart disease and nasopharyngeal and laryngeal cancers. Replacing solid fuels with cleaner and more efficient ones such as biogas, LPG and kerosene could largely eliminate the health risk and prevent 1.5 million deaths annually around the world.

Outdoor Air Pollution

Outdoor air is polluted by motor exhausts (NO_2, suspended particulate matter, lead oxides) and secondary contaminants like ozone or aldehydes generated by photochemical reactions of NO_2 with hydrocarbons in many cities. Sulfur dioxide (SO_2) and sooty dust are discharged in areas where coal is used and SO_2 in those areas where high sulfur petroleum is used. Nuclear power plant accident at Chernobyl in Russia, Bhopal MIC gas tragedy in India and the dioxin accident in Seveso, Italy are the serious air pollution accidents that have occurred in the past.

Air pollution is modified by the meteorological conditions. Wind helps to disperse and dilute pollutants. But in areas surrounded by mountains and tall buildings wind becomes weak and so dispersal is affected. Vertical diffusion of air is disturbed by temperature. Rapid cooling of lower layers of atmospheric air prevents vertical motion, traps water vapors and pollutants at lower levels and causes what is described as smog. Smog formation may be frequent in the winter than in summer or spring.

Adverse effects: Air pollution causes both immediate and delayed effects. Mostly, respiratory tract gets affected due to immediate effects, which can cause sudden death by suffocation. Delayed effects include chronic bronchitis, lung cancer, bronchial asthma, emphysema and respiratory allergies. Lead poisoning from automobile exhausts affects particularly children. Destruction of flora and fauna, damage to buildings and poor visibility also are caused by air pollution.

Some Known Pollutants

Nitric oxide (NO): This is oxidized to NO_2 within a few seconds. It has vasodilating action and actions on immunological mechanism. Involvement in atopic allergic conditions is also known.

Nitrogen oxide (NO_2): It is an insoluble gas and has properties similar to ozone. Indoor level is increased by smoking, heating and cooking and is suspected to cause asthma.

Diesel exhaust and sulfur dioxide: The diesel exhaust gas contains diverse carcinogenic substances such as benzopyrene, a polycyclic aromatic hydrocarbon (PAH), formaldehyde, nitrolene, diesel exhaust particles (DEPs), CO_2 and aliphatic hydrocarbons. The DEPs cause asthmatic conditions by producing superoxide (O_2^-) and hydroxyl (OH^-) radicals. Sulfur dioxide (SO_2), a water-soluble gas is discharged when coal and high sulfur petroleum are used as fuels. Sulfur dioxide in the air was the cause of London smog, Muse valley and Yokkaichi asthma. Now it has become a problem in countries in which use of coal is increased, e.g. China. Oxidation of SO_2 results in acid aerosols, which irritate respiratory passages and induce bronchial asthma (due to H^+ concentration in the aerosols).

Particulate matter: Suspended particulate matter of 10 microns or less in diameter are retained in pulmonary alveoli. Particles of various heavy metals, particles from the soil, asbestos, iron particles from spiked tires, pollen of Japanese cedar and cypress, and acid aerosols from NO_2 and SO_2 belong to suspended particulate matter group. Lead oxide, another particulate matter, can cause encephalopathy with malaise, tremor, impairment of attention, headache, hallucination and memory disorders. Lead poisoning in police men exposed to motor exhausts (due to leaded petrol) is known. Combustion of fossil fuels generates carcinogenic and mutagenic hydrocarbons (benzopyrene). Increase in lung cancer is related to release of carcinogens from factories. Tobacco smoke can pollute indoor air. In airtight houses, allergens such as mites, house dust and moulds are incriminated to cause asthma. Japanese cedar and cypress pollens cause pollinosis (allergic rhinitis) in slum dwellers.

Agricultural chemicals: Those like herbicides and pesticides infiltrate into residential areas and cause problems. Agricultural chemicals deposited on the ground will evaporate and become airborne when the temperature rises.

Monitoring of Air Pollution

In the monitoring of air pollution, levels of SO_2, smoke and suspended particles are usually used as indicators. The WHO has published approved methods of determining the concentration of common air pollutants and their health hazards in its publication 'Air Quality Guidelines for Europe'. In India, Central Pollution Control Board monitors air quality in major cities since 1990. The WHO also has established two international centers at London and Washington, three regional centers at Moscow, Nagpur and Tokyo, and 20 laboratories in various parts of the world to study and issue warning of air pollution as and when it occurs.

Measures to Reduce Indoor Air Pollution

Measures to reduce indoor air pollution and associated health effects include the following:

1. Changing to cleaner alternatives such as gas, electricity or solar energy.
2. Use of improved stoves or hoods that vent health-damaging pollutants to the outside.
3. Behavioral changes.

Millennium Development Goals (MDG) are guiding international action in this regard. Important agencies in fighting indoor pollution include the Partnership for Clean Indoor Air, the United Nations Environment Program, the United Nations Development Program and the World Bank as well as many research institutions and non-governmental agencies around the world.

Control of Air Pollution

Many engineering methods have been devised to control air pollution. Containment methods to prevent escape of toxic substances from the sources into the ambient air, replacement methods in which old processes causing air pollution are replaced by newer processes devoid of air pollution and dilution methods, which will dilute the concentration of pollutants, are some of them. Green belts between industrial area and residential area will serve the same purpose. Legislation is another strategy, which empowers authorities to monitor and take action against polluting sources like industries. The Air (Prevention and Control of Pollution) Act, 1981 has been enacted in India for this purpose.

❑ HUMIDITY

Humidity is the presence of water vapor in the air. It is measured as absolute humidity, relative humidity and specific humidity. Relative humidity is the most frequently used measurement of humidity because it is regularly used in weather forecasts. It indicates the likelihood of precipitation, dew or fog. In warm climates, more water molecules can evaporate and stay in the air in a vapor state.

Absolute Humidity

Absolute humidity refers to the mass of water in a particular volume of air. Absolute humidity is expressed as the number of kilograms of water vapor per cubic meter of air. In chemical engineering, it is defined as mass of water vapor per unit mass of dry air also known as the mixing ratio.

Relative Humidity

Relative humidity is defined as the ratio of the partial pressure of water vapor in a gaseous mixture of air and water vapor to the saturated vapor pressure of water at a given temperature. That is, a ratio of how much energy has been used to free water from liquid to vapor form to how much energy is left. Relative humidity is expressed as a percentage. It is calculated as follows:

$$RH = \frac{p(H_2O)}{p^*(H_2O)} \times 100\%$$

where, RH is the relative humidity of the gas mixture being considered;

$p(H_2O)$ is partial pressure of water vapor in the gas mixture;

$p^*(H_2O)$ is the saturation vapor pressure of water at the temperature of the gas mixture.

Falling rain may be cold enough to condense water vapor from warm, humid air, thus lowering the relative humidity. A hygrometer is used to measure the relative humidity.

Specific Humidity

Specific humidity is the ratio of water vapor to air (dry air plus water vapor) in a particular volume of air. Specific humidity ratio is expressed as a ratio of kilograms of water vapor, m_w, per kilogram of air, m_a.

Humidity is also measured on a global scale using remotely placed satellites. These satellites are able to detect the concentration of water in the troposphere at altitudes between 4 and 12 kilometers. Satellites that can measure water vapor have sensors that are sensitive to infrared radiation. Water vapor specifically absorbs and reradiates radiation in this spectral band. Satellite water vapor imagery plays an important role in monitoring climate conditions (like the formation of thunderstorms) and in the development of future weather forecasts.

Humidity and Air Density

Humid air is lighter, less dense, than dry air. This is due to the fact that a molecule of water weighs less than molecules of nitrogen (N_2) and oxygen (O_2). This may seem counterintuitive as water is commonly perceived to be much heavier than air. It is true that liquid water is heavier than air. However, the water that makes the air humid is not liquid; it is water vapor, which is lighter than nitrogen or oxygen gas.

Temperature and pressure have much more marked effects on the density of air; however, humid air is lighter than dry air at the same temperature and pressure because of this molecular difference.

Dew Point and Frost Point

Dew point is associated with relative humidity (if the dew point is below freezing, it is referred to as the frost point). Dew point is the temperature at which water vapor saturates from an air mass into liquid or solid usually forming rain, snow, frost or dew. Dew point normally occurs when a mass of air has a relative humidity of 100%. This happens in the atmosphere as a result of cooling through a number of different processes.

Effects on Human Body

The human body sheds heat by a combination of evaporation of perspiration, conduction to the surrounding air and thermal radiation. Under conditions of high humidity, the evaporation of sweat from the skin is decreased and the body's efforts to maintain an acceptable body temperature may be significantly impaired. Also, if the atmosphere is as warm as or warmer than the skin during times of high humidity, blood brought to the body surface cannot shed heat by conduction to the air and results a condition called hyperpyrexia. With so much blood going to the external surface of the body, relatively less goes to the active muscles, the brain and other internal organs. Physical strength declines and fatigue occurs sooner than it would otherwise. Alertness and mental capacity also may be affected. This resulting condition is called heat stroke or hyperthermia.

Recommendations for Comfort

The ASHRAE Standard 55–1992, Thermal Environmental Conditions for Human Occupancy, recommends relative humidity between 30% and 60% for comfort. Below 50% is preferred to control dust mites. In summer, air conditioning is used to remove high humidity from air. In winter, heating cold outdoor air can decrease indoor relative humidity levels to below 30% leading to discomforts such as dry skin and excessive thirst.

❑ TEMPERATURE

Effects of Cold

Cold causes non-freezing and freezing injuries.

Non-freezing Injuries

Chilblains: These are a mild cold injury caused by prolonged and repeated exposure, for several hours, to air temperatures from above freezing (0°C) to as high as 16°C. In the affected skin area there will be redness, swelling, tingling and pain.

Immersion foot: It occurs in individuals whose feet have been wet, but not freezing cold, for days or weeks. It can occur at temperatures up to 10°C. The primary injury is to nerve and muscle tissues. Symptoms include tingling and numbness, itching, pain and swelling of the legs, feet or hands. Blisters may develop. The skin may be red initially and turn to blue or purple as the injury progresses. In severe cases, gangrene may develop.

Trench foot: This is 'wet cold disease' resulting from prolonged exposure in a damp or wet environment from above the freezing point to about 10°C. Depending on the temperature, the onset of symptoms may range from several hours to many days, but the average is 3 days. Trench foot is more likely to occur at lower temperatures whereas an immersion foot is more likely to occur at higher temperatures and longer exposure times. A similar condition of the hands can occur if a person wears wet gloves for a prolonged period under cold conditions described above. Symptoms are similar to an immersion foot.

Freezing Injuries

Frostnip: This is the mildest form of a freezing cold injury. It occurs when ear lobes, nose, cheeks, fingers or toes are exposed to the cold. The top layers of the skin freeze. The skin of the affected area turns white and it may feel numb. The top layer of skin feels hard, but the deeper tissue still feels normal. Frostnip can be prevented by wearing warm clothing and footwear. It is treated by gentle rewarming (e.g. holding the affected tissue next to unaffected skin of the victim or of another person). As for all cold-induced injuries, never rub the affected parts because ice crystals in the tissue could cause damage if the skin is rubbed. Do not use very hot objects such as hot water bottles to rewarm the area or person.

Frostbite: This is a common injury caused by exposure to extreme cold or by contact with extremely cold objects (especially those made of metal). It may also occur in normal temperatures from contact with cooled or compressed gases. Frostbite occurs when tissue temperature falls below the freezing point (< 0°C) or when blood flow is obstructed. Blood vessels may be severely and permanently damaged and blood circulation may stop in the affected tissue. In mild cases, the symptoms include inflammation of the skin in patches accompanied by slight pain. In severe cases, there could be tissue damage without pain or there could be burning or prickling sensations resulting in blisters. Frostbitten skin is highly susceptible to infection and gangrene (local death of soft tissues due to loss of blood supply) may develop.

As first aid the victim should be moved to a warm area if possible. Rewarming the affected area on site should be avoided.

Constricting clothing or jewelry should be removed. The affected area is covered with a sterile dressing. Dry heat should not be applied to the affected area. Rubbing the area is harmful. Alcohol and smoking should be prohibited.

Hypothermia

In moderately cold environments, the body's core temperature does not usually fall more than 1°C–2°C below the normal 37°C because of the body's ability to adapt. However, in intense cold without adequate clothing, the body is unable to compensate for the heat loss and the body's core temperature starts to fall. The sensation of cold followed by pain in exposed parts of the body is one the first signs of mild hypothermia.

When the temperature continues to drop or the exposure time increases, the feeling of cold and pain starts to diminish because of increasing numbness (loss of sensation). If no pain can be felt, serious injury can occur without the victim noticing it.

Next, muscular weakness and drowsiness are experienced. This condition is called hypothermia and usually occurs when body temperature falls below 33°C. Additional symptoms of hypothermia include interruption of shivering, diminished consciousness and dilated pupils. When body temperature reaches 27°C, coma sets in. Heart activity stops around 20°C and the brain stops functioning around 17°C.

Hypothermia is a medical emergency. At the first sign, find medical help immediately. Wet clothing is removed first. The victim is placed between blankets so that the body temperature can rise gradually. Body-to-body contact can help warm the victim's temperature slowly. Rewarming the victim on site using hot water bottles or electric blankets should not be done. Warm, sweet (caffeine-free, non-alcoholic) drinks can be given unless the victim is rapidly losing consciousness, unconscious or convulsing.

Effects of Heat

Exposure to heat causes a wide spectrum of disorders such as heat stroke, heat hyperpyrexia, heat exhaustion, heat cramps and heat syncope.

Heat Stroke

Heat stroke is a form of hyperthermia with accompanying physical and neurological symptoms. Unlike heat cramps and heat exhaustion, heat stroke is a true medical emergency that can be fatal, if not properly and promptly treated.

In extreme heat, high humidity or vigorous exertion under the sun, the body is not able to dissipate the heat and the body temperature rises, sometimes up to 106°F or higher. A dehydrated person also may not be able to sweat fast enough to dissipate heat, which causes the body temperature to rise.

Infants, the elderly (often with associated heart diseases, lung diseases, kidney diseases or on certain medications that make them vulnerable to heat strokes) and athletes or outdoor workers physically exerting themselves under the sun are susceptible.

Symptoms: The symptoms of heat stroke can sometimes mimic those of heart attack or other conditions. Sometimes a person experiences symptoms of heart exhaustion before progressing to heat strokes. Symptoms of heat exhaustion may include nausea, vomiting, fatigue, weakness, headache, dizziness, muscle cramps and aches. However, some individuals can develop symptoms of heat stroke suddenly and rapidly without warning. Different people may have different symptoms and signs of heat stroke. But common symptoms and signs of heat stroke include high body temperature, the absence of sweating with hot red or flushed dry skin, difficulty in breathing, rapid pulse, strange behavior, hallucinations, confusion, agitation, disorientation, seizure and coma.

Treatment: As treatment first and foremost is cooling the victim. The victim is taken to a shady area. Cool or tepid water is applied to the skin (e.g. cool water from a garden hose). Fanning the victim to promote sweating and evaporation and placing ice packs under armpits and groins are done. Body temperature is monitored with a thermometer and cooling efforts are continued until the body temperature drops to 101°F–102°F.

Prevention: The most important preventive measures are avoiding dehydration and vigorous physical activities in hot and humid weather. In hot weather, workers should take plenty of fluids (such as water and buttermilk). Ingestion of alcohol, coffee and tea must be avoided as it may lead to dehydration. Wearing hats and light-colored, light and loose clothes may be beneficial.

Heat Exhaustion

Heat exhaustion is a milder form of heat-related illness that can develop after several days of exposure to high temperatures and inadequate or unbalanced replacement of fluids. Those most prone to heat exhaustion are elderly people, people with high blood pressure and people working or exercising in a hot environment.

Symptoms: Warning signs of heat exhaustion include heavy sweating, paleness, muscle cramps, tiredness, weakness, dizziness, headache, nausea or vomiting and fainting. The skin may be cool and moist. The victim's pulse rate will be fast and weak; breathing will be fast and shallow. If heat exhaustion is untreated, it may progress to heat stroke.

Treatment: Cool, non-alcoholic beverages, rest, cool shower bath or sponge bath, an air-conditioned environment and lightweight clothing are useful in treating the victims.

Heat Cramps

Heat cramps manifest as painful and spasmodic contractions of skeletal muscles and it occurs in individuals doing heavy muscular work in high temperature and humidity. The exact cause of heat cramps is unknown. These are probably related to electrolyte imbalance caused by excessive sweating. A large amount of sodium is excreted in sweat and drinking fluids with inadequate sodium content may result in a serious low-sodium condition called hyponatremia. Drinking salt-containing fluids like buttermilk or soda lemon salt may avert this condition.

Heat Syncope

Person standing in the sun collapses suddenly. But there is no rise in temperature. There is peripheral circulatory failure leading to reduced blood supply to the brain, which causes fainting. Schoolchildren may develop this condition during morning prayers. The patient should be taken to a shady area and made to lie with the head lowered.

❑ IONIZING RADIATION

Ionizing radiation comprises electromagnetic waves of extremely short wavelength and accelerated atomic particles (e.g. electrons, protons, neutrons and alpha particles). Ionizing radiation dislodges electrons from atoms by depositing strong local energy.

Sources

Sources of radiation are both natural and artificial.

Natural Sources

Cosmic rays, radium and other radioactive elements in the earth's crust, internally deposited ^{40}K, ^{14}C and other nuclides present normally in living cells, and inhaled radon and its daughter elements are the natural sources of radiation. Radiation received will be high in mountain sites, aircraft altitudes and in areas where earth is rich in radium (e.g. beach sand of Indian state of Kerala).

Artificial Sources

The artificial sources of radiation are the X-rays used in medicine, radioactive minerals in building materials (^{238}U, ^{232}Th, ^{40}K, ^{226}Ra), phosphate fertilizers and crushed rock, television sets, smoke detectors, radioactive fallout from atomic weapons (^{137}Cs, ^{90}Sr, ^{89}Sr, ^{14}C, ^{3}H, ^{95}Zr) and nuclear power stations (^{3}H, ^{14}C, ^{85}Kr, ^{129}I, ^{137}Cs).

Radiation Effects

X-rays and γ-rays are sparsely ionizing whereas charged particles are densely ionizing. Ionizing radiation produces ions and free radicals in the cells. It breaks chemical bonds and also causes other molecular alterations that may injure cells. Deoxyribonucleic acid (DNA) is the most critical target. When injured DNA is not repaired or misrepaired, it results in mutation. Number and structures of chromosomes are also altered. Chromosome aberration in blood lymphocytes is useful as a biological dosimeter in radiation accident victims. Large doses cause tissue atrophy. Rapidly multiplying cells are the most sensitive. Mutagenic effects are described as stochastic phenomena.

Skin, bone marrow and lymphatic tissues, intestines, gonads, respiratory tract, eye lens and many other tissues are affected by radiation (Table 25.1).

Heritable Effects

Heritable effects of irradiation are yet to be observed in humans. Human germ cells are no more radiosensitive than those of the mouse. From the existing evidence, it is estimated that less than 1% of all genetically determined diseases in humans is attributable to natural background irradiation.

Carcinogenic Effects

Carcinogenic effects of ionizing radiation have been documented extensively. Even though a molecular mechanism has not been elucidated, it is implicated in activating oncogenes and/or in the inactivation of tumor suppressor genes in many instances. The mechanism of carcinogenicity appears similar to that of chemical carcinogens. Not more than 3% of all cancers in population are attributable to natural background irradiation.

Prevention

Exposure should be kept as low as possible. Proper designing of facilities that deal with radiation, radiation protection program for workers by way of adequate training and supervision, and a well-developed and well-rehearsed emergency preparedness plan are important preventive steps. Safe disposal of radioactive wastes and monitoring of medical radiographic examinations and therapy are mandatory.

TABLE 25.1: Effects of radiation to the organs

Organ	Effects
Skin	A dose of 6 Sv* (600 rem†) or more causes erythema within a day followed by deeper or more prolonged erythema after 2–4 week. 10–20 Sv (1,000–2,000 rem) causes blistering, necrosis and ulceration in 2–4 week followed by atrophy. A second wave of ulceration months or years later also occurs.
Bone marrow and lymphatic tissues	Hematopoietic cells in bone marrow are killed in sufficient numbers causing profound leukopenia and thrombocytopenia in 3–5 week. Lymphocyte count comes down. Fatal infection and hemorrhage occur.
Intestine	10 Sv (1,000 rem) denude intestinal villi within days. Fatal dysentery-like syndrome results when large area of intestine is affected.
Gonads	Even a low dose of 0.15 Sv (15 rem) can cause oligospermia; 2–4 Sv can cause permanent sterility. 1.5–2.0 Sv (150–200 rem) affects ovary and causes temporary sterility and large dose can cause permanent sterility.
Respiratory tract	6–10 Sv causes acute pneumonitis in 1–3 month. Large exposure leads to respiratory failure in 1 week. Pulmonary fibrosis and cor pulmonale result months or years later.
Eye lens	5.5–14 Sv causes cataract after a few month.
Whole body radiation	Acute radiation syndrome characterized by malaise, anorexia, nausea and vomiting may be caused when major part of the body is exposed to more than 1 Sv. Subsequently after a latent period, hematological, gastrointestinal, cerebral or pulmonary diseases may be caused depending upon the location of exposure. Finally either recovery or death occurs.
Localized radiation	Some radiation effects are localized in organs such as thyroid (^{131}I) and bone (radium and strontium-90). Prenatal irradiation can cause malformation, mental retardation and childhood cancer.

*Sv, sievert; †rem, roentgen equivalent man.

❑ NON-IONIZING RADIATION

Ultraviolet (UV) radiation, visible light, infrared radiation and microwave radiation are the non-ionizing radiations.

Ultraviolet Radiation

Ultraviolet radiation is divided into three bands namely UVA (400–320 nm UVA is also called black light), UVB (320–280 nm) and UVC (280–100 nm).

Sources

Sunlight, tanning lamps, welding arcs, plasma torches, germicidal and black light lamps, electric arc furnaces, hot metal operations, mercury vapor lamps and lasers are the sources of UV radiation. Fluorescent lamps and some laboratory equipments are low-intensity sources.

Clinical Manifestations

As UV rays do not penetrate deeply into human tissues, it causes injuries only in skin and eyes. Sunburn and skin cancers due to UV radiation are common in fair-skinned people. Aging of the skin, solar elastosis, solar keratosis, photokeratitis (welder's flash), cortical cataract and pterygium are the other manifestations caused by UV radiation.

Prevention

Avoiding excessive exposure to sunlight by fair-skinned people and use of protective clothing, UV radiation screening lotions and UV radiation blocking sunglasses are the preventive steps. Workers' exposure is to be limited to 1.0 milliwatt/square centimeter (mW/cm^2) when exposure exceeds 1,000 seconds. Maintaining the protective ozone (O_3) layer of stratosphere by reducing greenhouse gases such as chlorofluorocarbons (CFCs) and other air pollutants is important. O_3 layer filters UV rays from the sun.

Infrared Radiation

Infrared radiation is electromagnetic waves in the wavelengths 7×10^{-5}–3×10^{-2} meter. Potentially hazardous sources are furnaces, ovens, welding arcs, molten glass and heating lamps. Burning of the skin and cataract formation in the eye lens are caused by infrared radiation. Glass blowers, blacksmiths, oven operators are prone to develop cataract. Exposure should not exceed 10 mW/cm^2.

Microwave and Radiofrequency Radiation

Wavelengths of microwave (MW) and radiofrequency (RF) radiation are between 3 kHz and 300 GHz. The sources of microwave radiation are radar, TV, radio, cellular phones and other telecommunication system, heating, welding and melting operations, wood and plastic processing, high temperature plasma and medical appliances like diathermy and hypothermia. Microwaves cause thermal injury to skin (burn) and other tissues. High intensity exposure (> 1.5 kW/m^2) can cause cataract. Microwave may interfere with cardiac pacemaker and other medical devices. Proper designing and shielding of the sources are imperative for prevention.

Extremely low frequency electromagnetic fields (ELF-EMFs) from solar activity, thunderstorms, electric power lines, transformers, motors, household appliances, video display tubes, medical devices like resonance imaging systems can affect nerves, neuromuscular, retina, heart and cardiac pacemakers. Occupational exposure can cause leukemia, brain cancer, miscarriages and birth defects. Areas containing EMFs stronger than 0.1 millitesla (mT) (transformers, accelerators, MRI systems) should exhibit warning placards. Wiring design changes may be necessary for preventing exposure.

Ultrasound

Ultrasound is not electromagnetic wave, but mechanical vibration at frequencies above audible range (> 16 kHz). The sources of ultrasound are cleaning, degreasing, plastic welding, liquid extracting, homogenizing and emulsifying operations, medical therapeutic operations such as lithotripsy and medical diagnostic ultrasonography (low power high frequency ultrasound).

Headache, earache, tinnitus, vertigo, malaise, photophobia, hyperacusia and peripheral neuritis can be caused by ultrasound. Diagnostic ultrasonography in pregnancy is known to cause adverse effects on the embryo. It is therefore recommended that exposure to ultrasound during pregnancy should be minimized in the following ways:

1. Using ultrasound only when medically indicated, i.e. only when a problem is suspected, rather than as a routine screening to determine the sex of the baby or check on its development.
2. Minimizing total exposure time (by choosing a skilled and knowledgeable operator).
3. Minimizing exposure intensity (i.e. avoiding Doppler, especially during the first trimester).
4. Informing individuals whether mechanical index (MI) or thermal index (TI) is greater than 1 and how this exposure compares with that found in normal diagnostic practice.

Visible Light

Too much light can affect retina, lens, iris and cornea, while too little light can cause eye strain.

❑ NOISE

Sounds that disturb human life are referred to as noise (Tables 25.2 and 25.3). From 20 Hz to 20 kHz is the perceivable range for human ear. Higher frequency waves are called ultrasonic waves, while low frequency ones are called infrasonic waves.

Noise in the Living Environment

Airports, high-speed railroad systems and trunk roads create high levels of sound. Residents in such areas are annoyed and consider the sound as nuisance even if they do not develop hearing impairment. Noise disturbs conversation and causes sleep disorders, difficulty in concentration and discomfort. A decrease in rapid eye movement (REM) sleep is reported as a sensitive indicator of road traffic noise exposure with a threshold level of L_{eq} 47.5 dB(A). Noise pollution has become a serious social problem over the world. The sense of 'noiseness' is dependent on factors such as individual disposition, age and taste of individuals, and also on the qualitative nature of the noise (music, natural sounds, household noise, traffic noise, factory noise, etc.). Nevertheless nuisance caused by noise in the population as a whole is well-recognized.

Noise in the Occupational Environment

Occupational exposure to noise is associated with hearing loss, which may be irreversible. Noise in the working environment may also affect autonomic nervous functions manifested as stress and changes in blood pressure.

Noise-induced disorders can be prevented by setting of tolerance standards of noise exposure and subdividing the working environment based on international standards such as those of International Organization for Standardization (ISO).

Infrasonic waves emanating from motor vehicles, railroads, dams, heat sources and compressors do not readily attenuate with distance. They cause autonomic imbalance such as sleep disorders, dizziness, irritability, headache and

TABLE 25.2: Sound levels of some noises

Noise	Decibel level
Speech 2–3 people	73
Speech radio	80
Music radio	85
Children shouting	79
Children crying	80
Vacuum cleaner	76
Piano	86
Jet take off	150

TABLE 25.3: Acceptable noise levels [dB(A)]

Source	Noise level
Residential	
Bedroom	25
Living room	40
Commercial	
Office	35–45
Conference	40–45
Restaurants	40–60
Industrial	
Workshop	40–60
Laboratory	40–50
Educational	
Classroom	30–40
Library	35–40
Hospitals	
Wards	20–35

Adapted from Basavanthappa's Community Health Nursing, 2nd edition gastrointestinal disorders. Prolonged exposure causes essential hypertension.

Noise pollution can also be harmful to wildlife. Perhaps the most sensational damage caused by noise pollution is the death of certain species of beached whales brought on by the extremely loud (up to 200 decibel) sound of military sonar.

Noise Mitigation and Control

There is also technology that has been applied with the aim of mitigating or controlling noise as much as possible provided that it has a sufficiently localized source. Controlling includes:

1. Roadway noise is the most widespread environmental component of noise pollution worldwide. There are a variety of effective strategies for mitigating adverse sound levels, which include use of noise barriers (e.g. growing stress), limitation of vehicle speeds, alteration of roadway surface texture, limitation of heavy duty vehicles, use of traffic controls that smooth vehicle flow to reduce braking and acceleration, innovative tire design and other methods. The US has developed a computer model for roadway noise that is capable of addressing local topography, meteorology, traffic operations and hypothetical mitigation.
2. Aircraft noise can be reduced to some extent by design of quieter jet engines. This strategy has brought limited, but noticeable reduction of urban sound levels. Reconsideration of operations such as altering flight paths and time of day runway use have demonstrated significant benefits for residential populations near airports. Federal Aviation Administration (FAA) sponsored residential retrofit (insulation) programs initiated in the 1970s have also enjoyed widespread success in reducing interior residential noise in thousands of affected residences across the US.
3. Scientific studies on industrial noise have emphasized redesign of industrial equipment, shock mounting assemblies and physical barriers in the workplace. Innovations have had considerable success; however, the costs of retrofitting existing systems are often rather high.

❑ SOIL

Soil can get contaminated in many ways. There are thousands of contaminant sources and pollutant types. The following list illustrates some of them:

1. Petroleum hydrocarbons from rupture of underground storage tanks [benzene, ethylbenzene, toluene, xylene, alkanes, alkenes, methyl tertiary butyl ether (MTBE)].
2. Spillage or leakage of solvents and dry cleaning agents (acetone, trichloroethylene, formaldehyde and perchloroethylene).
3. Leaching of contaminants from solid waste disposal sites (lead, mercury, chromium, cadmium, bacteria and hydrocarbons).
4. Water runoff, which carries pollutants and may deposit them at a point of percolation. Percolation into soils from use of pesticides and herbicides (wide variety of chemicals including DDT, lindane, organochlorines, organophosphates, carbamates, cyclodienes, etc.).
5. Deposition of dust from smelting operations and coal burning power plants (zinc, cadmium, lead, mercury).
6. Lead deposition from lead abatement or construction demolition.
7. Leakage of transformers [polychlorinated biphenyls (PCBs)].

Effects on Ecosystem

Soil contaminants can have significant deleterious consequences for ecosystems. There are radical soil chemistry changes, which can arise from the presence of many hazardous chemicals even at low concentration of the contaminant species. These changes can manifest in the alteration of metabolism of endemic microorganisms and arthropods resident in a given soil environment. The result can be virtual eradication of some of the primary food chain, which in turn can have major consequences for predator or consumer species. Even if the chemical effect on lower life forms is small, the lower pyramid levels of the food chain may ingest alien chemicals, which normally become more concentrated for each consuming rung of the food chain. Many of these effects are now well known such as the concentration of persistent DDT materials for avian consumers leading to weakening of egg shells, increased chick mortality and potentially species extinction.

Soil contaminants typically alter plant metabolism most commonly to reduce crop yields. This has a secondary effect upon soil conservation since the languishing crops cannot shield the earth's soil mantle from erosion phenomena. Some of these chemical contaminants have long half-lives and in other cases derivative chemicals are formed from decay of primary soil contaminants.

Effects on Health

There is a very large set of health consequences from exposure to soil contamination depending on pollutant type, pathway of attack and vulnerability of the exposed population. Chromium and many of the pesticide and herbicide formulations are carcinogenic to all populations. Lead is especially hazardous to young children in which group there is a high risk of developmental damage to the brain and nervous system, while to all populations kidney damage is a risk.

Chronic exposure to benzene at sufficient concentrations is known to be associated with higher incidence of leukemia. Mercury and cyclodienes are known to induce higher incidences of kidney damage, some are irreversible. Polychlorinated biphenyls and cyclodienes are linked to liver toxicity. Organophosphates and carbamates can induce a chain of responses leading to neuromuscular blockage. Many chlorinated solvents induce liver changes, kidney changes and depression of the central nervous system. There is an entire spectrum of further health effects such as headache, nausea, fatigue, eye irritation and skin rash for the above cited and other chemicals. Clearly at sufficient dosages a large number of soil contaminants cause death.

Many helminths, which cause disease in man, are transmitted from soil. The most common soil-transmitted helminths (STHs) are roundworm, whipworm and hookworms. *Ascaris lumbricoides* infect 1.221 billion, *Trichuris trichiura* 795 million and hookworms 740 million. *Strongyloides stercoralis* also is a common soil-transmitted helminth.

❑ WATER

Safe and wholesome water is the basic necessity for health and survival. Contaminated water is the cause for much of ill-health of mankind especially in developing countries.

Safe water is defined as the one that is free from pathogenic organisms and harmful chemicals, pleasant to the taste and usable for domestic purposes.

More than one tenth of global population still relied on unimproved water sources in 2010.

Rain reservoirs, rivers, streams, tanks, ponds and lakes provide surface water. Wells and springs provide ground water. Rainwater is almost free from pathogenic organisms, but may contain impurities like dust, soot, CO_2, and oxides of nitrogen and sulfur derived from atmosphere. Acid rain (formed due to oxidation of NO_2 and SO_2 to nitric acid and sulfuric acid respectively) may cause deleterious impact on plants, insects, etc. Surface water can get easily contaminated from natural as well as manmade sources. Ground water is better than surface water being usually free from contamination and pathogens, but may have a high mineral content, which renders it hard.

Sanitary well is the one that is located at a higher elevation, at least 15 m (50 feet) away from the source of contamination, has a brick lining up to a depth of 6 m (20 feet), a parapet wall up to 2–3 feet above the ground level, a cement concrete platform around extending at least 1 m (3 feet) in all directions, draining facilities and a covering for the top.

Water Pollution

Impurities derived from atmosphere, catchment area and the soil pollute water. Sewage, industrial and trade wastes, agricultural pollutants and physical pollutants also contaminate the water sources.

Indicators of Water Pollution

Total suspended solids, biochemical oxygen demand (BOD) at 20°C, level of chlorides, nitrogen and phosphorous, and absence of dissolved oxygen are used as indicators of water pollution.

Polluted water causes diseases due to biological agents and chemical substances present in it.

Biological agents that cause infectious diseases (transmitted through water) are the following.

Viral: Hepatitis A, poliomyelitis, rotaviral diarrhea.

Bacterial: Typhoid, bacillary dysentery, *Escherichia coli* diarrhea, cholera.

Helminthic: Roundworm, threadworm, hydatid disease.

Leptospiral: Leptospirosis (Weil's disease).

Waterborne creatures, snails and cyclops transmit schistosomiasis and guinea worm disease, respectively.

Vectors like mosquitoes, which breed in water, transmit diseases like malaria, filariasis, Japanese encephalitis, dengue, chikungunya, etc. Simulium flies, which breed in vegetations near lakes or rivers and tsetse flies that breed in thickets along rivers and streams transmit onchocerciasis and African trypanosomiasis, respectively.

Waterborne chemical pollutants such as detergent solvents, cyanides, heavy metals like mercury, minerals, organic acids, nitrogenous substances, bleaching agents, dyes, pigments, sulfides and ammonia. Toxic and biological organic compounds are all known to affect man's health.

High nitrate content in water causes methemoglobinemia in infants. Excess fluoride causes dental and skeletal fluorosis.

Hard water is claimed to have beneficial effects against cardiovascular diseases.

CHAPTER

26

Control of Biological Environment

The ecosystem is a naturally occurring community of organisms together with their environment, functioning as a unit. Disruption of ecosystems, either as a result of human activities or natural phenomena, can affect human health.

Pathogenic bacteria, viruses, fungi, parasites and the insect vectors in the environment are responsible for causing many diseases in man. Therefore, controlling the environment to prevent the occurrence of diseases from these biological agents forms an important public health activity.

❑ MOSQUITO CONTROL MEASURES

Now an integrated approach to control mosquito is resorted to. Special care is taken to prevent environmental pollution with toxic chemicals and to avoid insecticide resistance.

Antilarval Measures

Environmental Control

Elimination of breeding places called source reduction involves filling, leveling and drainage of breeding places and water management. Rendering the water unsuitable for breeding is also useful in source reduction, e.g. changing the salinity of water. Abolition of cesspools and open ditches and collection, removal and disposal of sewage and waste water are important to control *culex* mosquito. For the control of aedes, water holding containers like discarded tins, empty pots, broken bottles, coconut shells and other similar items should be removed. For the control of anopheles, their breeding places should be identified and abolished by filling or drainage and for the control of mansonoides, aquatic plants should be either removed or destroyed by herbicides.

Chemical Control

Mineral oils: Diesel oil, fuel oil, kerosene, other fractions of crude oils and mosquito larvicidal oil are sprayed over the water surface and the larvae die because they are not able to breathe through the layer of oil, which covers the water surface. As the life cycle of mosquito is about 8 days, oil is applied once a week. Application rate is 40–90 liters per hectare.

Paris green: The 2% dust of Paris green, prepared by mixing 2 kg of Paris green and 98 kg of soapstone powder or slaked lime is dusted by hand blowers or rotary blowers at the rate of 1 kg of actual Paris green per hectare of water surface. Paris green kills mainly anopheles larvae. The larvae are killed when Paris green is ingested by them as it is a stomach poison. In the usual dosage, Paris green does not harm fish, man or farm animals.

Synthetic insecticides: Organophosphorus compounds like fenthion, chlorpyriphos and abate are effective larvicides. Abate at 1 ppm level is very effective and least toxic. Organochlorine compounds (DDT, HCH) are not used because of their long residual effect, contamination of water and the development of resistance in the vector.

Biological Control

Larvivorous fish like *Gambusia affinis and Lebistes reticulatus* can be introduced in sewage ponds, ornamental ponds, cisterns, farm ponds and burrow pits to control the mosquito larvae.

Antiadult Measures

Residual Sprays

Dichlorodiphenyltrichloroethane (DDT), a residual insecticide, is sprayed 1–3 times a year on the walls and other surfaces where mosquitoes rest. When DDT resistance is observed, malathion, Propoxur or gamma HCH can be used. As mosquitoes can develop resistance, periodic investigations to find out the sensitivity of the mosquitoes should be conducted and only potent insecticides used.

Space Sprays

Pyrethrum extract is a nerve poison and it kills the mosquitoes on contact. After spraying at the dosage of 1 ounce of spray solution (0.1% of active principle) per 1,000 cubic feet of space, the doors and windows are kept closed for half an hour. Residual insecticides like malathion and fenitrothion are used for ultra low volume (ULV) fogging of space (Table 26.1).

Genetic Control

Genetic control is still in research stage. The endosymbiotic bacterium *Wolbachia* inhibits viral replication and dissemination in the main dengue vector, *Aedes aegypti*. This underscores the potential usefulness of *Wolbachia*-based control strategies in dengue.

Mosquito nets, screening of houses with wire meshes and repellents can be used to protect from mosquito bite.

❑ FLY CONTROL MEASURES

Environmental Control

Elimination of breeding places is the best method to control fly. Kitchen wastes, garbage and other refuse should be stored in bins with tight lids till disposal. Removal of refuse and their disposal by incineration, composting or sanitary land fill, provision of sanitary latrines, avoiding open air defecation, sanitary disposal of animal excreta (cattle dung) and improving general sanitation are necessary to prevent fly breeding.

TABLE 26.1: Dosage of residual sprays

Chemical	Dose	Frequency
DDT*	1–2 g/m²	Once in 6–12 month
Lindane	0.5 g/m²	Once in 3 month
Malathion	2 g/m²	Once in 3 month
OMS-33	2 g/m²	Once in 3 month

*DDT, dichlorodiphenyltrichloroethane

Insecticidal Control

Methoxychlor 5%, DDT 5%, Lindane 0.5% or chlordane 2.5% at 5 liters per 100 square meter of surface can be sprayed to kill susceptible flies. Resistant strains can be killed by diazinon 2%, dimethoate 2.5%, fenthion 2.5%, malathion 5% or ronnel 5%. Addition of sugar enhances effectiveness. Food or water should not be contaminated during spraying.

Solid or liquid baits containing diazinon, malathion, dichlorvos, ronnel or dimethoate also can be used to kill flies. Cheapest one is prepared by mixing three teaspoons of commercial formalin with one pint of water or milk and adding a little sugar.

Cords and ribbons impregnated with insecticides hung like festoons from ceilings are effective for 1–6 months. Space sprays of pyrethrin, DDT or HCH will produce only a temporary effect on fly population. Diazinon, dichlorvos and other insecticides used in breeding places to kill larvae of fly are not useful as they accelerate the development of resistance. Fly papers smeared with adhesive mixtures are not effective.

Screens with 14 meshes to the inch can be used in houses, hospitals, food markets and other places to protect from flies. Sustained health education to motivate people for the control of fly is very essential.

Control of Sandflies

A single application of 1–2 gram/square meter of DDT or 0.25 gram/square meter of Lindane will be effective in reducing sandflies. Houses, cattle sheds and other places should be sprayed. Removal of shrubs and vegetation within 50 yards of human habitations, filling up of cracks and crevices in walls and floors, locating cattle sheds and poultry houses away from human habitations all will help in the control of this vector.

❑ CONTROL OF LICE

Head and crab lice 0.5% malathion lotion is applied and left for 12–24 hours and then the hair is washed. It kills lice and nits. Carbaryl dust also is effective against lice.

Body Lice

Malathion powder or carbaryl dust can be sprayed or sprinkled to the inner surface of clothing as well as socks and on the body of persons. A single application can eradicate the infestation, but a second application may be needed after 7 days to kill the remaining lice. Personal hygiene is very important in the control of lice. A daily bath with soap, frequent washing of their long tresses by women, washing of clothing, towels and sheets in hot water with soap and ironing, autoclaving of clothes and bedding to destroy body louse are important in the control of lice.

❑ CONTROL OF RAT FLEAS

The 10% DDT is sprayed on floors and walls up to a height of about 1 feet. Or the insecticide can be sprayed over rat runs, under gunny bags and other areas where rats are frequent. Rodent burrows also should be sprayed with the insecticide. Animal hosts like cats, dogs and their quarters and premises should also be sprayed with the insecticides. When DDT resistance is observed, carbaryl or diazinon 2% or malathion 5% can be used. Repellents like diethyltoluamide and benzyl benzoate can be used to protect from flea bites. Rodent control should form part of flea control.

❑ CONTROL OF TICKS AND MITES

Insecticides like DDT, chlordane, dieldrin, lindane, malathion and toxaphene are effective against ticks and mites. They can be used as dusts or sprays. Animals like dogs and their premises should be treated with insecticidal sprays or dusts. Cracks and crevices in the ground particularly near buildings and paths should be filled up. Rodents and dog population should be reduced.

Clothing impregnated with repellants like indalone, diethyltoluamide and benzyl benzoate can protect workers from bites. Workers should also be instructed to search for ticks on their body and to remove them. Ticks should be removed without breaking the mouth parts.

❑ CONTROL OF RODENTS

1. Sanitation measures like proper storage, collection and disposal of garbage, proper storage of foodstuffs, rat proofing of buildings, godowns and warehouses, and destruction of rat burrows with plugging are important sanitary measures to control rats. Rat trapping also can be tried to control them.
2. Rodenticides: Barium carbonate is no more used now. Zinc phosphide mixed with wheat or rice flour in the ratio of 1 part to 10 parts of flour and few drops of edible oil is used as baits to kill rats. Rats are killed in 3 hours. While handling this rodenticide, rubber gloves should be worn as it is highly poisonous. Special care should be taken to avoid risk to man and domestic animals. Use of multiple dose poisons (e.g. warfarin, diphacinone) has been given up.
3. Fumigation: Calcium cyanide (cyanogas) is extensively used in India. It is pumped into rat burrows in powder form by a special foot pump. The 2 ounces of the poison is pumped into each burrow after closing the exit opening and then the burrow is sealed with wet mud. On contact with moisture, hydrogen cyanide gas is released, which kills rats as well as fleas.

❑ DISINFECTION PROCEDURES

Sterilization is the process, which destroys all forms life including spores. Disinfection is killing of infectious agents outside the body by chemical or physical agents.

Types of Disinfection

1. Concurrent disinfection is the procedure in which the infective discharges from the infected person and the soiled articles are disinfected immediately then and there. Urine, feces, vomit, contaminated linen, clothes, hands, dressings, aprons, gloves, etc. are disinfected throughout the course of an illness to prevent transmission to others.
2. Terminal disinfection is done after the patient has been discharged or after death.

Disinfection of water by chlorine, pasteurization of milk, hand washing before surgical procedures and application of antiseptic over the injection site before giving injections is examples of pre-current (prophylactic or preventive) disinfection.

Natural agents like sunlight and air are lethal to most bacteria and some viruses, but they cannot be totally depended upon.

Physical Agents

Burning

Burning of infective materials should be done in an incinerator. Dressings, rags, swabs and feces can be burnt. Burning of polyvinyl chloride (PVC) materials liberate toxic substances like dioxins. These toxic compounds cause impotence in males and are also carcinogenic.

Hot Air

Hot air oven (temperature 160°C–180°C for at least 1 hour to kill spores) is used to disinfect items like glassware, syringes, swabs, dressings, oils, Vaseline and sharp instruments. But plastic, rubber and other delicate articles cannot be sterilized by hot air.

Boiling

Water, small instruments, linen, gloves, etc. can be disinfected by boiling. Boiling for 5–10 minutes will kill bacteria but not spores or viruses. Contaminated linen, utensils and bed pans can be disinfected by boiling for 30 minutes.

Steam

Steam under pressure (temperature more than 100°C) is the most effective sterilizing agent. It destroys all forms of life including spores. Absolute sterility is obtained at 135°C. Items like linen, dressings, gloves, syringes, certain instruments and culture media can be sterilized using autoclaves, which generate steam at high temperature and pressure. However, sharp instruments and plastics cannot be sterilized in autoclaves.

Ionizing Radiation

Ionizing radiation (gamma radiation) is used to sterilize bandages, dressings, catgut and surgical instruments.

Chemical Agents

Crude phenol (a mixture of phenol and cresol) in 10% strength can be used to disinfect feces. At 5% strength it is used to mop floors and clean drains. Cresol (5%–10%) is used to disinfect feces and urine. Cresol emulsions such as Lysol, Izal and Cyllin are powerful disinfectants. The 2% Lysol is used to disinfect feces. Chlorhexidine (Hibitane) is a useful skin antiseptic and therefore used as effective hand lotions. The 1% creams and lotions of it are applied over burns and for hand disinfection. Dettol (5%) is used to disinfect instruments and plastic equipments (15 minute contact needed for disinfection). Cetrimide and Savlon are used to disinfect plastic appliances like Lippes loop (contact for 20 minute) and clinical thermometers (for 2 minute).

Bleaching powder (chlorinated lime) is widely used to disinfect water. Feces and urine can be disinfected by 5% solution of bleaching powder (contact for 1 hour). Sodium hypochlorite as 100–200 ppm solution is recommended for sterilizing infant feeding bottles. Chlorine tablets are used to disinfect water. One tablet with 4 mg of chlorine is enough to disinfect 1 liter of water (contact for ½ to 1 hour). Tincture of iodine is a good skin antiseptic. Lippes loop can be sterilized in aqueous solution of iodine. 1 drop of tincture of iodine can be added to 1 liter of water for disinfection in an emergency. Ethyl and isopropyl alcohols at 70% strength are good antiseptics and therefore are used commonly for skin disinfection and hand washing.

Formaldehyde gas is used to fumigate operation theaters, blankets, beds, books and other valuable items, which cannot be subjected to boiling. Lime as 10%–20% aqueous suspension is used to disinfect feces and urine (contact for 2 hour). Lime is also sprinkled in cattle sheds, stables and near urinals and latrines. Ethylene oxide, an explosive gas (now not encouraged) is used to sterilize fabrics, plastic equipments, cardiac catheters, books, etc. It destroys bacteria, spores and viruses.

❑ RECOMMENDED DISINFECTION PROCEDURES

Feces and urine can be disinfected by any one of the following disinfectants:

1. 50 g/L of 5% bleaching powder.
2. 100 mL/L of 10% crude phenol.
3. 50 mL/L of 5% cresol.
4. 100 mL/L of 10% formalin.

Quick lime can be used if the above are not available. If none is available boiling water may be added. After disinfection, emptied into water closet or buried.

Sputum collected in gauze or paper kerchiefs can be burnt. Boiling or autoclaving for 20 minutes at 20 pounds pressure can be done to destroy large amount of sputum. Or patient can spit in a sputum cup filled with 5% cresol and after a hour the contents can be emptied or disposed off.

Rooms can be exposed to direct sunlight and air. People must be prohibited for 48 hours if necessary. Bleaching powder at 25 ppm or more, formaldehyde solution (1% or more) or 2.5% cresol can be sprayed or used to mop the floors and hard surfaces. Rarely formaldehyde fumigation can be given to the room and it is kept closed for 6–12 hours. Formaldehyde gas can be generated by adding potassium permanganate to commercial formalin in large jars (170–200 g to 500 mL of formalin + 1 liter of water per 30 cubic meter).

❑ DISINFECTION OF WATER

Chlorination

Chlorine and its compounds are extensively used to disinfect water. For urban water supplies, chlorine gas can be used as it is cheap, quick in action, efficient and easy to apply. But it requires special equipment. Bleaching powder and perchloron containing 30% and 70% respectively of available chlorine are used for rural water supplies. As the available chlorine may get reduced on storage these disinfectants should be examined for available chlorine before using for disinfection. Chlorine compounds are stored in sealed containers without access to air in order to prevent loss of available chlorine. Chlorination of water leads to formation of toxic byproducts.

Chlorine kills pathogenic bacteria but has no effect on bacterial spores, certain viruses [polio, HA virus (HAV)], protozoal cysts and helminthic ova except in higher doses. It acts best at pH 7 and at higher pH values (> 8.5) it is unreliable.

Chlorine dioxide (ClO_2) is effective in destroying spores in doses that do not result in toxic byproduct formation. UV radiation is much more effective and reduces disinfection byproduct formation. Ozone with a CT (residual disinfectant concentration 'C' in mg/L and the disinfectant contact time 'T' in minutes) ranging from 1.7 to 6.3 can effectively inactivate bacterial spores including *Clostridium botulinum.*

Water to be disinfected should first be checked for its chlorine demand. By chlorine demand what is a meant is the amount of chlorine that is needed to oxidize the organic and inorganic materials present in the water. If organic matter in the water is high chlorine demand also will be high.

In chlorination of water supplies, chlorine should be added in such a way that there is residual chlorine (free chlorine) over and above the quantity needed to meet the chlorine demand of the particular water sample. For routine chlorination, residual chlorine of 0.2 ppm after 30 minutes of contact period is necessary to kill all the pathogenic bacteria. The amount of free and combined chlorine present 30 minutes after the addition of bleaching powder is found out by orthotolidine test.

Orthotolidine Test

The 0.1 milliliter of orthotolidine reagent is added to 1 milliliter of water. Chlorine reacts with the reagent and produces yellow color, which is matched against suitable standards or color disks. Reading taken within 10 seconds after the addition of reagent gives the amount of free chlorine and that taken after 15–20 minutes gives the amount of free and combined chlorine. A modified orthotolidine-arsenite (OTA) test can determine free and combined chlorine separately.

The volume of water is calculated and the dose of disinfectant is found out. The required quantity of disinfectant powder is made into a dilute solution and then added to the water source. The disinfectant solution is dispersed evenly in the water source by stirring with a stick. Bottom of the tank or well should not be disturbed. It should be ascertained, after half an hour, that there is at least 0.2 ppm of residual chlorine in the disinfected water source. The treated water should not be used for at least half an hour after the addition of disinfectant. Heavily polluted water can be subjected to super chlorination followed by dechlorination. By-products formed by chlorine with other substances in the water during chlorination have been found to be carcinogenic.

Break point chlorination: When chlorine is applied to water, first it reacts to remove bacteria. If chlorine is added further the residual chlorine gets reduced, because it is getting used to oxidize other organic matters present in the water. If chlorine addition is continued still further, then residual chlorine starts appearing again in the water sample. This point at which chlorine appears as residual chlorine is called the break point. This addition of chlorine beyond the break point is called break point chlorination. The residual chlorine beyond the break point is highly persistent and provides a safeguard against postcontamination.

Preparation of chlorine solution (1%): The 40 g of bleaching powder (3 heaped table spoon) is added to 1 liter of water.

Calculation of volume of water:

Circular well	: πr^2 × depth of water × 6.25
Square and rectangular well	: Length × breath × depth of water × 6.25
Tanks and ponds	: Length × breath × 1/3 depth of water at the deepest point in feet × 6.25

Normally a depth of 0–12 feet of water is taken for calculation and the above calculation gives the volume in gallons. Gallon when multiplied by 4.5 gives the volume in liters. To produce 1 ppm or 1 mg/L of water, 4 g of bleaching powder is to be added to 1,000 liters of clear water. Turbid water needs more bleaching powder.

Horrock's Apparatus

Horrock's water testing apparatus is designed to find out the dose of bleaching powder required for disinfection of water.

Contents

1. Six white cups (200 mL capacity each).
2. One black cup with a circular mark on the inside.
3. Two metal spoons (each holds 2 g of bleaching powder when filled level with the brim).
4. Seven glass stirring rods.
5. One special pipette.
6. Two droppers.
7. Starch-iodide indicator solution.
8. Instruction folder.

Procedure

1. Take one level spoonful (2 g) of bleaching powder in the black cup and make it into a thin paste with a little water. Add more water to the paste and make up the volume up to the circular mark with vigorous stirring. Allow to settle. This is the stock solution.
2. Fill the 6 white cups with water to be tested, up to about a centimeter below the brim.
3. With the special pipette provided add 1 drop of the stock solution to the 1st cup, 2 drops to the 2nd cup, 3 drops to the 3rd cup and so on.
4. Stir the water in each cup using a separate rod.
5. Wait for half an hour for the action of chlorine.
6. Add 3 drops of starch-iodide indicator to each of the white cups and stir again. Development of blue color indicates the presence of free residual chlorine.
7. Note the first cup, which shows distinct blue color. Supposing the 3rd cup shows blue color, then 3 level spoonfuls or 6 gram of bleaching powder would be required to disinfect 455 liters of water.

❑ WATER QUALITY STANDARDS

Physical Parameters

Turbidity

Less than 5 nephelometric turbidity units.

Color

Up to 15 true color units (TCU).

Taste and Odor

An unusual taste and odor is indicative of potentially harmful substances, but no guideline value is specified.

Temperature

Low temperature decreases the efficiency of disinfection, but high temperature may enhance the growth of microorganisms. No guideline has been specified in this regard.

Guideline values for naturally occurring chemicals that are of health significance in drinking water are given in Table 26.2.

Naturally occurring chemicals for which guideline values have not been established are detailed in Table 26.3.

TABLE 26.2: Guideline value

Chemical	μg/L	Remarks
Inorganic		
Arsenic	10 (A*, T†)	–
Barium	700	–
Boron	2,400	–
Chromium	50 (P‡)	For total chromium
Fluoride	1,500	Volume of water consumed and intake from other sources should be considered when setting national standards
Selenium	40 (P)	–

Contd...

Contd...

Chemical	μg/L	Remarks
Uranium	30 (P)	Only chemical aspects of uranium addressed
Organic		
Microcystin-LR	1 (P)	For total microcystin-LR (free plus cell-bound)

*A, provisional guideline value because calculated guideline value is below the achievable quantification level; ‡P, provisional guideline value because of uncertainties in the health database; †T, provisional guideline value because calculated guideline value is below the level that can be achieved through practical treatment methods, source protection, etc.

TABLE 26.3: Naturally occurring chemicals for which guideline values have not been established

Chemical	Reason for not establishing a guideline value	Remarks
Bromide	Occurs in drinking water at concentrations well below those of health concern	–
Chloride	Not of health concern at levels found in drinking water	May affect acceptability of drinking water
Hardness	Not of health concern at levels found in drinking water	May affect acceptability of drinking water
Hydrogen sulfide	Not of health concern at levels found in drinking water	May affect acceptability of drinking water
Iron	Not of health concern at levels causing acceptability problems in drinking water	May affect acceptability of drinking water
Manganese	Not of health concern at levels causing acceptability problems in drinking water	May affect acceptability of drinking water
Molybdenum	Occurs in drinking water at concentrations well below those of health concern	–
pH	Not of health concern at levels found in drinking water	An important operational water quality parameter
Potassium	Occurs in drinking water at concentrations well below those of health concern	–

Contd...

Contd...

Chemical	Reason for not establishing a guideline value	Remarks
Sodium	Not of health concern at levels found in drinking water	May affect acceptability of drinking water
Sulfate	Not of health concern at levels found in drinking water	May affect acceptability of drinking water
Total dissolved solids	Not of health concern at levels found in drinking water	May affect acceptability of drinking water

Adapted from WHO guidelines for drinking water quality, 4th edition, 2011

Guidance levels for common natural and artificial radionuclides for members of the public are detailed in Table 26.4.

Fecal Contaminants

Presumptive coliform test, test for fecal streptococci and *Clostridium perfringens* and colony counts identify fecal pollution and general contamination.

TABLE 26.4: Guidance levels for common[*] natural and artificial radionuclides for members of the public

Radioactive isotope	Radionuclide	Guidance level[†] in (Bq/L)
Naturally occurring radioactive isotope that starts the uranium decay series[‡]	Uranium-238	10
Naturally occurring radioactive isotopes belonging to the uranium decay series	Uranium-234	1
	Thorium-230	1
	Radium-226	1
	Lead-210	0.1
	Polonium-210	0.1
Naturally occurring radioactive isotope that starts the thorium decay series	Thorium-232	1
Naturally occurring radioactive isotopes belonging to the thorium decay series	Radium-228	0.1
	Thorium-228	1

Contd...

Contd...

Radioactive isotope	Radionuclide	Guidance level† in (Bq/L)
Artificial radionuclides that can be released to the environment as part of the fission products found in reactor emissions or nuclear weapons tests	Cesium-134§	10
	Cesium-137§	10
	Strontium-90§	10
Artificial radionuclide that can be released to the environment as a fission product; it is also used in nuclear medicine procedures and thus can be released into water bodies through sewage effluent	Iodine-131§,‖	10
Radioactive isotope of the hydrogen produced artificially as a fission product from nuclear power reactors and nuclear weapons tests; it may be naturally present in the environment in a very small amount and presence in a water source suggests potential industrial contamination	Tritium	10,000
Naturally occurring radioactive isotope widely distributed in nature and present in organic compounds and in the human body	Carbon-14	100
Artificial isotope formed in nuclear reactors that also exists in trace quantities in natural uranium ores	Plutonium-239§	1
Artificial isotope byproduct formed in nuclear reactors	Americium-241§	1

*This list is not exhaustive. In certain circumstances, other radionuclides should be investigated; †Guidance levels are rounded to the nearest order of magnitude; ‡Separate guidance levels are provided for individual uranium radioisotopes in terms of radioactivity (i.e. expressed as Bq/L). The provisional guideline value for total content of uranium in drinking-water is 30 μg/L based on its chemical toxicity, which is predominant compared with its radiological toxicity; §These radionuclides either may not occur in drinking water in normal situations or may be found at doses that are too low to be of significance to public health. Therefore, they are of lower priority for investigation following an exceedance of a screening level; ‖Although iodine and tritium will not be detected by standard gross activity measurements and routine analysis for these radionuclides is not necessary, if there are any reasons for believing that they may be present, radionuclide specific sampling and measurement techniques should be used. This is the reason for including them in this table (*Adapted from* WHO guidelines for drinking water quality, 4th edition 2011).

CHAPTER

27

Environmental Sanitation

❑ SANITATION

The term sanitation was used in a restricted sense to sanitary disposal of human excreta in the past. The term actually covers the whole field of controlling the environment, which is necessary to prevent diseases and promote health. National Sanitation Foundation of USA defines sanitation as "Sanitation is a way of life. It is the quality of living that is expressed in the clean home, the clean farm, the clean business, the clean neighborhood and the clean community." The term environmental sanitation has been defined as "The control of all those factors in man's physical environment, which may cause deleterious effects on physical development, health and survival." Developed countries have been able to control the environmental factors such as food, water, housing, clothing and sanitation, and raise the standard of life of people thereby improving the health of the people there. But developing countries still struggle to improve the environmental factors responsible for much of ill health.

Improved sanitation is regarded as a sociocultural and economic yardstick for any nation. However, improved sanitation is not available for 2.6 billion globally as of 2004.

The sanitation coverage in India during 2000–2001 was 21.9%. It gradually increased to 70.23% in 2010–2011. Below poverty line (BPL) households and 3.54 crore above poverty line (APL) households have been provided with sanitation facilities in rural India. Sikkim has become the first Nirmal State in the country achieving

100% total sanitation coverage. Total sanitation campaign (TSC) aims to achieve universal rural sanitation coverage by 2012.

❑ DISPOSAL OF WASTES

Solid Wastes Disposal

Garbage (food wastes), rubbish (paper, plastic, wood, metal, throw-away containers, glass, etc.), demolition products (bricks, masonry, pipes, etc.), sewage treatment residue, dead animals, manure and other discarded materials constitute solid wastes (refuse).

Refuse is preferably stored, before disposal, in galvanized steel dustbins fitted with a cover. Paper sacks are used for this purpose in the west. Public bins without cover are kept in an elevated place in the streets for the public to throw their domestic wastes.

Refuse collection ideally should be done house to house, but it is not done in India. People invariably litter the streets with refuse making its collection a difficult proposition. Refuse collection vehicles take the wastes to the place of disposal. Open carts should be replaced by closed mechanized carriers for proper disposal.

Solid wastes finally are disposed of in any one of the following methods.

Dumping

Dumping is the most unsanitary method according to WHO expert committee. Refuse is simply dumped in low-lying areas. It is the easiest method of disposal of solid wastes, but has many drawbacks. It is exposed to flies and rodents. It is a source of foul smell and ugly sight. Wind may disperse the loose wastes. Surface and ground water may get polluted.

Controlled Tipping (Sanitary Land Filling)

Controlled tipping is the most satisfactory method of refuse disposal. Refuse is placed in a trench or prepared area and covered with earth. Chemical, bacteriological and physical changes convert the refuse into an innocuous mass over a period of 4–6 months.

Incineration

Burning the wastes in incinerators is the method of choice, where land availability is a constraint. But organic wastes and plastics may release toxic chemicals like dioxins and furans when burnt. Therefore, refuse should be sorted out into different components to remove organic and PVC materials before incineration.

Composting

Refuse and night soil are dumped together in alternate layers. Bacterial action results in the formation of humus like material called compost, which is used as manure. Two methods followed for composting are:

1. Bangalore method (anaerobic method): Refuse and night soil are placed in alternate layers and the top refuse layer is covered with excavated earth. In 4–6 months, decomposition is complete. Trench pits for composting should be located far away from city limits (not loss than a ½ mile). This method is not recommended by Environmental Hygiene Committee for larger municipal towns.
2. Mechanical composting (aerobic method): The refuse is first cleared of materials like rags, bones, metal, glass and others, which may interfere with the grinding operation and then pulverized in pulverizes. The pulverized refuse is then mixed with sewage sludge or night soil in a rotating machine and incubated. Composting process is complete in 4–6 weeks.

Manure Pits

In rural areas digging manure pits to dump solid wastes is a practical solution. Garbage, dung, straw and leaves are dumped into the pits and covered with earth after each day's filling.

Burial

Trenches can be used to dump solid wastes generated in small camps. After filling, it is covered with earth. After 4–6 months the contents can be used as manure.

Excreta Disposal

Open air defecation is very common in India. Human excreta, when not disposed by sanitary methods, becomes a health hazard. It pollutes soil and water, contaminates food and acts as breeding place for house flies, all leading to the spread of many fecal-borne diseases like typhoid, diarrhea, jaundice, hookworm disease, etc. Proper disposal of human excreta is, therefore, an important environmental sanitation measure in the prevention and control of communicable diseases.

Disease causing pathogens are transmitted to a new susceptible host from the night soil of a sick person through contaminated water, soiled fingers, flies and polluted soil (Fig. 27.1).

The most effective step in preventing the transmission of fecal-borne diseases is segregation of the feces and its sanitary disposal. Sanitary latrine acts as the sanitation barrier and prevents the contact of the susceptible host with the disease causing germs in the feces (Fig. 27.2).

Methods of Excreta Disposal

Very primitive to advanced methods of excreta disposal are being followed in India.

Conservancy system: This is the most primitive method of excreta disposal. Humans (scavengers) are employed to remove fecal matter from enclosures (service latrines) used for defecation. The Environmental Hygiene Committee has recommended doing with human scavenging system and going for sanitary latrines.

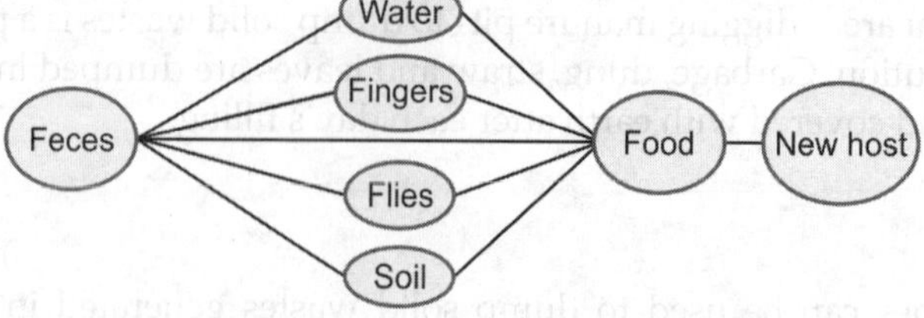

Figure 27.1: Transmission of fecal-borne diseases

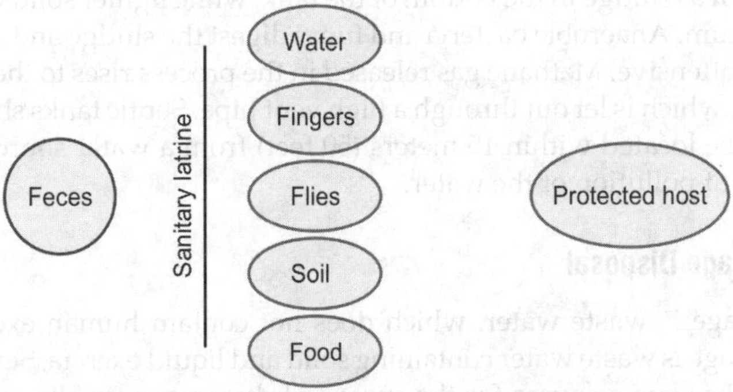

Figure 27.2: Sanitation barrier to fecal-borne diseases

Sanitary latrines: They are as follows.

Bore-hole latrine: A hole, 13–16 feet deep and 12–16 inches in diameter, with a concrete squatting plate, is used for defecation. When the hole is full up to 20 inches from the brim it is closed with earth and another hole used. Anaerobic digestion converts the night soil into an innocuous mass. Smell and fly nuisance cannot be avoided in this type of latrine and is not recommended now.

Dug-well latrine: A bigger pit, 10–12 feet deep and 30 inches in diameter with a concrete squatting plate placed over, forms this type of latrine. When the pit is filled up a new pit is prepared. Smell and fly nuisance will be there.

Water-seal latrine: This is the modern sanitary method of excreta disposal. This consists of a latrine pan to receive night soil, urine and wash water, a squatting plate with foot rest and an 'S' trap – a bent pipe, which will hold water in its bend (water seal). The water seal, seals off night soil from flies and also eliminates smell nuisance by preventing the escape of foul gases. A connecting pipe takes the night soil and flush water to a dug well 10–12 feet deep, 30 inches in diameter. When the pit fills up, another can be dug up nearby and the connecting pipe directed into it. A super structure for privacy around the squatting plate is erected.

Septic tank: It can be used in the place of dug well, in urban areas where land is a constraint, for the disposal of excreta. It is a masonry tank with two chambers. The flushed out night soil settles down as sludge in the bottom of the tank, while lighter solids float as scum. Anaerobic bacteria and fungi digest the sludge and make it inoffensive. Methane gas released in the process rises to the surface, which is let out through a high vent pipe. Septic tanks should not be located within 15 meters (50 feet) from a water source for fear of pollution of the water.

Sewage Disposal

Sullage is waste water, which does not contain human excreta. Sewage is waste water containing solid and liquid excreta. Sewage can become a source for the spread of diseases, specially enteric and helminthic when it is allowed to pollute soil and water supplies, contaminate food and stagnate to facilitating fly and mosquito breeding. Safe disposal of sewage, therefore, is an important environmental sanitation measure to prevent disease spread.

Sewage Treatment

Sewage must be treated to make it inoffensive and safe before disposal.

Sewage is first allowed to pass through a metal screen. Screening removes large floating objects like pieces of wood, rags, dead animals, etc.

Sewage then goes to grit chamber. Here, heavier solids like sand and gravel settle down, while organic matters pass through. Next sewage is let into primary sedimentation tank, which is a large tank. Sewage flows slowly across the tank and spends 6–8 hours in the tank. Suspended matter, 50%–70% of solid matter, settles down. Sludge formed in the tank bed is removed by mechanically operated devices without disturbing the operation in the tank. Microorganisms convert organic substances into simple substances and ammonia. Scum formed, on the surface, from fat and grease, is removed. If organic trade waste is present, the sewage is treated with chemicals like lime, aluminum sulfate and ferrous sulfate, which precipitate the animal proteins quickly.

The effluent from primary sedimentation tank still contains organic matter and microorganisms. It is subjected to aerobic oxidation in either trickling filter bed or by activated sludge process. In trickling filter method, the effluent is sprinkled on the surface of the filter bed. As the effluent percolates through the filter bed, it gets oxidized by the bacterial flora in the zoogleal layer formed by algae, fungi, protozoa and bacteria. The oxidized sewage is let into secondary sedimentation tanks.

In larger cities, activated sludge process is employed to oxidize the sewage. The effluent from primary sedimentation tank is mixed with sludge—a rich culture of aerobic bacteria, drawn from final settling tank. Organic matter gets oxidized to CO_2, nitrates and water by aerobic bacteria. Typhoid and cholera bacilli are destroyed in the process and coliforms greatly reduced.

The oxidized sewage is next let into secondary sedimentation tank and detained for 2–3 hours. The sludge that forms in this tank is aerated and inoffensive, rich in bacteria, nitrogen and phosphates. This aerated sludge is let into sludge digestion tanks.

In sludge digestion tanks, aerated sludge undergoes anaerobic autodigestion by which complex solids are broken down into water, CO_2, methane and ammonia. Sludge digestion taken 3–4 weeks or longer for completion. Alternatively aerated sludge can be disposed into sea by pumping. Composting with refuse also can be done.

The supernatant effluent is disposed by letting into rivers and streams (disposal by dilution) or it can be used for irrigation purposes. Untreated sewage is sometimes discharged into sea. But raw sewage should never be discharged into rivers.

A cheap method of sewage treatment is the use of what are called oxidation ponds for oxidation. Oxidation ponds are open, shallow pools, 3–5 feet deep, with an inlet and an outlet. Organic matter in the sewage is oxidized by bacteria to CO_2, ammonia and water. Algae present in the pond utilize CO_2, water and inorganic minerals, with the help of sunlight, for their growth. In sunlight, algae liberate O_2, which is used for oxidation. Aerobic oxidation takes place in sunlight in the day, while in the night, in the bottom layers, anaerobic oxidation takes place. The supernatant effluent may be used either for irrigation of vegetable crops or discharged into river or other water courses after appropriate treatment.

❑ WASTES FROM HEALTHCARE ACTIVITIES (CENTRAL POLLUTION CONTROL BOARD)

Approximately 20% of hospital wastes are considered hazardous materials that may be infectious, toxic or radioactive.

1. Infectious wastes—cultures and stocks of infectious agents, wastes from infected patients, wastes contaminated with blood and its derivatives, discarded diagnostic samples, infected animals from laboratories and contaminated materials (swabs, bandages) and equipment (disposable medical devices, etc.).
2. Anatomic—recognizable body parts and animal carcasses.
3. Sharps—syringes, disposable scalpels and blades, etc.
4. Chemicals—like solvents and disinfectants.
5. Pharmaceuticals—expired, unused and contaminated; whether the drugs themselves (sometimes toxic and powerful chemicals) or their metabolites, vaccines and sera. Chemicals and pharmaceuticals amount to about 3% of waste from healthcare activities.
6. Genotoxic waste—highly hazardous, mutagenic, teratogenic or carcinogenic such as cytotoxic drugs used in cancer treatment and their metabolites.
7. Radioactive wastes—such as glassware contaminated with radioactive diagnostic material or radiotherapeutic materials.
8. Wastes—with high heavy metal content such as broken mercury thermometers.

Infectious and anatomic wastes together represent the majority of the hazardous waste up to 15% of the total waste from healthcare activities.

Sharps represent about 1% of the total waste from healthcare activities.

Genotoxic waste, radioactive matter and heavy metal content represent about 1% of the total waste from healthcare activities.

The major sources of healthcare waste are hospitals and other healthcare establishments, laboratories and research centers, mortuary and autopsy centers, animal research and testing laboratories, blood banks and collection services and nursing homes for the elderly.

High-income countries can generate up to 6 kilograms of hazardous waste per person per year. In the majority of low-income countries, healthcare waste is usually not separated into hazardous or non-hazardous waste. In these countries, the total healthcare waste per person per year is anywhere from 0.5–3 kilograms.

Health Impacts

Healthcare waste is a reservoir of potentially harmful microorganisms, which can infect hospital patients, healthcare workers and the general public. Other potential infectious risks include the spread of, sometimes resistant microorganisms from healthcare establishments into the environment. These risks have so far been only poorly investigated. Wastes and byproducts can also cause injuries, e.g. radiation burns or sharps-inflicted injuries; poisoning and pollution, whether through the release of pharmaceutical products, in particular, antibiotics and cytotoxic drugs, through the waste water or by toxic elements or compounds such as mercury or dioxins.

Disposal of Cytotoxic Waste

Cytotoxic waste is highly hazardous and should never be land filled or discharged into the sewerage system. Disposal options include the following.

Return to Original Supplier

Safely packaged, but outdated drugs and drugs that are no longer needed should be returned to the supplier. This is currently the preferred option for countries that lack the facilities for incineration. Drugs that have been unpacked should be repackaged in a manner as similar as possible to the original packaging and marked outdated or not for use.

Incineration at High Temperatures

Full destruction of all cytotoxic substances may require temperatures up to 1,200°C; incineration at lower temperatures may result in the release of hazardous cytotoxic vapors into the atmosphere.

Modern double-chamber pyrolytic incinerators are suitable, provided that a temperature of 1,200°C with a minimum gas residence time of 2 seconds or 1,000°C with a minimum gas residence time of 5 seconds can be achieved in the second chamber. The incinerator should be fitted with gas-cleaning equipment. Incineration is also possible in rotary kilns designed for thermal decomposition of chemical wastes, in foundries or in cement kilns, which usually have furnaces operating well in excess of 850°C. Incineration in most municipal incinerators, in single-chamber incinerators or by open-air burning is inappropriate for the disposal of cytotoxic waste.

Treatment of Hospital Waste

Treatment of waste is required:

- To disinfect the waste, so that it is no longer the source of infection
- To reduce the volume of the waste
- Make waste unrecognizable for esthetic reasons
- Make recycled items unusable.

General Waste in Hospital

The 85% of the waste generated in the hospital belongs to this category. The safe disposal of this waste is the responsibility of the local authority.

Biomedical Waste in Hospital

The 15% of hospital waste are biomedical waste.

Methods of Treatment in Hospital

Deep burial: The waste under category 1 and 2 only can be accorded deep burial and only in cities having less than 500,000 population.

Autoclave and microwave treatment: Standards for the autoclaving and microwaving are also mentioned in the Biomedical Waste (Management and Handling) Rules, 1998. All equipment installed/shared should meet these specifications. The waste under category

3, 4, 6, 7 can be treated by these techniques. Standards for the autoclaving are also laid down.

Shredding: The plastic (IV bottles, IV sets, syringes, catheters, etc.), sharps (needles, blades, glass, etc.) should be shredded, but only after chemical treatment/microwaving/autoclaving. Needle destroyers can be used for disposal of needles directly without chemical treatment.

Secured landfill: The incinerator ash, discarded medicines, cytotoxic substances and solid chemical waste should be treated by this option.

Incineration: The incinerator should be installed and made operational as per specification under the BMW rules, 1998 and a certificate may be taken from CPCB/State Pollution Control Board and emission levels, etc. should be defined. In case of small hospitals, facilities can be shared. The waste under category 1, 2, 3, 5, 6 can be incinerated depending upon the local policies of the hospital and feasibility. The polythene bags made of chlorinated plastics should not be incinerated. It may be noted that there are options available for disposal of certain category of waste. The individual hospital can choose the best option depending upon the facilities available and its financial resources. However, it may be noted that depending upon the option chosen, correct color of the bag needs to be used.

Safety Measures

All the generators of biomedical waste should adopt universal precautions and appropriate safety measures, while doing therapeutic and diagnostic activities and also while handling the biomedical waste. It should be ensured that:

- Drivers, collectors and other handlers are aware of the nature and risk of the waste
- Written instructions provided regarding the procedures to be adopted in the event of spillage/accidents
- Protective gears provided and instructions regarding their use are given
- Workers are protected by vaccination against tetanus and hepatitis B.

Training

- Each and every hospital must have well planned awareness and training program for all categories of personnel including administrators (medical, paramedical and administrative)
- All the medical professionals must be made aware of Biomedical Waste (Management and Handling) Rules, 1998
- To institute awards for safe hospital waste management and universal precaution practices
- Training should be conducted to all categories of staff in appropriate language/medium and in an acceptable manner.

❑ E-WASTE

E-waste contains over 1,000 different substances and chemicals, many of which are toxic and are likely to create serious problems for the environment and human health if not handled properly (Table 27.1).

E-waste in India

Even though the recycling operation is covered under various labor and industrial laws in India, almost none of them are implemented in the 'informal' sector. Applicable laws include the Factories Act, which lays down stringent requirements for industrial operations including some concerning health and safety conditions as well as working hours. There are requirements of worker compensation and medical insurance under the Employees State Insurance (ESI) Act. The ESI Act also covers areas such as maternity benefits and hospital care. The Provident Fund Act and The Workmen's Compensation Act provide saving to protect against old age and joblessness. There are also threshold limit values (TLVs) set for the concentration of chemicals in the air for worker exposure. Many of the small-scale enterprises recycling e-wastes are illegal or semilegal and because of this, checks are difficult. In order to implement laws, information on the dangers in the workplace needs to be disseminated and labor unions must deal with issues of worker safety adequately. Finally, a significant number of workers are children. Many policy-makers understand child labor as a consequence of poverty and do not take initiatives to curb it. For a manufacturer, however, child labor is merely a cheap source of work.

E-waste Management

Searching for cheaper ways to get rid of the wastes, traders began shipping hazardous waste to developing countries. International outrage following these irresponsible activities led to the drafting and adoption of strategic plans and regulations at the Basel Convention. The Convention Secretariat, in Geneva, Switzerland, facilitates and implements the plans and regulations of the Convention and related agreements. It also provides assistance and guidelines on legal and technical issues, gathers statistical data and conducts training on the proper management of hazardous waste.

TABLE 27.1: Effects of e-waste constituents on health

Source of e-waste and the constituent	Health effects
Solder in printed circuit boards, glass panels and gaskets in computer monitors—lead	Causes damage to central and peripheral nervous systems, blood systems and kidney Affects brain development in children Lead tends to accumulate in the environment and has high acute and chronic effects on plants, animals and microorganisms
Chip resistors and semiconductors—cadmium	Toxic irreversible effects on human health Accumulates in kidney and liver Causes neural damage Teratogenic
Relays and switches, printed circuit boards—mercury	Chronic damage to the brain, kidneys and developing fetus Respiratory and skin disorders due to bioaccumulation in fishes
Corrosion protection of untreated and galvanized steel plates, decorator or harder for steel housings—hexavalent chromium	Asthmatic bronchitis DNA* damage

Contd...

Contd...

Source of e-waste and the constituent	Health effects
Cabling and computer housing—plastics including PVC†	Burning produces dioxin It causes reproductive and developmental problems Immune system damage Interfere with regulatory hormones
Plastic housing of electronic equipments and circuit boards—brominated flame retardants	Disrupts endocrine system functions
Front panel of CRTs‡—barium	Short-term exposure causes: Brain swelling Muscle weakness Damage to heart, liver and spleen
Motherboard—beryllium	Carcinogenic (lung cancer) Inhalation of fumes and dust causes chronic beryllium disease or berylliosis Skin disease such as warts
Toners	Inhalation is the primary exposure pathway Acute exposure may lead to respiratory tract irritation Carbon black has been classified as a class 2B carcinogen, possibly carcinogenic to humans Reports indicate that color toners (cyan, magenta and yellow) contain heavy metals
Phosphor and additives	The phosphor coating on CRTs contain heavy metals such as cadmium and other rare earth metals, e.g. zinc and vanadium as additives These metals and their compounds are very toxic This is a serious hazard posed for those who dismantle CRTs by hand

*DNA, deoxyribonucleic acid; †PVC, polyvinyl chloride; ‡CRTs, cathode-ray tube.

The Basel Convention brought about a respite to the transboundary movement of hazardous waste. India and other Countries have ratified the Convention. However, United States (US) is not a party to the ban and is responsible for disposing hazardous waste, such as, e-waste to Asian countries even today.

In the European Union where the annual quantity of electronic waste is likely to double in the next 12 years, the European Parliament recently passed legislation that will require manufacturers to take back their electronic products when consumers discard them, this is called extended producer responsibility. It also mandates a timetable for phasing out most toxic substances in electronic products.

In industries, management of e-waste should begin at the point of generation. This can be done by waste minimization techniques and by sustainable product design. Waste minimization in industries can be done by adopting:

- Inventory management
- Production-process modification
- Volume reduction
- Recovery and reuse.

Inventory Management

Proper control over the materials used in the manufacturing process is an important way to reduce waste generation (Freeman, 1989). By reducing both the quantity of hazardous materials used in the process and the amount of excess raw materials in stock, the quantity of waste generated can be reduced. This can be done in two ways, i.e. establishing material-purchase review and control procedures and inventory tracking system.

Developing review procedures for all material purchased is the first step in establishing an inventory management program. Procedures should require that, all materials be approved prior to purchase. In the approval process, all production materials are evaluated to examine, if they contain hazardous constituents and whether alternative non-hazardous materials are available.

Another inventory management procedure for waste reduction is to ensure that only the needed quantity of a material is ordered. This will require the establishment of a strict inventory tracking system. Purchase procedures must be implemented, which ensure that materials are ordered only on an as-needed basis and that only the amount needed for a specific period of time is ordered.

Production-process Modification

Changes can be made in the production process, which will reduce waste generation. This reduction can be accomplished by changing the materials used to make the product or by the more efficient use of input materials in the production process or both. Potential waste minimization techniques can be broken down into three categories:

- Improved operating and maintenance procedures
- Material change
- Process-equipment modification.

Improved operating and maintenance procedures: Improvements in the operation and maintenance of process equipment can result in significant waste reduction. This can be accomplished by reviewing current operational procedures or lack of procedures and examination of the production process for ways to improve its efficiency. Instituting standard operation procedures can optimize the use of raw materials in the production process and reduce the potential for materials to be lost through leaks and spills. A strict maintenance program, which stresses corrective maintenance, can reduce waste generation caused by equipment failure. An employee-training program is a key element of any waste reduction program. Training should include correct operating and handling procedures, proper equipment use, recommended maintenance and inspection schedules, correct process control specifications and proper management of waste materials.

Material change: Hazardous materials used in either a product formulation or a production process may be replaced with a less hazardous or non-hazardous material. This is a very widely used technique and is applicable to most manufacturing processes. Implementation of this waste reduction technique may require only some minor process adjustments or it may require extensive new process equipment. For example, a circuit board manufacturer can replace solvent-based product with water-based flux and simultaneously replace solvent vapor degreaser with detergent parts washer.

Process-equipment modification: Installing more efficient process equipment or modifying existing equipment to take advantage of better production techniques can significantly reduce waste generation. New or updated equipment can use process materials more efficiently producing less waste. Additionally, such efficiency reduces the number of rejected or off-specification products, thereby reducing the amount of material, which has to be reworked or disposed off. Modifying existing process equipment can be a very cost-effective method of reducing waste generation. In many cases the modification can just be relatively simple changes in the way the materials are handled within the process to ensure that they are not wasted. For example, in many electronic manufacturing operations, which involve coating a product, such as electroplating or painting, chemicals are used to strip off coating from rejected products so that they can be recoated. These chemicals, which can include acids, caustics, cyanides, etc. are often a hazardous waste and must be properly managed. By reducing the number of parts that have to be reworked, the quantity of waste can be significantly reduced.

Volume Reduction

Volume reduction includes those techniques that remove the hazardous portion of a waste from a non-hazardous portion. These techniques are usually to reduce the volume and thus the cost of disposing of a waste material. The techniques that can be used to reduce waste-stream volume can be divided into two general categories: source segregation and waste concentration. Segregation of wastes is in many cases a simple and economical technique for waste reduction. Wastes containing different types of metals can be treated separately so that the metal value in the sludge can be recovered. Concentration of a waste stream may increase the likelihood that the material can be recycled or reused. Methods include gravity and vacuum filtration, ultra filtration, reverse osmosis, freeze vaporization, etc.

For example, an electronic component manufacturer can use compaction equipments to reduce volume of waste cathode-ray tube.

Recovery and Reuse

This technique could eliminate waste disposal costs, reduce raw material costs and provide income from a salable waste. Waste can be recovered on-site or at an off-site recovery facility or through inter industry exchange. A number of physical and chemical techniques are available to reclaim a waste material such as reverse osmosis, electrolysis, condensation, electrolytic recovery, filtration, centrifugation, etc. For example, a printed-circuit board manufacturer can use electrolytic recovery to reclaim metals from copper and tin-lead plating bath.

However, recycling of hazardous products has little environmental benefit if it simply moves the hazards into secondary products that eventually have to be disposed off. Unless the goal is to redesign the product to use non-hazardous materials, such recycling is a false solution.

Sustainable Product Design

Minimization of hazardous wastes should be at product design stage itself keeping in mind the following factors.

1. Rethink the product design: Efforts should be made to design a product with fewer amounts of hazardous materials. For example, the efforts to reduce material use are reflected in some new computer designs that are flatter, lighter and more integrated. Other companies propose centralized networks similar to the telephone system.
2. Use of renewable materials and energy: Biobased plastics are plastics made with plant-based chemicals or plant-produced polymers rather than from petrochemicals. Biobased toners, glues and inks are used more frequently. Solar computers also exist, but they are currently very expensive.
3. Use of non-renewable materials that are safer: Because many of the materials used are non-renewable, designers could ensure the product is built for reuse, repair and/or upgradeability. Some computer manufacturers such as Dell and Gateway lease out their products thereby ensuring they get them back to further upgrade and lease out again.

❑ SANITATION IN SLAUGHTERHOUSE

Proper fencing, pest (insects, rodents and birds) control measures and liquid and solid waste disposal are the main environmental hygiene activities in slaughterhouses (Tables 27.2 and 27.3).

TABLE 27.2: Wastewater treatment systems

Category	Essential treatment
Large slaughterhouse	Self-cleaning type screening, anaerobic treatment, aerobic treatment and filter press for dewatering of sludge
Medium slaughterhouse	Two-stage screening (bar type), anaerobic pond and polishing pond
Small slaughterhouse	Two-stage screening (bar type), anaerobic pond and polishing pond

TABLE 27.3: Sanitation standards in slaughterhouse

Category of slaughterhouse/unit (parameters)	Limit not to exceed (mg/L)
Large slaughterhouse* (capacity above 70 TLWK†/day)	
Biochemical oxygen demand (BOD_5) at 20°C	100
Suspended solids	100
Oil and grease	10
Medium‡ and small§ slaughterhouse (capacity above 70 TLWK/day)	
BOD_5 at 20°C	500
Meat processing industry||	
Frozen meat	
BOD_5 at 20°C	30
Suspended solids	50
Oil and grease	10
Raw meat from own slaughterhouse	
BOD_5 at 20°C	30
Suspended solids	50
Oil and grease	10
Raw meat from other slaughterhouse: Disposal via screen and septic tank¶	
Seafood industry	
BOD_5 at 20°C	30

Contd...

Contd...

Category of slaughterhouse/unit (parameters)	Limit not to exceed (mg/L)
Suspended solids	50
Oil and grease	10

*Large slaughterhouse, large animals greater than 40,000 and goats/sheeps 600,000 or daily live weight killed greater than 70 tonnes; †TLWK, tonne of live weight killed; ‡Medium slaughterhouse, large animals around 10,001–40,000 and goats/sheeps 100,001–600,000 or daily live weight killed 15–70 tonnes; §Small slaughterhouse, large animals greater than 10,000 and goats/sheeps upto 100,000 or daily live weight killed upto 5 tonnes; ||The industrials having slaughterhouse along with meat processing units will be considered in meat processing category for fixing standard; ¶In case of disposal into municipal sewer where sewage is treated, the industries shall install screen and oil and grease separation units.

Adapted from Central Pollution Control Board, Ministry of Environment and Forests, GOI.

Insect Control

Biological control (using natural enemies of the pests), sanitation and water management programs, physical methods like burning and use of sticky adhesives, disrupting the breeding cycle by release of sterilized males or genetically modified species, use of chemical attractants to trap or confuse the breeding pattern are all the different methods that can be employed in the control of insects. Chemical insecticides are to be avoided if possible.

Rodent Control

Preventing access to food supplies will force rats to migrate in search of foods elsewhere. Use of baits and traps also will be useful. Biological control with cats and dogs should not be permitted in the production areas.

Bird Control

Preventing access to buildings is the best way to control birds. Toxicants, shooting and trapping may also be used to control birds.

Personal hygiene practices like hand washing before work, after using toilets, after touching dirty objects and materials and after smoking and eating should be stressed for the workers handling the food products. Hand washing facilities must be sufficient. Practices like scratching the skin or the hair, correcting clothes and picking the nose will transfer bacteria to the hands and thence to meat handled by hand. Use of special bacteriostatic soap and use of nail brush are recommended.

Alkaline Hydrolysis

Slaughterhouse waste was processed in rendering houses and meat and bone meal was used as a component in animal meals before the appearance of bovine spongiform encephalopathy. However, the emergence of mad cow disease resulted in the prohibition of the use of meat and bone meal in animal nutrition. The rendering houses have remained functional for carcasses and slaughterhouse waste using incarceration as the only proper method prescribed for final sanitation of meat and bone meal. However, slaughterhouse waste is a highly valuable raw material for anaerobic digestion. This work emphasizes the use of alkaline hydrolysis as a pretreatment in the production of biogas for the first and second category of slaughterhouse waste. During alkaline hydrolysis, slaughterhouse waste is mixed with alkali NaOH/KOH and boiled for 3–6 hours at 150°C with a pressure of 4 bars. The chemical bonds of the large protein molecules, nucleic acids (DNA and RNA), lipids, viruses and prions break into smaller molecules which react with NaOH/KOH to form Na/K-salts. Fatty acids react with alkalis to form soaps. The resulting chemical compound is a neutral or partially alkaline solution of organic substances suitable for anaerobe microbiological decomposition or a valuable raw material for anaerobic digestion.

Disposal

Methods of waste disposal are given in Table 27.4.

Diseases Caused due to Dead Bodies

Cholera

Contact with the body leads to exposure to *Vibrio cholerae* and requires careful washing using soap and water.

TABLE 27.4: Method of waste disposal

Type of waste	Method of disposal
Water consisting of inedible offals, animal tissue, organs, body parts, carcasses, etc.	Rendering (in large slaughterhouse), rendering or controlled incineration (in medium slaughterhouse), burial (in small slaughterhouse)
Stomach/intestinal contents, dungs, etc.	Composting (all types)
Sludge from wastewater treatment system	Composting (all types)

Adapted from Central Pollution Control Board, Ministry of Environment and Forests, GOI.

Ebola

Ebola is spread through bodily secretions such as blood, saliva, vomit, urine and stool but can easily be killed with soap and water. Those dealing with the disposal of bodies require high levels of protection.

Typhus and Plague

To avoid infestation with the fleas and lice that spread these diseases, protective clothing should be worn. Body bags should be used to store the bodies prior to burial or cremation. Cremation sites should be located at least 500 meters downwind of dwellings. The resultant ashes should be disposed of according to the cultural and religious practice of the community.

❑ ACTION IN MEDICAL EPIDEMICS

Where possible, in the case of a medical epidemic, body handling should be left to specialist medical staff. Rather than using lime for disinfection purposes which has a limited effect on infectious pathogens, it is better to use chlorine solution or other medical disinfectants. Any vehicles used to transport bodies to burial or cremation sites during epidemics should also be disinfected after use. It is important to make communities aware of the risks of contagion from practices such as traditional washing of the dead. Also, any large gathering, including a funeral, can be a way of spreading an epidemic. Consequently, burial or cremation should take place soon after death at a site near the place of death with limits placed on the size of crowd.

❑ GLOBAL ENVIRONMENTAL PROBLEMS

In this scientific era man has been able to conquer many of the diseases. Now, he enjoys a better standard of life overall. At the same time, it is also found that many of man's activities have led to damage of not only local ecology but also of global environment. Population explosion and the concomitant over exploitation of the resources of the earth result in degradation of the environment. The ecological disturbances have reached such a stage now that it requires action at the global level.

Disruption of the stratospheric ozone by CFCs is an important environmental problem. As ozone layer gets depleted, UVB radiation to earth is increased. UVB is known to cause skin cancer, cataract and reduced immune response in humans besides its ill-effects on the ecosystem particularly on ocean and terrestrial plants.

Methane, CO_2 and CFCs generated during human activities prevent radiation of heat from the earth and thereby increase the temperature on the earth. Consequent elevation of sea level in coastal areas, ill-effects on agriculture, change in geographic distribution of insect–transmitted infectious diseases all can cause deleterious effects on society, economy and health.

Tropical forest is being denuded due to over exploitation for construction materials, fuels and farming. This reduces the environment preserving ability of forests. Erosion of top soil and floods, global warming and extinction of many species are the adverse consequences.

Acidification of lakes and marshes by acid rain (SO_2 and NO_2 converted to sulfuric acid and nitric acid respectively) kill living things including fish. Ago forests get damaged directly by acid rains and indirectly through acidification of soil. Acid water can damage concrete, lime stone and marble.

Various human activities pollute oceans. Pollutants from mountains, forest and farm lands, factory wastes, sewage, sea dumping of construction wastes and discharge from ships all pollute oceans causing change in the ecosystem of the oceans. Occurrence of large red tides in coastal regions and an increase in anaerobic environment causing blue tides are the result of ocean pollution.

Hazardous wastes generated in developed countries are often transferred to developing countries for economic reasons.

Nuclear disasters can affect areas much beyond the place of occurrence. Chernobyl power plant accident in 1986 in Russia caused radiation pollution over all of Europe far beyond Soviet borders.

Therefore, it can be easily inferred that global environmental problems are the result of expansion of socioeconomic activities that take place at high speed. Cooperation of all nations is essential to control the global environmental problems. International conference on environmental issues at Rio de Janeiro was an important milestone in the efforts to control global environmental problems. All the participating countries accepted to cooperate in the action plan to harmonize development with preservation. The International Council of Scientific Unions proposed the Agenda of Science of Environment and Development into 21st century. World Climate Research Program, International Geosphere–Biosphere Program and Human Dimension of Global Environmental Change are the other programs that work on the global environmental problems.

CHAPTER

28

Occupational Health

❑ OCCUPATIONAL ENVIRONMENT

Workers represent half the world's population and are the major contributors to economic and social development. Their health is determined not only by workplace hazards but also by social and individual factors and access to health services. Despite the availability of effective interventions to prevent occupational hazards and to protect and promote health at the workplace, large gaps exist between and within countries with regard to the health status of workers and their exposure to occupational risks. Still only a small minority of the global workforce has access to occupational health services.

Occupational health deals with all aspects of health and safety in the workplace and has a strong focus on primary prevention of hazards. The objective of the occupational health service is to safeguard the health of workers wherever they work. Any occupational environment will be made up of:

- Physical, chemical and biological agents
- Machines
- Human beings.

Physical factors (heat, cold, humidity, radiation, light, noise, vibrations, dust and ionizing radiation) and chemical agents (toxic dusts, gases and variety of chemicals) in working environment can affect the health of the workmen. According to WHO, every year atleast 200,000 people die from cancer related to their workplace. Lung cancer, mesothelioma and bladder cancer are among the most common types of occupational cancers.

Biological agents like bacteria and virus may also pose hazard to them in certain occupations.

Unguarded machines, moving parts, poor installation of the plant and lack of safety measures, may cause accidents. Unphysiological postures for long hours cause fatigue, diseases of joints and muscles affecting the workmen's efficiency and health.

Man-to-man relationship in the working environment is also crucial to the health of workmen. Service conditions, job satisfaction, security, worker's participation, welfare conditions, trade union activities and many such factors influence the health of the workmen. A good domestic environment of the workmen is also equally important for their health and efficiency.

❑ OCCUPATIONAL HAZARDS

The workmen will encounter any of the five types of hazards, depending upon the occupation. They are physical, chemical, biological, mechanical and psychosocial hazards.

Physical Hazards

Heat

Heat in industries may cause burns, heat exhaustion, heat stroke, etc. Radiant heat and stagnant heat are encountered in foundries and jute, and textile industries respectively. Mines also have high temperatures.

Cold

Cold conditions may cause chilblains, immersion foot, frostbite, etc.

Light

Light in a working place should be optimal. Poor light can cause eyestrain, headache, lacrimation and congestion, while excess light causes discomfort, annoyance and visual fatigue and even accidents due to blurring of vision.

Noise

Noise is produced in many industries. Exposure to excessive noise may result in either temporary or permanent loss of hearing. It may also cause nervousness, fatigue and interference in communication.

Exposure to vibration for long periods may induce spasm in blood vessels of fingers and may also affect the joints of the hands, elbows and shoulders.

Ultraviolet Radiation

Ultraviolet radiation from arc welding may cause intense conjunctivitis and keratitis in the eyes.

Ionizing Radiation

Ionizing radiation from X-rays and radioactive isotopes (cobalt 60, phosphorus 32) can cause genetic changes, cancer, leukemia, sterility and even death in extreme cases.

Chemical Hazards

When skin is exposed to direct contact with chemicals, dermatitis, eczema, ulcers and even cancer may be caused. Some chemicals get absorbed systemically through the skin and cause adverse effects.

Inhalation of dust (0.1–150 microns) emanating from the industrial floor, gases released or leaked during many processes and fumes and dusts of metals and their compounds used in industrial processes may affect the health of workmen, depending upon the duration and severity of exposure. Ingestion of chemicals through contaminated hands, foods or cigarettes may also cause ill health in them.

Biological Hazards

Individuals handling animal products (hair, wool, hides) and agricultural workers may be exposed to diseases like brucellosis, leptospirosis, anthrax, hydatidosis, tetanus, etc.

Mechanical Hazards

Accidents in the shop floor are due to protruding or moving parts.

Psychosocial Hazards

Lack of job satisfaction, frustration, poor interpersonal relationships and insecurity of the job affect workmen psychologically and lead to psychosomatic illness in them.

Psychological problems like; hostility, aggressiveness, anxiety, depression, alcoholism, drug abuse, sickness, absenteeism and psychosomatic problems like; headache, pain in shoulders, back and neck, propensity to peptic ulcer, hypertension and heart disease can be caused by bad working environment.

Pneumoconiosis

Pneumoconiosis is the accumulation of dust in the lungs and the tissue reaction to its presence. The lung changes in pneumoconiosis range from simple deposition of dust, as in the case of siderosis (deposition of iron dust in lungs, clearly observed by X-ray examination, but with no clinical manifestations) to conditions with impairment of lung function, such as byssinosis (caused by cotton and flax dust) and to the more serious fibrotic lung diseases such as silicosis (caused by free crystalline silica dust). These lung diseases may cripple the workmen by reducing their working capacity. Some of these conditions are described below.

Silicosis

Silicosis is the commonest and one of the most serious occupational diseases. It is irreversible fibrosis of the lungs caused by inhalation of free crystalline silica dust (silica dioxide). It is estimated that about 3 million people working in various types of mines, ceramics, potteries, foundries, metal grinding, stone crushing, agate grinding, slate pencil industry, etc. are occupationally exposed to free silica dust and are at potential risk of developing silicosis. Extremely high exposures are associated with much shorter latency and more rapid disease progression. Silica exposure also predisposes to development of pulmonary tuberculosis, which is an important public health problem in the country.

Respirable silica dust may be invisible to the naked eye and is so light that it can remain airborne for a long time. It can thus travel long distances in the air and so affect populations not otherwise considered to be at risk.

Remedial Measures

Action should be taken before exposure happens. As there is no effective treatment for this condition, proper dust control measures, personal protective measures and periodic examination of workers are essential to control this disease. Silicosis is a notifiable disease under the Factories Act 1948 and Mines Act 1952. Inhaled crystalline silica (in the form of quartz or cristobalite) from occupational sources is classified by the International Agency for Research on Cancer (IARC) as a Group 1 human lung carcinogen.

Anthracosis

Exposure to coal dust causes anthracosis. It is a common affliction of coal miners and others, who work with coal. Inhaled coal dust progressively buildup in the lungs leading to inflammation and fibrosis and in the worst case necrosis. Progressive massive fibrosis is marked by lung dysfunction, pulmonary hypertension and cor pulmonale and can cause premature death. There is no cure for anthracosis and treatment generally involves providing symptomatic relief. It is notifiable under the Mines Act 1952.

Byssinosis

Byssinosis is an occupational lung disease caused by exposure to cotton, flax and hemp dust. Maximum numbers of workers with byssinosis are reported in the cotton textile industry. In India, there are about 1.07 million workers engaged in the manufacture of cotton textiles.

The workers engaged in the initial processes of textile manufacturing (blow, card, frame and ring frame) are exposed to cotton dust and develop the disease after some years of exposure.

The epidemiological studies conducted by National Institute of Occupational Health (NIOH) recently showed a very high prevalence of the disease especially in blow (30%) and card (38%) sections. These prevalence figures were same as reported in UK and other countries of the world.

Smoking, impaired lung function and a history of respiratory allergy increase a textile worker's risk of developing byssinosis. Byssinosis does not lead to permanently disabling lung disease.

It manifests as chronic cough, progressive dyspnea, chronic bronchitis and emphysema. Reducing exposure is essential. Any worker who has symptoms of byssinosis or who has breathing problems should be transferred to a less-contaminated area.

Prevention

Eliminating exposure to textile dust is the surest way to prevent byssinosis. Using exhaust hoods, improving ventilation and employing wetting procedures are very successful methods of controlling dust levels to prevent byssinosis. Protective equipment required during certain procedures also prevents exposure to levels of contamination standard for cotton dust exposure.

Bagassosis

Bagassosis, an extrinsic allergic alveolitis, develops in people who inhale sugarcane dust (bagasse). It is caused by a thermophilic actinomycete. Initially it manifests as acute bronchiolitis characterized by breathlessness, cough, hemoptysis and fever. Early treatment will cure the disease. But repeated exposure results in significant pulmonary fibrosis. Terminal complications of pulmonary fibrosis include respiratory failure and cor pulmonale.

Farmer's lung, caused by spores of thermophilic actinomycetes (*Micropolyspora faeni, Thermoactinomyces vulgaris*) from mouldy grains, straw, hay, suberosis due cork dust, malt workers' lung from mouldy barley *(Aspergillus)* and wheat disease from wheat flour *(Sitophilus granarius)* are the other extrinsic allergic alveolitis conditions. When the moisture content of hay or grain dust is over 30%, thermophilic actinomycetes grow rapidly and they, when inhaled, cause acute symptoms like respiratory difficulty in farmer's lung. Recurrent attacks may lead to damage of lungs with resultant cor pulmonale.

Prevention

Prevention of this condition can be effected by dust control, personal protection and periodic medical examination and by keeping the moisture content of bagasse below 20% along with spraying of 2% propionic acid.

Asbestosis

Exposure to asbestos (silicates) causes asbestosis, lung cancer and mesothelioma of pleura and peritoneum. In India, the total use of asbestos is 1.25 lakh tonnes, out of which more than 1.0 lakh tonnes are being imported. Significant occupational exposure to asbestos occurs mainly in asbestos cement factories, asbestos textile industry and asbestos mining and milling. The severity of asbestosis is generally related to the amount and duration of exposure to asbestos.

Inhalation of asbestos causes asbestosis. Currently about 125 million people around the world are exposed to asbestos at work and at least 107,000 people die each year from asbestos related diseases according to World Health Organization (WHO).

Prevention

Reducing the level of exposure to asbestos is the best prevention against asbestosis. A worker's exposure to asbestos may not exceed 0.1 fiber per cubic centimeter of air. Regulated areas for asbestos work, appropriate training and protective gear such as face masks are important preventive aspects. Asbestos in good condition, do not pose any threat to health. Only damaged asbestos fibers get released into the air. Repair or removal of an asbestos product is best done by a professional.

The WHO, in collaboration with the International Labor Organization and with other intergovernmental organizations and civil society, works with countries toward elimination of asbestos-related diseases.

OTHER OCCUPATIONAL HAZARDS

Lead Poisoning

Lead poisoning occurs in battery and glass manufacturing industries, rubber industry, in ship building yards, in printing press and pottery industries. Exposure to lead is more than any other toxic metal in industrial workers. Non-occupational exposure to lead occurs from automobile exhausts, lead pipes used for water supply and from paints.

Lead enters the body through inhalation, ingestion and skin contact. Average adult population will have 150–400 mg of body store and the normal blood level is about 25 µg/100 mL. Clinical symptoms are seen when the blood level rises to 70 µg/100 mL. Lead poisoning due to inorganic lead is manifested as abdominal colic, loss of appetite, basophilic stippling of RBCs, anemia and wrist and foot drop. Organic lead poisoning leads to central nervous system (CNS) symptoms such as insomnia, headache, mental confusion and delirium.

Diagnosis is made by measurement of urinary coproporphyrin (CPU) (< 150 µg/L in unexposed persons) and urinary aminolevulinic acid (ALAU) (> 5 mg/L in the exposed) in urine and measurement of lead in blood and urine. Acceptable blood lead concentration in healthy person is less than 5 µg/dL for children and less than 25 µg/dL for adults. Urinary excretion of lead is less than 80 µg/L in adults and children and in occupational exposure it should be less than 120 µg/L.

Prevention

Prevention can be effected by substitution, exhaust ventilation, personal protection, good housekeeping and periodic examination of workmen, personal hygiene and health education. The chelating agent d-penicillamine promotes excretion of lead in urine and is therefore given to remove lead from the body. Lead poisoning is a notifiable and compensatable disease in India since 1924.

Occupational Cancers

Gas workmen, coke oven workers, tar distillers, oil refiners, dyestuff makers, road makers and workers dealing with mineral oil, pitch, etc. are prone to develop skin cancers. Workmen in gas industry, asbestos industry, in nickel, arsenic and chromium plants and in uranium mines are vulnerable to lung cancers. Bladder cancers are reported in industries dealing with aromatic amines (dyes, rubbers, gas amines and electric cable industries). Exposure to benzol, X-rays and radioactive substances are associated with leukemia (blood cancer).

Occupational Dermatitis

Occupational dermatitis is caused by irritant chemicals (acids, alkalis, dyes, solvents, grease, tar, pitch, etc.) in industrial workers. Allergic dermatitis is also seen due to sensitizing agents.

Occupational Radiation

Radiation hazard is an important problem for persons working in atomic power plants, X-ray units, radiation therapy units, nuclear installation, etc. Acute burns, dermatitis and blood dyscrasias, malignancies, and genetic effects on chronic exposure are the adverse effects of exposure to radiation.

Agricultural workers are exposed to variety of diseases. They are prone to get zoonotic diseases, accidents, toxicity due to fertilizers and insecticides and farmers' lung.

Occupational Accidents

Accidents in industries are common. It may vary from very minor ones to even fatal accidents. Temporary and permanent disabilities are caused in significant numbers. Human factors like inexperience, poor vision and hearing, carelessness, overconfidence, slow cerebration, etc. are responsible for 85% of accidents. Bad working environment like poor illumination, humidity, noise and unsafe machines are also important causes for accidents.

Noise in the Occupational Environment

Continuous exposure to noise levels above 90 dBA can produce adverse auditory and non-auditory health effects.

Occupational exposure to noise is associated with hearing loss, which may be irreversible at 4,000 Hz. Noise also affects autonomic nervous functions manifested as stress and changes in blood pressure.

Noise-induced disorders can be prevented by setting of tolerance standards of noise exposure and subdividing the working environment based on international standards such as those of International Organization for Standardization (ISO).

Production Efficiency is Affected in a Noisy Environment

The combined effect of heat (35°C) and noise (100 dB) caused higher error rate in the work and also decreased accuracy in reasoning ability. The combined effect of noise (100 dB) and illumination (300 lux) affected accuracy score.

Infrasonic waves emanating from motor vehicles, railroads, dams, heat sources and compressors do not readily attenuate with distance. They cause autonomic imbalance such as sleep disorders, dizziness, irritability, headache and gastrointestinal disorders. Prolonged exposure causes essential hypertension.

❑ PREVENTION OF OCCUPATIONAL DISEASES

Medical Measures

Preplacement examination of employees, periodic medical examinations, proper medical and healthcare services, notification of occupational diseases, adequate supervision of working environment, maintenance of records of occupational health service, health education and counseling are all important measures for prevention.

Biological Measures

Periodic examination of blood or urine specimens to detect excessive absorption of a potentially toxic substance is important.

Health Protection Measures

Nutritional program/supplements, mental health, measures for women and children, maternal and child health (MCH) and family welfare services and recreation facilities are to be provided.

Personal Protective Measures

Masks, aprons, gloves, helmets, safety shoes, gumboots, goggles, screens, earplugs, earmuffs and barrier creams are to be provided.

Engineering Measures

Proper designing of industrial houses, good housekeeping, proper ventilation, mechanization, substitution, dust control measures, adequate enclosures around accident prone machines, isolation of offensive processes, protective devices for workmen and environmental monitoring are all needed for safeguarding the health of industrial personnel.

Adequate legislation to take care of violation of industrial norms by unscrupulous industrialists is also needed to protect workmen from hazards. WHO estimates that only 10%–15% of workers have access to a basic standard of occupational health services.

A WHO Global Plan of Action on Workers Health has been developed with the objective of:

1. Providing a framework for concerted action by all health and non-health actors for protecting and promoting the health of workers.
2. Establishing political momentum for primary prevention of occupational and work-related diseases.
3. Ensuring coherence in the planning, delivery and evaluation of health interventions at the workplace.

Global Plan of Action by WHO deals with all aspects of workers' health including primary prevention of occupational hazards, protection and promotion of health at work, employment conditions and a better response from health systems to workers' health. It is underpinned by certain common principles. All workers should be able to enjoy the highest attainable standard of physical and mental health and favorable working conditions. The workplace should not be detrimental to health and well-being. Primary prevention of occupational health hazards should be given priority. All components of health systems should be involved in an integrated response to the specific health needs of working populations.

Countries and member States should formulate their national policy frameworks to promote workers' health, strengthening their Ministries of Health and integrating workers' health concerns into national health strategies. They also need to minimize the gaps between different groups of workers in terms of levels of risk and health status. High-risk economic sectors and vulnerable working populations, such as younger and older workers, need special consideration and protection.

The WHO also assists countries to develop national occupational health profiles, policies and action plans and to create the capacity to implement the plans. WHO has a particular focus on strengthening capacity building activities, developing and disseminating practical solutions and to enhance work addressing selected priority groups, such as healthcare workers. In order to expand the coverage of workers by occupational health services, WHO is supporting the development of basic occupational health services.

The WHO has developed a work plan for the period 2006–2010 in collaboration with the WHO Network of Collaborating Centers and supports the implementation of the Global Strategy on Occupational Health for all.

A paradigm shift from the labor approach to the public health approach has been suggested (Table 28.1).

❑ ERGONOMICS

Ergonomics is the science that deals with the designing of work systems and environments, which will reduce strain and stress and thereby enhance performance. Jobs, systems, products and environments are matched with the physical and mental abilities of people in order to improve efficiency, safety and well-being. Ill-designed furniture, machines and environment can cause physical ailments and accidents, whereas ergonomically-designed system

TABLE 28.1: Difference between labor approach and public approach

Labor approach	Public approach
Occupational health	**Workers' health**
Employees with labor contract	All workers
Employer's responsibility	Responsibility of everybody
Only at the workplace	Beyond the workplace
Only work-related health issues	All health determinants
Negotiation between workers and employers	Wider social dialogue with stakeholders, insurance, health and environment authorities
	Health protection not subject to collective negotiation

is easy to use and causes less fatigue and ill health. Knowledge of anatomy and physiology, psychology and technology are integrated to create ergonomic designs with the involvement of experts from several disciplines. Ergonomics can be applied to both specific occupational groups and the general public. Public utility services like transport systems (buses, cars), furnitures, kitchen utensils, floor covers, commonly used tools, containers used for carrying and storing can beneficially use ergonomics principles. Designs must fit the anthropometry, strength and endurance of the entire population. Designs for the public use will require more sophisticated considerations than that for specific occupational groups, as the user population in specific jobs is better defined in terms of physical and psychological capacities.

❑ EMPLOYEES' STATE INSURANCE SCHEME

Employees' State Insurance (ESI) is an important insurance scheme for industrial workers. This is governed by the ESI (Amendment) Act 1984. The Central and State Governments and employers and employees of various establishments, finance this scheme.

This scheme aims to accomplish the task of protecting employees against the hazards of sickness, maternity, disablement and death due to employment injury and to provide medical care to insured persons and their families.

This scheme covers small power using factories employing 10–19 persons, non-power using establishments employing 20 or more persons, shops, hotels and restaurants, cinema halls and theaters, road motor transport establishments and newspaper establishments.

SECTION

8

Healthcare System in India

CHAPTER

29

Healthcare Delivery System

❑ HEALTH CARE IN INDIA

Health care in India is provided by means of a three-tier integrated system of primary, secondary and tertiary healthcare institutions. Primary health care (PHC) is essential health care, affordable and accessible, given to all with their active participation and it is provided in primary healthcare institutions like primary health centers and subcenters. Secondary health care is essentially a curative service and it is provided by district hospitals and community health centers, which are the first level referral centers. Tertiary health care is super specialty care provided in regional and central level institutions, which offer specialized treatments like kidney transplant, bypass heart surgery, etc. Health care in India is provided by the following sectors:

1. Public health sector:
   - Primary health centers and subcenters
   - Community health centers
   - Rural hospitals
   - District hospitals
   - Specialist hospitals
   - Teaching hospitals
   - Employees State Insurance Scheme (ESIS)
   - Central Government Health Scheme (CGHS)
   - Defense health services
   - Railway health services
   - National health programs.

2. Private sector:
   - General practitioners
   - Private hospitals, polyclinics, nursing homes, etc.
3. Indigenous systems of medicine.
4. Voluntary health agencies.

At village level, Accredited Social Health Activist (ASHA) and Integrated Child Development Services Scheme (ICDS) are in operation.

Accredited Social Health Activist

The ASHA is a literate (up to class 8) woman resident of the village, married/widowed/divorced, preferably in the age group of 25–45 years, selected by a rigorous process. ASHA will have to undergo series of training episodes to acquire the necessary knowledge, skills and confidence for performing her roles.

The ASHAs will receive performance-based incentives for promoting universal immunization, referral and escort services for reproductive and child health (RCH), other healthcare programs, and construction of household toilets. Empowered with knowledge and a drug kit to deliver first-contact health care, every ASHA is expected to be a fountainhead of community participation in public health programs in her village. She will create awareness on health and its social determinants, mobilize the community toward local health planning, increased utilization and accountability of the existing health services. She will counsel women on birth preparedness, importance of safe delivery, breastfeeding and complementary feeding, immunization, contraception and prevention of common infections including reproductive tract infection/sexually transmitted infections (RTIs/STIs), and care of the young child. ASHA will mobilize the community and facilitate them in accessing health and health-related services available at anganwadi/subcenters/PHCs such as immunization, antenatal check up (ANC), postnatal check up, supplementary nutrition, sanitation and other services being provided by the government.

One subcenter is established for every 5,000 population in plains and for every 3,000 population in hilly, tribal and backward areas. Subcenters are manned by one male and one female multipurpose health worker. Maternal and child health (MCH) care, family planning and immunization are looked after by these peripheral level health workers.

❑ PRIMARY HEALTH CENTER

A PHC to provide primary health care is established for every 30,000 population in plains and for every 20,000 population in hilly, tribal and backward areas. PHCs are manned by a medical officer and the supportive staffs such as pharmacist, nurse, block extension educator, health assistant (male and female), lab technician, etc.

Functions of PHC

- Medical care
- Family planning and MCH
- Safe water supply and sanitation
- Prevention and control of locally endemic diseases
- Collection and reporting of vital statistics
- Health education
- Implementation of national health programs
- Referral services
- Training of health guides, health workers, local dais and health assistants
- Laboratory services.

District, specialist and teaching hospitals provide secondary and tertiary care to the community. The current opinion is that these institutions should involve not only in providing curative services but also in providing promotive and preventive services as well.

Employees State Insurance Scheme

Employees State Insurance Scheme (ESIS) provides medical care, sickness benefits, maternity benefits, employment injury benefits for workers besides pension for dependants in case of death of a worker due to employment injury.

Central Government Health Scheme

The Central Government Health Scheme (CGHS) was started in 1954 with the objective of providing comprehensive medical care to the central government employees, both serving and pensioners and their dependant family members. The scheme is also providing service to members and former member of Parliament, judges of Supreme Court and High Court, freedom fighters, former Governors and former Vice Presidents of India.

Defense

Defense medical services cater to the health and medical care needs of defense personnel.

Railway

Railway health service provides comprehensive health care to railway employees.

General Services

General private practitioners constitute 70% of the medical care in India.

Ayurveda, Siddha and Homeopathy practitioners mostly serve rural people. But it is disturbing to learn that many of them practice modern medicine and thereby cause considerable harm to rural societies.

❑ CENTRAL BUREAU OF HEALTH INTELLIGENCE

Central Bureau of Health Intelligence (CBHI) established in 1961 is the national nodal institute in the Directorate General of Health Services, Ministry of Health and Family Welfare, Government of India. CBHI headquarters is located at Nirman Bhavan, New Delhi.

Objectives

Broad objectives of the CBHI are as follows:

1. Maintain and disseminate:
   a. National health profile.
   b. Health sector policy reform options database.
   c. Inventory and geoinformatics system (GIS) mapping of government health facilities in India, etc.
2. Review the progress of health sector millennium development goal (MDG) in India.
3. Annual road safety profile of India.
4. Facilitate capacity building and human resource development.
5. Need-based operational research for efficient health information system (HIS) as well as use of Family of International Classification in India and Southeast Asia Region.

The CBHI has four divisions, which are as follows:

1. Policy and infrastructure—headed by a Joint Director.
2. Training, collaboration and research headed by a Joint Director.
3. Information and evaluation headed by a Joint Director.
4. Administration—headed by Director/Deputy Director Administration

The CBHI has six health information field survey units (FSUs) located in different Regional Offices of Health and Family Welfare (ROHFW) of Government of India (GOI) at Bengaluru, Bhopal, Bhubaneswar, Jaipur, Lucknow and Patna; each headed by a Deputy Director with technical and support staff, who function under the supervision of Regional Director (HFW/GOI).

Regional health statistics training Center (RHSTC) of CBHI at Mohali, Punjab (near Chandigarh) and other training centers are as follows:

1. Medical Record Department and Training Center of Safdarjung Hospital, New Delhi.
2. JIPMER Puducherry conducts CBHI in service training courses.

❑ VOLUNTARY HEALTH AGENCIES

Voluntary health agencies also contribute significantly to health care in India. They supplement the work of government agencies, do pioneering work in healthcare research, provide health education, demonstrate innovative methods, guard the work of government agencies and help in advancing health legislation.

Indian Red Cross Society, Hindu Kusht Nivaran Sangh, Indian Council for Child Welfare, Tuberculosis association of India, Bharat Sevak Samaj, Central Social Welfare Board, the Kasturba Memorial Fund, Family planning Association of India, All India women's conference, All India Blind Relief Society, Indian Medical Association, All India Dental Association, The Trained Nurses Association of India are some important voluntary agencies contributing for the health care in India. International agencies like Rockefeller Foundation, Ford Foundation and CARE are also doing significant healthcare work in India. WHO, UNICEF, SIDA, DANIDA, Damien Foundation, World Bank, USAID are some of the other international organizations that help in different health programs in India.

World Health Organization

The World Health Organization (WHO), an agency of the United Nations, acts as a coordinating authority on international public health. It was established on 7th April 1948; the date celebrated every year as World Health Day. Geneva, Switzerland has its headquarters (HQ). WHO inherited the mandate and resources of its predecessor, the Health Organization of the League of Nations. The organization is financed by contributions from member states and from donors.

Infrastructure

World Health Assembly is WHO's supreme decision-making body and the member countries appoint delegates to it. All UN member states are eligible for WHO membership. WHO has 193 member states. Taiwan's membership is opposed by the Chinese.

The WHO assembly generally meets in May each year. It appoints the Director General for a five-year term, supervises the financial policies of the organization and reviews and approves the proposed program budget.

Executive Board

The World Health Assembly elects 34 members, who are technically qualified in the field of health for 3-year term to an Executive Board. The main functions of the board are to give effect to the decisions and policies of the assembly, to advise it and generally to facilitate its work.

Secretariat

The day-to-day work of WHO is carried out by its secretariat, which has some 8,500 health and other experts and support staff, working at HQ, in the six regional offices and in the individual representation offices in 147 countries. WHO also employs goodwill ambassadors.

Regional Offices

The WHO maintains six regional offices, they are:

1. Africa HQ: Brazzaville, Congo.
2. America HQ: Washington, DC, USA.
3. Eastern Mediterranean HQ: Cairo, Egypt.
4. Europe HQ: Copenhagen, Denmark.
5. Southeast Asia HQ: New Delhi, India.
6. Western Pacific HQ: Manila, Philippines.

The regional committee is incharge of setting the guidelines for the implementation of all the health and other policies within its region. It also serves as a progress review board for the actions of WHO within the region. The Regional Director directly supervises all the WHO representatives heading WHO country offices within their region, who are not nationals of the respective countries.

Country Offices

The WHO operates 147 country and liaison offices in all its regions. The country offices act as the primary adviser of that country's government in matters of health and pharmaceutical policies. Liaison offices are headed by a liaison officer, who is national from that particular country.

Mission

The constitution of WHO states that its mission is, "the attainment by all people of the highest possible level of health."

Functions

The WHO implements a six point agenda:

1. Promoting development.
2. Fostering health security.
3. Strengthening health systems.
4. Harnessing research, information and evidence.
5. Enhancing partnerships.
6. Improving performance.

The WHO fulfils its objectives through its core functions detailed below:

1. Providing leadership on matters critical to health and engaging in partnerships, where joint action is needed.
2. Shaping the research agenda and stimulating the generation, translation and dissemination of valuable knowledge.
3. Setting norms and standards, and promoting and monitoring their implementation.
4. Articulating ethical and evidence-based policy options.
5. Providing technical support, catalyzing change and building sustainable institutional capacity.
6. Monitoring the health situation and assessing health trends.

The WHO coordinates international efforts to monitor outbreaks of infectious diseases and also aids in preventing and treating such diseases. It supports the development and distribution of safe and effective vaccines and pharmaceutical diagnostics and drugs. WHO aims to eradicate polio within the next few years.

The WHO also carries out campaigns to boost consumption of fruits and vegetables worldwide and to discourage tobacco consumption. The WHO has recently banned the recruitment of cigarette smokers in its offices. WHO also conducts research on whether or not the electromagnetic field surrounding cell phones has a negative influence on health.

The WHO acts as a check on the power of the drug policy-making Commission on Narcotic Drugs as an additional responsibility.

The WHO publishes, the World Health Report, International Travel and Health, International Health Regulations, The International Classification of Diseases (ICD), International Pharmacopoeia, journals such as bulletin of the World Health Organization, Eastern Mediterranean Health Journal, Pan American Journal of Public Health, Weekly Epidemiological Record, WHO Drug Information and also regional publications.

The WHO also maintains a model list of essential and affordable medicines that countries' healthcare systems should make available to people.

The WHO holds partnerships with many private sectors such as Program for Appropriate Technology in Health (PATH), International AIDS Vaccine Initiative (IAVI), etc.

United Nations Children's Fund

The United Nations Children's Fund was established in 1946. In 1953, its name was shortened from United Nations International Children's Emergency Fund to United Nations Children's Fund. But it is still known by the popular acronym 'UNICEF' based on the old name. UNICEF provides long-term humanitarian and developmental assistance to children and mothers in developing countries.

Infrastructure

The GQ of UNICEF is in New York. Its supply division is in Copenhagen, which serves as the primary point of distribution for such essential items as lifesaving vaccines, antiretroviral medicines for children and mothers with HIV, nutritional supplements, emergency shelters, educational supplies and more.

Executive Board

The 36 member Executive Board establishes policies, approves programs and oversees administrative and financial plans. The Executive Board is made up of government representatives who serve 3-year terms.

The UNICEF works in over 191 countries and territories. Eight regional offices guide and provide technical assistance to country offices. Country offices carry out UNICEF's mission with the cooperation of the host governments.

The UNICEF is not active in Bahamas, Brunei, Cyprus, Latvia, Liechtenstein, Malta, Mauritius, Monaco and Singapore.

Funding

Government contributes two third of the organization's resources. Private groups and some 6 million individuals contribute the rest through the National Committees. UNICEF is known for its 'Trick-or-Treat for UNICEF' program in which children collect money for UNICEF from the houses they trick-or-treat at a Halloween night.

Functions

The UNICEF is currently focused on five primary priorities:

1. Child survival and development.
2. Basic education and the gender equality (including girls' education).
3. Child protection from violence, exploitation and abuse.
4. HIV/AIDS and children.
5. Policy advocacy and partnerships for children's rights.

Related areas of UNICEF action include early childhood development, adolescence development and participation and life skills-based education.

Education

The aim of UNICEF is to get more girls into school, ensure that they stay in school and that they are equipped with the basic tools they need to succeed in later life. As part of its ongoing efforts to ensure every girl and boy their right to an education, UNICEF's acceleration strategy tried to speed up progress in girls' enrollment in 25 selected countries during the 2002–2005 period.

Immunization Plus

Every year, more than 2 million children die from diseases that could have been prevented by inexpensive vaccines. The plus in the program is the additional immunizations made possible during interventions.

Child Protection and Well-being

Violations of the child's right to protection take place in every country and are massive, under-recognized and under-reported.

The UNICEF's child protection programs help in preventing and responding to violence, exploitation and abuse against children including commercial sexual exploitation, trafficking, child labor and harmful traditional practices such as female genital mutilation/cutting and child marriage. These programs also target children who are uniquely vulnerable to these abuses, such as when living without parental care, in conflict with the law and in armed conflict. UNICEF supports the international Child Rights Information Network. In 2007, UNICEF published 'an overview of child well-being in rich countries,' which showed that UK and USA are at the bottom in a group of 21 economically advanced nations for overall child well-being.

HIV/AIDS

The UNICEF is running several programs dedicated to control both online and offline child pornography in order to prevent the transmission of AIDS.

Early Childhood

Every child must be ensured of the best start in life. It is no exaggeration to say that their future and indeed the future of their communities, nations and the whole world depend on it. UNICEF applies a holistic, evidence-based approach to early childhood. Preventive and curative health care including immunization, adequate nutrition, safe water and basic sanitation must be provided an essential condition.

The UNICEF Innocenti Research Centre in Florence, Italy, established in 1988, conducts research to improve international understanding of the issues relating to children's rights, to promote economic policies, that advance the cause of children and to help facilitate the full implementation of the United Nations Convention on the Rights of the Child in industrialized and developing countries.

The UNICEF has been criticized for having political bias. But unlike NGOs, UNICEF is an intergovernmental organization and thus, is accountable to governments. These gives it a unique reach and access in every country in the world, but this also sometimes hampers its ability to speak out on rights violations.

United Nations Development Program

The United Nations Development Program (UNDP), established in 1965, is the largest multilateral source of development assistance in the world.

Infrastructure

Headquartered in New York City, the UNDP has country offices in 166 countries, where it works with local governments to meet development challenges and develop local capacity. The UNDP is an executive board within the United Nations General Assembly.

In 1997, United Nations Development Group (UNDG) was created to improve the effectiveness at the country level. The UNDG brings together the operational agencies working on development.

The UNDP coordinates UN's activities in the field of development through its leadership of the UNDG and through the resident coordinator system and it is funded entirely by voluntary contributions from member nations.

Functions

The UNDP provides expert advice, training and grant support to developing countries with emphasis on assistance to the least-developed countries. To accomplish the millennium developmental goals and encourage global development, UNDP focuses on poverty reduction, HIV/AIDS, democratic governance, energy and environment and crisis prevention and recovery. UNDP also encourages the protection of human rights and the empowerment of women in all of its programs.

Besides, UNDP publishes an annual human development report based on the human development index since 1990 to measure and analyze developmental progress. In addition to a global report, UNDP also publishes regional, national and local human development reports.

International Labor Organization

The International Labor Organization (ILO) founded in 1919, is a specialized agency of the United Nations that deals with labor issues. It became a member of the UN system after the formation of the UN at the end of World War II.

Infrastructure

International Labor Organization's (ILO) headquarters is in Geneva, Switzerland. Its Secretariat is known as the International Labor Office. Its constitution, as amended to date, includes the Declaration of Philadelphia (1944) on the aims and purposes of the organization.

Functions

The primary goal of the ILO today is to promote opportunities for women and men to obtain decent and productive work in conditions of freedom, equity, security and human dignity. In working towards this goal, ILO works on four thematic groupings or sectors:

1. Standards of fundamental principles and rights at work.
2. Employment.
3. Social protection.
4. Social dialogue.

International labor conference

The ILO hosts the International Labor Conference in Geneva every year in June. At the conference, conventions and recommendations are crafted and adopted by majority decision. The conference also makes decisions on the ILO's general policy, work program and budget.

International labor standards

As already mentioned, one of the principal functions of the ILO is setting international labor standards, sometimes referred to as the International Labor Code, through the adoption of conventions and recommendations covering a broad spectrum of labor-related subjects.

The ILO has a specialist program addressing child labor the International Program on the Elimination of Child Labor (IPEC).

ILOAIDS

Under the name ILOAIDS, the ILO has created the Code of Practice on HIV/AIDS and the world of work as a document. ILOAIDS provides principles for policy development and practical guidelines for programs at enterprise, community and national levels, which includes prevention of HIV, management and mitigation of the impact of AIDS on the world of work, supporting workers infected and affected by HIV/AIDS and elimination of stigma and discrimination on the basis of real or perceived HIV status.

❑ FORD FOUNDATION

The Ford Foundation was chartered on January 15, 1936 by Edsel Ford and two Ford motor company executives as a charitable foundation to receive and administer funds for scientific, educational and charitable purposes, all for the public welfare. It is based in New York City and aims to promote democracy, reduce poverty, promote international understanding and advance human achievement. The Ford Foundation is an independent, nonprofit, non-governmental organization.

The foundation makes grants through its New York headquarters and through 12 international field offices. In fiscal year 2006, it approved $530 million in grants for projects that focused on strengthening democratic values, community and economic development, education, media, arts and culture, and human rights.

❑ ROCKEFELLER FOUNDATION

The Rockefeller Foundation was established by John D Rockefeller along with his son and their principal business and philanthropic advisor, Frederick T Gates, in New York in 1913.

International Health Commission

In 1913, the foundation set up the International Health Commission (later board), the first appropriation of funds for work outside the US, which launched the foundation into international public health activities. This expanded the work of the Sanitary Commission worldwide, working against various diseases in 52 countries from 6 continents and 29 islands, bringing international recognition of the need for public health and environmental sanitation. Its early field research on hookworm, malaria and yellow fever provided the basic techniques to control these diseases and established the pattern of modern public health services.

The commission established and endowed the world's first school of hygiene and public health at Johns Hopkins University and later at Harvard and then spent more than $25 million in developing other public health schools in the US and in 21 foreign countries. In 1913 it also began a 20-year support program of the Bureau of Social Hygiene, whose mission was research and education on birth control, maternal health and sex education.

China Medical Board

In 1914 the foundation set up the China Medical Board, which established the first public health university in China, the Peking Union Medical College in 1921. This was subsequently nationalized when the communists took over the country in 1949. In the same year, it began a program of international fellowships to train scholars at the world's leading universities at the postdoctoral level, a fundamental commitment to the education of future leaders.

Activities

The overall philanthropic activity of the foundation has been divided into five main subject areas, viz. medical, health and population sciences, agricultural and natural sciences, arts and humanities, social sciences and international relations.

It has supported United Nations programs throughout its history, such as the recent First Global Forum on Human Development organized by the United Nations Development Program (UNDP) in 1999.

❑ CARE

Cooperative for Assistance and Relief Everywhere (CARE) is one of the largest international relief and humanitarian organizations in the world with programs in nearly 70 countries. Worldwide staffing exceeds 12,000; most of whom come from the nation in which they work. CARE is a non-governmental organization and a private voluntary organization, which was founded in 1945 by Wallace Campbell to provide relief to survivors of World War II.

Mission

The Mission of CARE is to serve individuals and families in the poorest communities in the world for strengthening their capacity for self-help, providing economic opportunity, delivering relief in emergencies, influencing policy decisions at all levels and addressing discrimination in all its forms.

The emergency relief during and after disasters is being continuously provided by CARE. But presently it focuses on addressing underlying causes of poverty. In areas such as health, education and economic development, CARE works to empower women, because experience has shown that women's gains yield dramatic benefits for families and communities. CARE also advocates for policies that defend human rights and promote the eradication of poverty.

As of 2007, CARE operates programs in many countries in Africa, Asia, Latin America, Middle East and Eastern Europe.

CARE in India

CARE works in 28 Indian states. It helps more than 6.5 million people in more than 100,000 villages across 10 Indian states to get education, work and health care and gives basic education to uneducated children.

The most successful project of CARE is the Girl's Primary Education (GPE) Project in Uttar Pradesh. 90 community schools were set up through 'Mother's Groups' where girls can get primary school education. CARE focuses on health and nutrition; prevention, awareness and treatment of HIV and AIDS; basic education; helping people to earn a living, learn new skills, and preparing for and responding to disasters.

During the 2004 tsunami, CARE worked in four districts of Tamil Nadu and helped people to get their lives back on track by rebuilding homes that were destroyed during the tsunami. It also helped people to find work by giving out tools and new boats, and trained people in new skills. CARE's Credit and Savings for Household Enterprise (CASHE) project has helped millions of poor Indians to start their own businesses.

CHAPTER

30

National Health Programs in India

❑ NATIONAL HEALTH PROGRAMS

Many National Health Programs are directly run by the Ministry, Government of India, in addition to the regular medical and healthcare delivery systems. In this task, Government of India is assisted by various international and foreign agencies. Notable among them are WHO, UNICEF, UNFPA, World Bank, SIDA, DANIDA, NORAD and USAID. These programs, implemented to combat communicable, non-communicable and other major diseases, can have a bearing on the reduction of mortality and morbidity. They also will have a salutary effect on the efforts to improve the quality of life of the common man by reinforcing the delivery of primary, secondary and tertiary health care throughout the country. The programs are described below.

National Vector-borne Diseases Control Program

The National Health Policy (2002) has set the goals for reduction of mortality because of malaria and other vector-borne diseases by 50% by the year 2010; elimination of kala-azar by the year 2010 and elimination of lymphatic filariasis by the year 2015.

The Directorate of National Vector-borne Diseases Control Program (NVBDCP) is the national nodal agency for prevention and control of major vector-borne diseases of public health importance namely malaria, filaria, kala-azar, Japanese encephalitis and dengue/dengue hemorrhagic fever (DHF).

Malaria

Malaria is still a major health problem in India. In 2011, there were 575,349 cases and 157 deaths.

The biggest burden of malaria in India is borne by the most backward, poor and remote parts of the country, with greater than 90%–95% cases reported from rural areas and less than 5%–10% from urban areas; however, the low malaria incidence in urban areas may be due to almost non-existing surveillance. Orissa, with a population of 36.7 million, contributes about 25% of the total annual malaria cases, more than 40% of *Plasmodium falciparum* malaria cases and nearly 20%–30% of deaths caused by malaria in India. Meghalaya, Mizoram, Maharashtra, Rajasthan, Gujarat, Karnataka, Goa, southern Madhya Pradesh, Chhattisgarh and Jharkhand are the other states where more cases are reported.

The problem of malaria is now plagued by vector resistance to insecticides especially in sub-Saharan Africa and India and parasite resistance to chloroquine and recently to artemisinin.

National Malaria Eradication Program

A nationwide Malaria Control Program was launched in 1953. Enthused by the excellent results achieved through Malaria Control Program, the National Malaria Eradication Program (NMEP) was launched by the Government in 1958. The NMEP had spectacular success initially and the incidence of malaria could be brought down from 75 million with 0.8 million deaths to 0.1 million with no deaths by 1965. Thereafter, the program received a setback due to a combination of factors like financial, logistics, administrative and technical nature and there was resurgence of the disease during early 70s. Therefore, the Modified Plan of Operation (MPO) was launched in 1977 to tackle the situation. The objectives of the MPO were:

1. Effective control of malaria to reduce malaria morbidity.
2. Preventing deaths due to malaria.
3. Consolidation of gains achieved so far.

The main strategies adopted were:

1. Early case detection and prompt treatment.
2. Vector control by house spraying in rural areas with annual parasite incidence of two and above with appropriate

insecticides and by recurrent antilarval measures in urban areas.
3. Health education and community participation.

Role of primary health centers
Primary health centers were involved in collection and examination of blood smears in fever cases through peripheral level workers. Drug distribution centers and fever treatment depots were established in rural and remote areas. Active and passive surveillance was being carried out to keep track of the malaria problem.

Resurgence of malaria in 1994 gave birth to malaria action program. 'Antimalaria month' is being observed during the month of June to create awareness in the community. The incidence was reduced from 6.47 million in 1976 to around 2.5–3 million cases annually till 1996. Since 1997, declining trend has been recorded. Annual parasitic incidence (API) declined to greater than 2 for the first time in 2002 and since then it is reported to be greater than 2.

The state governments are responsible for planning, implementation, supervision and monitoring of the program. North eastern (NE) states are being provided 100% support for program implementation including operational cost.

Enhanced malaria control project
Under the Enhanced Malaria Control Project (EMCP) with World Bank assistance additional support for control of malaria in 100 districts predominantly inhabited by tribes in eight states (Andhra Pradesh, Chhattisgarh, Gujarat, Jharkhand, Madhya Pradesh, Maharashtra, Orissa and Rajasthan) is being provided since September 1997.

The EMCP lays emphasis on:

1. Early diagnosis and prompt treatment.
2. Selective vector control.
3. Innovative ecofriendly methods like introduction of medicated mosquito nets, larvivorous fishes, bio larvicides, etc.
4. Epidemic planning and rapid response including intersectoral coordination.
5. Institutional and human resources development through training/reorientation training, strengthening management

information system (MIS), information, education and communication (IEC) and operational research.

Role of primary health care

The project is being implemented through the primary healthcare system.

For effective implementation of the project, additional inputs are being provided to the identified districts in the form of commodities (synthetic pyrethroids, mosquito bed nets, newer drugs, rapid diagnostic kits, etc.) and cash grant. IEC and training activities are also covered under the project.

Since the implementation of EMCP in 1997, the reported malaria cases in the country declined to 1.82 million cases in 2004 as against over 2.66 million cases in 1997; a decline of about 32%. The number of *Plasmodium falsiparum* cases has also declined from 1.04 million in 1997 to 0.89 million in 2004, a decline of 15%.

Intensified Malaria Control Project

Since 27 June 2005 Intensified Malaria Control Project (IMCP) was implemented in NE states (except Sikkim), selected high-risk areas of Orissa, Jharkhand and West Bengal. The objectives were:

1. Increasing access to rapid diagnosis and treatment in remote and inaccessible areas through community participation.
2. Reducing malaria transmission risk by use of insecticide treated bed nets.
3. Enhancing awareness about malaria control and promoting community, NGO and private sector participation.

Now, the control program of malaria is an integral component of National Rural Health Mission (NRHM) and is implemented under the overall umbrella of NRHM. The program will be monitored at the national level through the mechanisms established under NRHM. Directorate of NVBDCP is the nodal agency for policy recommendation and issuance of technical guidelines, whereas the state government health institution is the primary implementing agencies. Assistance by GOI whether cash or commodity or otherwise will be based on the approved program implementation plan (PIP) of the state governments, commonly known as record of proceedings (ROP) of the National Program Coordination Committee (NPCC).

Strategies

Strategies during 11th five year plan (2007–2012):

1. Focused interventions in high malaria endemic areas.
2. Linkage with NRHM and use of NRHM institutions for prevention and control of vector-borne diseases (VBD) (especially involvement of village health and sanitation committees (VHSCs) for indoor residual spray (IRS).
3. Early diagnosis and treatment by:
   a. Strengthening of human resources for surveillance and laboratory support.
   b. Introduction and scale up of rapid diagnostic kit (RDK).
   c. Introduction and scale up of artemisinin-based combination therapy (ACT) for Pf cases.
   d. Geographical information system (GIS) mapping for focused intervention in high risk prioritized districts.
   e. Up scaling use of bed nets, preferably long lasting insecticidal nets (LLINs).
   f. Intensive monitoring and supervision.
   g. Intensified information, education and communication (IEC) and behavior change communication (BCC) activities involving community.

Filariasis

Filariasis has been reported from over 250 districts in 20 states and UTs wherein over 500 million people live.

The National Filaria Control Program (NFCP) was launched in 1955. NFCP activities were mainly confined to urban areas. The program has been extended to rural areas also since 1994 and the activities are carried out through primary health centers in endemic states. At present, about 52 million urban populations are being protected through recurrent antilarval measures by 206 control units and 199 filarial clinics. Delimitation of the problem is being done by 27 filarial survey units.

Control strategies

The main control strategies under the program are:

1. Recurrent antilarval measures at weekly intervals.

2. Environmental methods including source reduction by filling ditches, pits, low-lying areas, deweeding, desilting, etc.
3. Biological control of mosquito breeding through larvivorus fish.
4. Antiparasitic measures through 'detection' and 'treatment' of microfilaria carriers and disease person with diethylcarbamazine citrate by filarial clinics in towns covered under the program.

The National Health Policy (2002) has envisaged elimination of lymphatic filariasis by the year 2015. In the year 2004, 202 endemic districts in 20 states in the country with a target population of 407 million were brought under a revised single dose mass drug administration (MDA) strategy. Under this strategy, single dose of diethylcarbamazine citrate (DEC) tablets is administered to all individuals living at risk of filariasis excluding pregnant women, children below 2 years of age and seriously ill persons. The coverage of target population was 87.89% in 2011.

Kala-azar

An estimated 165.4 million population is at risk of contracting kala-azar in four eastern states of India namely Bihar, Jharkhand, Uttar Pradesh and West Bengal. Kala-azar is endemic in 48 districts and sporadic in a few other districts. Mostly poor socioeconomic groups of population primarily living in rural areas are affected. In 2012, 16,125 cases with 22 deaths (Bihar 20; Jharkhand and Uttrakhand 1 each) have been reported so far. The disease shows a declining trend since 2007.

A centrally sponsored control program was launched in 1990-91 in endemic areas. Under this, medicines for kala-azar treatment, insecticides and technical support are being provided by the central government. The state governments implement the program through primary healthcare system and district/zonal and state malaria control organizations and also provide other costs involved in strategy implementation. With the launching of the control program, kala-azar incidence has come down.

Strategies: These are as follows:

1. Vector control through indoor residual spray with DDT up to 6 feet height from the ground twice annually.
2. Early diagnosis and complete treatment.
3. Information, education, communication.
4. Capacity building.

Kala-azar Elimination Initiative

National Health Policy goal aims at elimination of Kala-azar by the year 2010. Elimination program is 100% centrally supported (except regular staff of state governments and infrastructure). In addition to medicines and insecticides, cash assistance is being provided to endemic states since December 2003 to facilitate effective strategy implementation.

Japanese Encephalitis

First case of Japanese encephalitis (JE) was reported in 1955. Now outbreaks have been reported from different parts of the country. The state of Uttar Pradesh reported the highest number of cases (3,145) followed by Assam (1,343) and Bihar (745) in 2012 so far.

State and central governments take efforts to contain JE outbreaks by instituting various public health measures.

Preventive measures: The preventive measures are as follows:

1. Reducing the vector density: The reduction in mosquito breeding requires ecomanagement, as the role of insecticides is limited.
2. Taking personal protection against mosquito bites using insecticide-treated mosquito nets.
3. It is not recommended as an outbreak control measure, as it takes at least 1 month after second dose to develop antibodies at protective levels and the outbreaks are usually short-lived.
4. Piggeries may be kept away (4–5 km) from human dwellings.

Challenges: Challenges in the control of JE are:

1. Outdoor habit of the vector.
2. Scattered distribution of cases spread over relatively large areas.

3. Role of different reservoir hosts.
4. Specific vectors for different geographical and ecological areas.
5. Immune status of various population groups is not known; making it difficult to delineate vulnerable population groups.

Strategies: Major strategies for the control of JE:

1. Strengthening case management at PHCs, CHCs and hospitals through training of medical and nursing staff.
2. Sentinel, serological and clinical surveillance in endemic and their adjoining areas.
3. As there is no specific treatment of JE, clinical management is supportive.
4. Vector control measures mainly fogging during outbreaks and space spraying.
5. Development of better vaccine production facilities to enable vaccination of all children below 15 years.

Technical support: Technical support is provided on request by the state health authorities, for outbreak investigations and control. Central government has launched a vaccination program against JE during 2006 for children between 1 and 15 years of age in 11 districts of five states namely UP, Bihar, Assam, Karnataka and West Bengal. Altogether 86 JE endemic districts in the states of Assam, Andhra Pradesh, Bihar, Haryana, Goa, Karnataka, Kerala, Maharashtra, Tamil Nadu, Uttar Pradesh and West Bengal have been covered.

A single dose of live-attenuated SA14-14-2 vaccine (0.5 mL subcutaneously) is administered. Vaccine should be used within 2 hours after reconstitution.

Dengue

Dengue is prevalent throughout India in most of the metropolitan cities and towns. Outbreaks have also been reported from rural areas of Haryana, Maharashtra and Karnataka. All age groups and both the sexes are affected. Deaths are more in children during DHF outbreaks. During 2009, up to 29.04.09, 899 cases with four deaths have been reported. Recently there has been an upsurge in the incidence of cases. In 2012 till September, 17, 104 cases with 100 deaths have been reported.

Treatment and prevention

As there is no specific treatment and vaccine for dengue, the emphasis is on avoidance of mosquito breeding conditions in homes, workplaces and minimizing the man-mosquito contact. Community awareness and participation as well as intersectoral collaboration are crucial for effective control of dengue. In addition, enactment and enforcement of appropriate civic bye-laws and building bye-laws should also be stressed upon in all urban areas to prevent mosquitogenic conditions in line with the Delhi, Mumbai, Goa, Chandigarh, etc.

An intensive IEC campaign is launched for preventing and containing all vector-borne diseases including dengue. The services of voluntary health agencies including the Indian Medical Association are being utilized for spreading the message of prevention and control.

Early reporting of the suspected dengue fever is important for control. Management of dengue fever is symptomatic and supportive. In dengue shock syndrome, replacement of plasma losses, correction of electrolyte and metabolic disturbances and blood transfusion are recommended.

Government of India assistance

The Government of India provides need-based support to states, which includes insecticides, larvicides as well as cash assistance for IEC activities and capacity building through trainings. In addition, technical support in the form of guidelines, advisories and epidemiological investigations and feedback are also provided.

Six-nation initiative to fight dengue

ICMR is embarking upon a new research initiative 'Eco-bio-social aspects of dengue in Asia' project to eradicate dengue. Assisted by the Special Program for Research and Training in Tropical diseases, Geneva and the International Development Research Center (IDRC), Canada, the initiative focuses on better understanding of ecological, biological and sociological aspects to prevent dengue. Scientists from India, Thailand, Sri Lanka, Philippines, Indonesia and Myanmar will develop and evaluate community-based ecosystem management interventions in 2008–2009 to reduce transmission below threshold level for epidemic outbreak. WHO, World Bank, UNICEF and UNDP fund the program.

Chikungunya

Chikungunya re-emerged in the country during 2006 in epidemic form after a quiescence of about three decades. Andhra Pradesh, Karnataka, Maharashtra, Tamil Nadu, Madhya Pradesh, Gujarat, Kerala, Andaman and Nicobar Islands, GNCT of Delhi, Rajasthan, Pondicherry, Goa, Orissa, West Bengal, Lakshadweep and Uttar Pradesh were affected. During 2009, 73288 suspected chikungunya fever cases from 13 states have been reported. Since then there has a decline in the incidence (in 2010–48,126 cases; in 2011–20,402 cases; in 2012 up to October–13,704 cases). Government of India continuously monitors the situation and emphasizes for implementation of strategic action plan by the state governments. Government of India has identified 13 apex referral laboratories for advanced diagnosis and regular surveillance of dengue and chikungunya fever cases and 137 sentinel surveillance hospitals for proactive surveillance. National Institute of Virology, Pune has been entrusted to supply test kits to these institutes.

Control

For control of epidemics, vector control is considered to be one of the important strategies to interrupt or reduce transmission. Adult mosquitoes can be controlled by the use of chemical insecticides. However, rapid and effective source reduction for elimination of breeding sites of vector mosquitoes will achieve the same results. Moreover, larval control is more economical and provides sustainable control by eliminating the source of newly emergent adult mosquitoes. Surveillance and IEC activities are essential component of control strategy.

National Leprosy Eradication Program

The National Leprosy Eradication Program (NLEP) is a centrally sponsored health scheme of the Ministry of Health and Family Welfare, Government of India. The program is headed by the Deputy Director of Health Services (leprosy) under the administrative control of the Directorate General Health Services, Government of India. While the NLEP strategies and plans are formulated centrally, the program is implemented by the states/UTs. The program is also supported as partners by the World

Health Organization, The International Federation of Antileprosy Associations (ILEP) and few other non-government organizations (NGOs).

Government of India launched the National Leprosy Eradication Program in 1983 with the objective of eliminating the disease by the end of the century in the country by reducing the caseload to one or less/10,000 population.

Multidrug Therapy

The program was expanded with World Bank assistance and the whole country was brought under multidrug therapy (MDT) and the program was implemented through 490 district leprosy societies. The first phase of the World Bank supported National *Leprosy Elimination Project* began in 1993-94 and ended in March 2000. The second phase of the project was started in April 2001, which ended successfully in December 2004. During the second phase, NLEP was decentralized to states/districts and leprosy services were integrated with the general healthcare system. Since then, free MDT is available at all subcenters, PHCs and government hospitals and dispensaries on all working days. Since 2005, national program continues with GOI funds.

Modified Leprosy Elimination Campaigns

Five nationwide Modified Leprosy Elimination Campaigns (MLEC) were conducted from 1998 to 2003 to create mass community awareness about leprosy and to undertake a case detection drive along with prompt treatment with MDT. More than 9.90 lakh leprosy cases were detected and treated (with MDT) during these campaigns.

Global Alliance for Elimination of Leprosy

WHO formed a Global Alliance for Elimination of Leprosy for enhancing the opportunities to eliminate leprosy by the year 2005. The members of global alliance are leprosy-affected endemic countries, WHO and ILEP agencies.

The National Health Policy, 2002 had set the goal of elimination of leprosy (i.e. to reduce the number of cases to less than 1/10,000 population) by the year 2005. India has achieved this goal of elimination of leprosy as a public health problem at the national level in the month of December 2005, when the recorded prevalence rate in the country was 0.95/10,000 population. By March 2007, the prevalence rate of leprosy in the country had declined to 0.72/10,000 population. By March 2009, 32 states/ union territories (UTs) have achieved the goal of leprosy elimination. Only three states/UT viz. Bihar, Chhattisgarh, Dadra and Nagar Haveli are yet to achieve elimination. At the end of March 2009, there were 86,331 leprosy cases on record. As a result of intensive IEC activities, public awareness about the disease and its curability has increased significantly and the stigma and discrimination against leprosy-affected persons has declined appreciably. Concerted community mobilization is still required to reduce it further.

As on 31st March 2012, 445 districts out of total 642 have Annual New Case Detection rate (ANCDR) less than 10/100,000 population and 74 districts have ANCDR greater than 20/100,000. Only 11 districts in Chhattisgarh , Gujarat, Maharashtra, West Bengal, Dadra and Nagar Haveli, Orissa and Delhi have reported an ANCDR greater than 50/100,000 population. There were 642 cases totally.

The program will continue the efforts to achieve elimination of leprosy in the remaining states and districts through existing MDT services, capacity building of health service staff and strengthening of monitoring and supervision of the program. Enhancing disability prevention and medical rehabilitation services by involving more medical colleges and PMR institutions and intersectoral collaboration for rehabilitation of leprosy-disabled persons will also be focused.

Voluntary organizations

A total of 285 voluntary organizations functioned in the field of leprosy in India. Many international voluntary organizations (ILEP agencies) such as Leprosy Mission, German Leprosy Relief Association, Damien Foundation, Lepra India, Italian Leprosy Relief Association, Swiss Emmaus, etc. also helped in the implementation of the program through their own centers or through the local NGOs.

The Central Leprosy Division of Directorate General of Health Services, Ministry of Health and Family Welfare, Government of India in association with Novartis Comprehensive Leprosy Care Association (NCLCA) and Tata Department of Plastic Surgery, JJ Hospital recently released new guidelines on disability, prevention and medical rehabilitation (DPMR) for National Leprosy Eradication Program in India.

National Tuberculosis Control Program

Tuberculosis is a major public health problem in India. India accounts for one fifth or 26% of the global TB incidence, (WHO 2012) and is estimated to have the highest number of active TB cases amongst all the countries of world. Every year there are approximately 1.9 million new cases of which approximately 8 lakhs are smear positive and therefore infectious. Two persons die from TB in India every three minutes; more than 1,000 people every day.

National Tuberculosis Control Program (NTCP) was launched in 1962 and implemented through a network of district tuberculosis centers (DTC). Even after 30 years of implementation of the program, no significant epidemiological impact was observed. Therefore, in 1992, the NTCP was reviewed by a committee of experts.

Objectives

Based on the findings of this review committee, a revised strategy for National TB Control Program, Revised National TB Control Program (RNTCP) was launched in the country on 26th March 1997 with the following objectives:

1. To achieve and maintain a cure rate of at least 85% among newly detected infectious TB cases.
2. To achieve and maintain detection of at least 70% of such cases in the population.

By 23rd March 2006, the entire country has been covered under RNTCP. The program is being implemented with assistance from

World Bank, Department for International Development (DFID), United States Agency for International Development (USAID), Global Drug Facility (GDF) and Global Fund to Fight AIDS, Tuberculosis and Malaria (GFATM).

Directly Observed Treatment, Short-course

The five principal components of directly observed treatment, short-course (DOTS) are:

1. Political and administrative commitment.
2. Case detection by sputum smear microscopy.
3. Uninterrupted supply of high-quality anti-TB drugs.
4. Standardized treatment regimens with directly observed treatment for at least the first 2 months.
5. Systematic monitoring and accountability.

Overall, the performance of the RNTCP has been excellent with cure/treatment completion rate consistently above 85% and death rate reduced to less than 5%. Every month, more than 100,000 patients are placed under treatment. In 2006 alone, India placed around 14 lakh cases on DOTS. The program envisages to develop an effective partnership with the healthcare provider outside the public health system including NGOs, private practitioners, corporate sectors, etc. Treatment of multidrug-resistant TB (MDR-TB) patients by 'DOTS-Plus' strategy has been launched in the states of Gujarat and Maharashtra in early 2007 and will be extended to the entire country in a phased manner.

Consultants have been hired by WHO to work under the direction of respective state governments to ensure effective implementation and monitoring of RNTCP.

Government of Denmark has agreed to provide a grant of approximately 31.95 crores for implementation of RNTCP in 14 tribal districts of Orissa. The service delivery has already started in some of the affected districts.

RNTCP during the 12th five year plan (2012–2017) aims to achieve 'universal access' to quality-assured TB diagnosis and treatment. This requires broad and concerted efforts and support from all stakeholders with substantial enhancement of commitment and financing at all levels.

The national guidelines on pediatric TB diagnosis and management has been updated based on the recent evidence and advances in pediatric TB diagnosis and treatment in consultation with Indian Academy of Pediatrics during January – February 2012.

National AIDS Control Program

AIDS has emerged as one of the most serious public health problems in India. The total number of people living with HIV/AIDS in 2007 was estimated to be 2.31 million, females constituting around 39% of the burden (0.9 million). Children below 15 years constitute 3.5% of the total estimated cases. While Manipur and Nagaland have the highest HIV prevalence in the country, number of people living with HIV/AIDS is the highest in Andhra Pradesh and Maharashtra. The most important mode of transmission in India is heterosexual transmission (85.8%).

There are an estimated 22 million at risk people in the country. National AIDS Control Program (NACP) was launched in 1987. National AIDS Control Organization (NACO) was set up to monitor this program in 1992 by the Ministry of Health and Family welfare.

Phases of Implementation

The program has been implemented in phases. During phase I (1992–99), the emphasis was on awareness campaigns and environment building activities in the state. In phase II (1999–2004), the focus was shifted to changing the behavior particularly of high- risk groups through intervention in order to prevent contracting of HIV/AIDS. Phase III began in January 2007. Since more than 99% of population is uninfected, India has an opportunity to prevent an explosive epidemic (as witnessed in Sub-Saharan Africa or Southeast Asian countries) by adequately investing in prevention and treatment. Accordingly, during phase III, two third of the resources and efforts have been committed to prevention with the remaining dedicated to care, support and treatment.

Under NACP phase III, districts have been categorized according to the level of infection and the risk. Out of the total 611 districts, 163 districts with high prevalence are in category A; 59

districts with concentrated epidemic in category B; 278 districts with increased prevalence of vulnerable population, in category C and 111 districts in category D. This categorization based on vulnerability enables to prepare need-based plans.

Objectives

1. To reduce new infections by 60% in high prevalence states so as to obtain the reversal of the epidemic.
2. To reduce the same by 40% in the vulnerable states so as to stabilize the spread of the epidemic.

The program is being implemented under five components:

Priority targeted intervention for populations at high risk

High-risk groups like female sex workers (FSW), injecting drug users (IDU) and men having sex with men (MSM) are targeted. Peer counseling, condom promotion, treatment of sexually transmitted infections, etc. are provided. These people will be supported to organize themselves into community-based organizations (CBOs), i.e. organizations managed by the target beneficiaries themselves so as to ensure sustain ability and reduce their continued dependence on NGOs for accessing critical services. The target is to bring 50% of interventions under CBO management during III phase.

Preventive interventions for the general population

Under this component, conducting IEC and awareness campaigns, provision of voluntary testing and counseling services, ensuring safety of blood and blood products for transfusion and prevention of occupational exposure are undertaken.

1. Information, education and communication (IEC) activities include multimedia campaigns and special communication packages for sex workers, IDUs, truckers street children, etc. focused radio programs to provide information about prevention and control of HIV/AIDS and field publicity units like song and drama division in rural areas. Over 4,000 universities had covered over 3.5 million students under 'University Talks AIDS' programs. AIDS hotlines with 1,097 toll free numbers have been established in 65 major cities in the country.

2. Integrated counseling and testing services (ICTC) and prevention of parent to child transmission centers (PPTCT) are being established. Community health centers, 24-hour PHCs and private sector hospitals will be equipped with testing and counseling facilities. In hard-to-access areas and tribal areas, mobile ICTCs will be made available to provide counseling and testing services. To prevent mother to child transmission, T-cell (CD4) count of all pregnant HIV positive women will be done in the nearest antiretroviral therapy yes (ART) center.
3. STI Services: STI clinics will be established in district hospitals and medical colleges by the end of financial year 2006–07. The STI services are also being provided at subdistricts level under the RCH program. 5,000 preferred private service providers will also be involved particularly in category A and B districts. The ICMR STD network will also be utilized to monitor drug resistance and deciding on syndromic protocol.
4. Blood safety: The blood safety component of the program ensures supply of adequate and safe blood in the country. It is mandatory to test all donated blood for hepatitis B and C, HIV, syphilis and malaria.
5. Low-cost care for people living with HIV/AIDS: Drugs for management of opportunistic infections in HIV/AIDS patients are ensured. Community care centers in high prevalent states provide palliative care to terminally ill AIDS patients.
6. ART centers in 29 states of country provide antiretroviral drugs.
7. The National Pediatric ART Initiative launched on 30th November 2006, provides specific pediatric formulations to enhance the coverage of children.

Prevention will go hand-in-hand with access to prophylaxis, management of opportunistic infections and ART.

Institutional strengthening

As on March, 2007, a total of 794,000 personnel were trained, including specialist doctors of medical colleges, general DMOs, nurses, IEC officers, counselors, NGOs, laboratory technicians, blood bank officials and district nodal officers.

Building capacity for monitoring and evaluation program activities

An independent national monitoring and evaluation (M and E) agency was selected. Each state AIDS prevention and control society (SACS) was asked to have its own monitoring and evaluation (M and E) officer.

Development of indigenous vaccine and operational research are the main activities under research priorities of the program.

Intersectoral collaboration

This component aims at promoting collaboration amongst the public, private and voluntary sectors. A high level national council on AIDS has been constituted under the chairmanship of the Prime Minister with representation of 33 ministries and departments to ensure mainstreaming of involvement of people living with HIV/AIDS prevention activities in ongoing programs of ministries concerned and departments.

Reviews indicate that most of the targets set for NACP III are likely to be achieved by mid 2012 in terms of scale-up of coverage of high-risk group (HRG), safe blood supply, testing services, scale-up of ART and various interventions with community ownership and following principles such as greater involvement of people living with HIV/AIDS (GIPA).

National AIDS Control Organization (NACO) has started discussions with various partners to collect suggestions and advice for the implementation of the National AIDS control program phase IV.

Integrated Disease Surveillance Project

Integrated Disease Surveillance Project (IDSP) was launched in November 2004. It is intended to detect early warning signals of impending outbreaks and help to initiate an effective response in a timely manner.

Pilot project has also been started by IDSP for strengthening community-based disease surveillance in three states (Maharashtra, Orissa and Karnataka). Dashamantapur (Koraput-Orissa), Semiliguda (Koraput-Orissa), Akkalkuwa (Nandurbar-Maharashtra) and Taloda (Nandurbar-Maharashtra) have started community-based surveillance activities. Seven infectious disease hospitals, one each in four metros and Bengaluru, Ahmedabad and Hyderabad have been given funds for strengthening reporting from ID Hospitals. IDSP is supporting activities related to avian influenza under IDSP with total outlay of ₹ 20.85 crores for 3 years (2006–09) for human component. A networking model has been developed with 10 laboratories and additionally ICMR with its four branch laboratories.

National Program for Control of Blindness

Main causes of blindness include cataract, refractive errors, corneal blindness, childhood blindness, glaucoma and diabetic retinopathy. National Program for Control of Blindness (NPCB) was launched as a 100% centrally sponsored program in the year 1976 with the goal of reducing the prevalence of blindness to 0.3% by 2020. Rapid survey on avoidable blindness conducted during 2006–07 showed a reduction in the prevalence rate of blindness from 1.1% (2001–02) to 1% (2006–07).

Regional Institute of Ophthalmology was established; medical colleges and district hospitals and block-level primary health centers were upgraded; mobile units were developed and the required ophthalmic manpower in eye care units for provision of various ophthalmic services was recruited. The program also extended assistance to voluntary organizations for providing eye -care services including cataract operations and eye banking.

Services available under the program include free cataract surgery for the poor, detection and correction of refractive errors in children and treatment of corneal blindness by corneal transplantation from donated eyes.

Now, the program implementation is decentralized and the activities are coordinated by state/district blindness control societies throughout the country. During the year 2005–06, more than 48 lakh cataract operations were performed. 90% of them were implanted with intraocular lenses (IOL). 2.94 crore students were screened for refractive errors, 7.26 lakh refractive error cases were detected and 3.50 lakh poor children were given free glasses. Nearly 25,000 eye donations take place annually in the country.

During the 10th five year plan, emphasis is being given to develop capacities for treatment of childhood blindness, glaucoma and diabetic retinopathy through training of eye surgeons and supply of ophthalmic equipments.

Revised Blindness Control Program

During the 11th five year plan period, the scope of the scheme has been expanded.

The stress was on technology upgradation during this plan period. The highlights are as follows:

1. Supply of good screening and diagnostic tools and equipments.
2. Dedicated OPD, eye ward and eye OT units.
3. Fully trained surgical team.
4. Modern surgical tools and intraoperative patient care apparatus.
5. Full asepsis to prevent postoperative infection.
6. Quality presterilized drugs and surgical consumables.
7. Training for sponsored candidates from all over the country.

During 12th plan period, it is proposed to modify the pattern of assistance to effectively reduce prevalence of blindness and develop infrastructure and eye care services delivery system.

New initiatives in 12th plan are:

1. Free glasses for people above 40 years to correct presbyopic vision.
2. Observation of eye testing fortnight for school children during June each year when most schools are on vacation.
3. Multipurpose mobile ophthalmic units in all districts the entire country to conduct:
   a. Screening eye camp.
   b. School eye screening .
   c. On the spot refraction and free spectacles.
   d. Screening for diabetic retinopathy, glaucoma.
   e. Activity for improving the performance of eye banks.
   f. Special campaigns for creating mass awareness.
4. Construction of dedicated ophthalmic units.

5. Grant-in-aid for NGO eye units in district hospitals.
6. Involvement of private practitioners.
7. Training of human resources-eye surgeons, paramedical ophthalmic assistants (PMOAs), auxiliary nurse midwives (ANMs), accredited social health activists (ASHAs).

Vision Centers

During this plan period, it is envisaged to set up 3,000 'vision centers' with basic screening equipment catering to every 5,000 population; develop a network of 30 eye banks and 130 eye donation centers to facilitate collection and processing of donated eyes and provide non-recurring assistance to 40 voluntary organizations for strengthening and expanding eye care services in rural areas.

National Iodine Deficiency Disorders Control Program

Iodine deficiency is seen in various parts of the country. Out of 282 districts covering all the states/union territories surveyed, 241 districts are found to be endemic, where the prevalence of iodine deficiency disorders is more than 10%. It is estimated that more than 6.1 crores people are suffering from goiter and 88 lakh people are mental/motor handicaps.

Objectives

Since 1962, the Government of India is implementing the National Iodine Deficiency Disorders Control Program (NIDDCP) (formerly known as the National Goiter Control Program) with the following objectives:

1. To undertake surveys to assess the magnitude of iodine deficiency disorders (IDDs).
2. To supply iodized salt in place of common salt.
3. To conduct resurveys to assess the impact of control measures after every 5 years.
4. To undertake monitoring the quality of iodized salts and assess urinary iodine excretion pattern.
5. To conduct health education and publicity.

The annual production of iodized salt is about 48 lakh metric tonnes (MT). The Government has banned the sale of non-iodized salt in the entire country for direct human consumption under Prevention of Food Adulteration Act, 1954 from 17th May 2006. For effective implementation of NIDDCP at the state level, 29 states/UTs have established IDD control cells.

As a newer initiative, neonatal screening for thyroid stimulating hormone (TSH) and screening of children for growth disorder, school performance, subclinical hypothyroidism, etc. are being undertaken in GBT hospital in Delhi. It is likely to be extended as a universal neonatal TSH screening in future.

National Mental Health Program

The WHO report on global burden of diseases has projected mental illness to be the fourth major cause of morbidity. Epidemiological studies in India indicate that the prevalence rate of mental and behavioral disorder is 80.6% for urban sector and 48.9% in the rural sector.

The National Mental Health Program was started in 1982 for providing community-based mental health care using the existing public health infrastructure. The program also includes strengthening of departments of psychiatry in medical colleges (70 medical colleges have been covered), modernization of mental hospitals (23 mental hospitals have been funded), focusing on IEC and public education, research and training.

Objectives

1. To ensure availability and accessibility of minimum mental health care for all in the foreseeable future, particularly to the most vulnerable and underprivileged sections of population.
2. To encourage application of mental health knowledge in general health care and in social development.
3. To promote community participation in the mental health services development and to stimulate efforts towards self-help in the community.

District Mental Health Program

A model delivery of community-based mental health care at the level of district evolved by National Institute of Mental Health and Neurosciences (NIMHANS), Bengaluru, was adapted as the District Mental Health Program (DMHP) and it was implemented in 27 districts across 22 states/UTs in the year 1996. Now it is under implementation in 123 districts throughout the country. A sum of ₹ 70 crores has been earmarked for implementation of the national mental health program during the year 2007-08.

Components

Components of district mental health program are:

1. Training programs of all workers in the mental health team at the identified nodal institute in the state.
2. Public education in the mental health to increase awareness and reduce stigma.
3. For early detection and treatment, the OPD and indoor services are provided.
4. Providing valuable data and experience at the level of community to the state and center for future planning, improvement in service and research.

Pilot Project on Micronutrient Malnutrition

The pilot project against micronutrient malnutrition is being implemented since 1995 in Assam and four other states namely Bihar, Orissa, West Bengal and Gujarat. This project has been merged with NIDDCP.

Objectives

The objectives of the program are:

1. To assess the magnitude of fluorosis and dental caries.
2. To assess and improve iron and vitamin A status in school going children, adolescent boys and girls, non-pregnant women, adult males and geriatric population.

3. To launch extensive information, education and communication strategies through mass media to improve the dietary habits of the population.
4. To study zinc level in various food products and soil.

The program is being implemented in one district of each of the five states. In Assam, Kamrup district was taken up for activities to be undertaken namely advocacy and sensitization meetings with people involved in policy making with elected members, teachers, social workers, etc. A baseline survey was conducted to assess the socioeconomic status, food intake pattern, estimation of hemoglobin (HB), soil zinc, fluorine in drinking water, etc. Training was also organized at block level, prior to field activity surveys. Based on the results of the survey, the IEC strategy is being developed in the local languages.

National Cancer Control Program

In India it is estimated that there are 2–2.5 million cancer patients at any given point of time with about 0.7 million new cases coming every year and nearly half die every year. Two third of the new cancers are presented in advance and incurable stage at the time of diagnosis. More than 60% of these affected patients are in the prime of their life between the ages of 35 and 65 years, with increasing life expectancy and changing lifestyles concomitant with development, the number of cancer cases will be almost three times the current number.

Cancers of the head and neck in both sexes and of the uterine cervix in women are the most common malignancies seen in the country. The age-adjusted incidence rate per 100,000 for all types in India in urban areas range from 106 to 130 for men and 100 to 140 for women, but still lower than USA, UK and Japan rates. 50% of all male cancers and 25% of all female cancers are tobacco related. 34% of all cancers are tobacco related. Seven-fold increase in tobacco-related cancer morbidity is predicted in future.

Government of India has launched the National Cancer Control Program in 1975 and revised its strategies in 1984–85 stressing on primary prevention and early detection of cancer.

Objectives

1. Primary prevention: Health education and prevention of intake of tobacco.
2. Secondary prevention: Early detection of common cancers such as of cervical, oral and breast and other tobacco-related cancers.
3. Tertiary prevention: Strengthening the existing institutions for comprehensive therapy including palliative care.

The program was revised in December 2004. Under the revised program there are five schemes:

1. Recognition of new Regional Cancer Centers (RCCs).
2. Strengthening of existing RCC.
3. Development of oncology wing in Government institutions (medical colleges as well as government hospitals).
4. District cancer control program spread over a period of 5 years.
5. Decentralized NGO scheme for IEC activities.

Under the 10th five year plan, the major focus has been on correcting the geographical imbalance in the availability of cancer treatment facilities in the country.

❑ GUINEA WORM DISEASE ERADICATION

Guinea worm disease has been eradicated in India. The eradication has been certified by International Commission for Certification of Dracunculiasis Eradication, WHO in its meeting at Geneva during February 15th–17th, 2000.

India Yaws-free

India took up Yaws Eradication Program (YEP) in 1996–97. National Institute of Communicable Diseases (NICD) implemented the program. The project was first taken up in Koraput district of Orissa in 1996–97 and in 1999 it was extended to all endemic districts of the state.

Yaws has been eliminated from India as no case has been reported for the past 3 years. If there is no incidence for next 2 years, than it will mean the disease has been eradicated.

The Central Rural Sanitation Program

Rural sanitation is a state subject. The Central Rural Sanitation Program (CRSP) was launched in 1986 by the central government to supplement the efforts of the states through technical and financial assistance.

Objectives

1. To bring about an improvement in the general quality of life in the rural areas.
2. To accelerate sanitation coverage in rural areas.
3. To generate felt demand for sanitation facilities through awareness creation and health education.
4. To cover schools/anganwadis in rural areas with sanitation facilities and promote hygiene education and sanitary habits among students.
5. To encourage cost-effective and appropriate technologies in sanitation.
6. To eliminate open defecation, to minimize risk of contamination of drinking water sources and food.
7. To convert dry latrines into sanitary latrines and eliminate manual scavenging practice, whenever in existence in rural areas.

Strategies

1. Community-led, people-centered and demand-driven approach.
2. Alternate delivery mechanisms would be adopted.
3. Rural school sanitation is a major component.
4. Involvement of Panchayat Raj institutions, cooperatives, women groups, self-help groups, NGOs, etc.

Components

- IEC activities
- Rural sanitary marts and production centers
- Construction of individual household latrines

- Women sanitary complex
- School sanitation
- Administrative charges.

Implementing Agencies

At the district level, District Water and Sanitation Mission is the implementing agency. Both the Total Sanitation Campaign (TSC) and Swajaldhara should be implemented by the same agency. At the state level, the State Water and Sanitation Mission constituted for sector reform should supervise. In states where water supply and sanitation are handled by two different departments, separate institutional setup may also be made subject to the condition that officials handling water supply should be actively associated with the institutional setup. NGOs have to be actively involved in IEC activities as well as in hardware activities.

Maintenance

Individual household latrines

All the members of the family should be trained in the proper upkeep and maintenance of the sanitation facilities. Individual household latrines are maintained by the households themselves.

Community sanitary complexes

The cost of maintaining community sanitary complexes may be met by the panchayats, voluntary organizations, charitable trusts and self-help groups (SHGs).

Institutions/organizations

Institutions/organizations operating and maintaining the sanitary complexes may charge suitable user charges to meet the operation and maintenance cost fully.

School/anganwadi

The departments concerned should provide adequate funds for the maintenance of toilets in these institutions.

Total sanitation campaign

Total Sanitation Campaign (TSC), as a part of reform principles, was initiated in 1999 when Central Rural Sanitation Program was restructured making it demand-driven and people-centered. It follows a principle of 'low to no subsidy,' where a nominal subsidy in the form of incentive is given to rural poor households for construction of toilets. TSC is a comprehensive program to ensure sanitation facilities in rural areas with broader goal to eradicate the practice of open defecation.

Total Sanitation Campaign gives strong emphasis on information, education and communication (IEC), capacity building and hygiene education for effective behavior change with involvement of PRIs, CBOs, NGOs, etc. The key intervention areas are individual household latrines (IHHL), school sanitation and hygiene education (SSHE), community sanitary complex, anganwadi toilets supported by rural sanitary marts (RSMs) and production centers (PCs). The revised approach is expected to generate demand for sanitary facilities.

To improve the implementation of TSC, Government of India has separately launched an award scheme the 'Nirmal Gram Puraskar' (NGP) for fully, sanitized and open defecation-free gram panchayats, block and districts. In the first year of its institution, only 40 PRIs were awarded NGP on 24th February 2005. In the second year the number of awarded PRIs/blocks and organization have increased to 772.

The sanitation coverage in India during 2000–01 was a mere 21.9%. It gradually increased to 70.23% in 2010–11. Sikkim has become the first Nirmal State in the country achieving 100% total sanitation coverage.

Nirmal Bharat Abhiyan (NBA): Total sanitation campaign (TSC) renamed as 'Nirmal Bharat Abhiyan' (NBA) with an objective to accelerate sanitation coverage in the rural areas comprehensively has been launched since 1st April, 2012. The goal is to achieve 100% access to sanitation for all rural households in the country by 2022. Nirmal Bharat Abhiyan is currently being implemented in 607 rural districts across the country. Implementation of NBA is proposed with Gram panchayat (GP) as the base unit with a vision of Nirmal Bharat by 2022 with all GPs in the country attaining nirmal status. Individual household latrine in both below poverty line (BPL) and identified above poverty line (APL) households within a gram panchayat, solid and liquid waste management for proposed and existing gram panchayats, provision of sanitation facilities in all Government schools and Anganwadi centers and appropriate convergence with Mahatma Gandhi National Rural Employment Guarantee Scheme (MGNREGS) are to be taken up. The incentive amount has been increased from ₹ 3,200 to ₹ 4,600 and the minimum beneficiary share shall be ₹ 900 in cash or labor. Apart from that an amount of ₹ 4,500 can also be dovetailed from MGNREG Act. In the 12th plan an outlay of ₹ 34,377 crores has been provided for rural sanitation as compared to ₹ 6,540 crores in the 11th plan.

National Program for Prevention and Control of Deafness

Hearing loss is the most common sensory deficit in humans today. According to WHO, approximately 63 million people are suffering from significant auditory impairment with a prevalence of 6.3% in Indian population. National Sample Survey Organization (NSSO) survey estimates that 291 persons per one lakh population suffer from severe to profound hearing loss (NSSO, 2001). Of these, a large percentage is children between the ages of 0–14 years. With such a large number of hearing-impaired young Indians, severe loss of productivity both physical and economic may be the consequences. An even larger percentage of our population suffers from milder degrees of hearing loss and unilateral (one sided) hearing loss.

A pilot phase has been implemented in 25 districts derived from 10 states and one union territory till March 2008. It is proposed to expand the program to 203 districts by the end of 11th five year plan. In the current year (2008–09), 35 new districts have been included in the program.

Capacity building at the district hospitals to ensure better care and state of the ART department of ENT at the medical colleges are envisaged under the project.

Objectives

1. To prevent the avoidable hearing loss because of disease or injury.
2. Early identification, diagnosis and treatment of ear problems that are responsible for hearing loss and deafness.

3. To medically rehabilitate persons of all age groups suffering from deafness.
4. To strengthen the existing intersectoral linkages for continuity of the rehabilitation program for persons with deafness.
5. To develop institutional capacity for ear care services by providing support for equipment, material and training personnel.

Components of the Program

1. Manpower training and development for prevention, early identification and management of hearing impaired and deafness cases. Training would be provided to all from medical college level ENT and audiology specialists to grass root-level workers.
2. Capacity building for the district hospital, CHC and PHC in respect of ENT/audiology infrastructure.
3. Providing service including rehabilitation: Screening camps for early detection of hearing impairment and deafness, management of hearing and speech-impaired cases and rehabilitation (including provision of hearing aids), at different levels of healthcare delivery system.
4. Awareness generation through IEC activities: For early identification of hearing impaired, especially children, so that timely management of such cases is possible and to remove the stigma attached to deafness.
5. Monitoring and evaluation.

National Program for Prevention and Control of Diabetes, Cardiovascular Diseases and Stroke

The National Program for Prevention and Control of Diabetes, Cardiovascular Diseases and Stroke (NPDCS) has been launched from 4th January 2008.

Objectives of the Pilot Phase

1. Risk reduction for prevention of non-communicable diseases (NCDs) (diabetes, CVD and stroke).
2. Early diagnosis and appropriate management of diabetes, cardiovascular diseases and stroke.

Strategies

- Health promotion for the general population
- Disease prevention for the high-risk groups
- Orienting the public health delivery system
- Setting up special clinics
- Specific interventions at the tertiary level to enhance capacity to respond to the needs of NCD
- Specific intervention for rheumatic fever/rheumatic heart disease.

Health promotion for the general population

Health promotion activities target healthy, risk-free population and involves development of an effective communication strategy to modify individual, group and community behavior through media. It also focuses on community mobilization and participation and mainstreaming the health promotion agenda to reach until the village level. The interventions involve at various settings of community, school and workplace.

Community-based interventions

This involves health education regarding benefits of physical activities, dietary changes, mainstreaming the agenda of health promotion into the activities of village health and sanitation committees (VHSCs), gram panchayats, self-help groups and faith-based organizations will be part of the strategy for health promotion.

Workplace interventions

This is done by identifying peer educators and providing initial training. The trained educators introduce health promotion for their respective organizations.

School-based interventions

Here the intervention involves evaluation of the existing school health program components viz. physical education, nutrition and food services, health promotion for school personnel, health education and health services followed by activities to make health promotion, a defined agenda in the school curriculum.

Disease prevention for the high risk

Interventions aim at early diagnosis and appropriate management for reducing morbidity and mortality targeting people, who suffer from elevated risks demonstrated through hypertension, obesity, high blood lipid and glucose levels and those who have suffered from a previous cerebral or coronary event and are at the high risk.

Orienting the public health delivery system

Healthcare providers at all levels will be mobilized and trained to involve in risk detection and screening viz. blood pressure checks, recommending lifestyle modifications, dissemination of information and referring for further management. System strengthening will be at all levels; the primary, secondary and tertiary levels.

Setting up special clinics

Special clinic for diabetes/cardiovascular disease/stroke will be established at the district hospital. Services of private practitioners may be taken for this clinic as a visiting consultant. The clinic will do the screening and will also provide the management. Difficult and complicated cases will be referred to tertiary care center or the nearby medical college.

The resources of private sector will be harnessed; low yield technologies and cost-effective interventions will be used.

Specific interventions at the tertiary level to enhance capacity to respond to the needs of NCD

It has been established that prompt intervention to manage a cardiac event can reduce mortality to a large extent. Identification of a referral center and strengthening the linkage to the nearest referral center at the tertiary/secondary level and also strengthening the center through provision of necessary infrastructure and manpower.

Specific intervention for rheumatic fever/rheumatic heart disease

Rheumatic fever affects children and, if early detection and treatment is given, it does not affect the heart. If not detected and treated early it will affect the heart that will require prolonged cardiac care and also surgical interventions. Specific activities for creation of public awareness, reorientation of primary healthcare providers for early detection and referral will be taken up.

National program for prevention and control of non-communicable diseases

India is experiencing a rising burden of non-communicable diseases (NCDs). According to a WHO report (2002), cardiovascular diseases (CVDs) will be the largest cause of death and disability in India by 2020. Overall, NCDs are emerging as the leading cause of deaths in India accounting for over 42% of all deaths (Registrar General of India).

It is estimated that the overall prevalence of diabetes, hypertension, ischemic heart diseases (IHD) and stroke is 62.47, 159.46, 37.00 and 1.54 respectively per 1,000 population of India. There are an estimated 25-lakh cancer cases in India. According to the National Commission on Macroeconomics and Health (NCMH) Report (2005), the crude incidence rate (CIR) for cervix cancer, breast cancer and oral cancer 21.3, 17.1 and 11.8 (among both men and women) per 100,000 populations respectively.

Preventable risk factors

The main preventable risk factors for NCDs are tobacco consumption, poor dietary habits, sedentary lifestyle, stress, etc. national family health survey III (2005–06) reported that the prevalence of current tobacco use was 57% among men and 10.8% among women. Over 8 lakh deaths occur every year due to diseases associated with tobacco use. The cancer registry data reveals that 48% of cancers in males and 20% in females are tobacco related and are totally avoidable. Common cancers caused by smoking tobacco are lung, larynx, pharynx and esophagus, while cancers of the mouth, tongue and lips are due to chewing and smoking tobacco.

The central government proposes to supplement the efforts of states by providing technical and financial support through National Program for Prevention and Control of Cancer, Diabetes, Cardiovascular Disease and Stroke (NPCDCS). The NPCDCS program is divided into two components which are as follows:

1. Cancer.
2. Diabetes, CVDs and stroke.

These two components have been integrated at different levels as far as possible for optimal utilization of the resources. The activities at state, districts, CHC and subcenter level have been planned under the program and will be closely monitored through NCD cell at different levels.

The NPCDCS aims at integration of NCD interventions in the NRHM framework for optimization of scarce resources and provision of seamless services to the end customer/patients as also for ensuring long-term sustain ability of interventions. Thus, the institutionalization of NPCDCS at district level within the district health society, sharing administrative and financial structure of NRHM becomes a crucial program strategy for NPCDCS. The NCD cell at various levels will ensure implementation and supervision of the program activities related to health promotion, early diagnosis, treatment and referral and further facilitates partnership with laboratories for early diagnosis in the private sector. Simultaneously, it will attempt to create a wider knowledge base in the community for effective prevention, detection, referrals and treatment strategies through convergence with the ongoing interventions of National Rural Health Mission (NRHM), National Tobacco Control Program (NTCP) and National Program for Health Care of Elderly (NPHCE), etc. and build a strong monitoring and evaluation system through the public health infrastructure.

Objectives

1. Prevent and control common NCDs through behavior and lifestyle changes.
2. Provide early diagnosis and management of common NCDs.
3. Build capacity at various levels of health care for prevention, diagnosis and treatment of common NCDs.
4. Train human resource within the public health setup viz. doctors, paramedics and nursing staff to cope with the increasing burden of NCDs.
5. Establish and develop capacity for palliative and rehabilitative care.

Strategies

The strategies to achieve the above objectives are as follows:

1. Prevention through behavior change.
2. Early diagnosis.

3. Treatment.
4. Capacity building of human resource.
5. Surveillance, monitoring and evaluation.

National Program for the Health Care of the Elderly

The National Program of the Health Care of the Elderly (NPHCE) is an articulation of the international and national commitments of the government as envisaged under the UN Convention on the Rights of Persons with Disabilities (UNCRPD), National Policy on Older Persons (NPOP) adopted by the Government of India in 1999 and section 20 of 'The Maintenance and Welfare of Parents and Senior Citizens Act, 2007' dealing with provisions for medical care of senior citizen.

Surveillance

The increase in human longevity in 20th century has resulted in the increase of old age population all over the world. India is no exception to this. In India, the population over the age of 60 years has tripled in the last 50 years. In 2001, the proportion of older people was 7.7%, which increased to 8.14% in 2011 and will be 8.94% in 2016. According to 2001 census, there were 75.93 million Indians above the age of 60 years (38.22 million males and 37.71 million females).

Along with rising numbers, the expectancy of life at birth is also consistently increasing indicating that a large number of people are likely to live longer than before.

The national sample surveys of 1986–87, 1995–1996 and 2004 have shown that the burden of morbidity in old age is enormous. Non-communicable diseases are extremely common in older people irrespective of socioeconomic status. The treatment/management of these chronic diseases is also costly for the elderly whose income decreases postretirement and more so for the elderly in the unorganized sector and dependent elderly women. It is also seen that many older people take ill health in their stride as a part of 'usual/normal ageing'. This observation has a lot of significance, as self-perceived health status is an important indicator of health service utilization and compliance to treatment interventions.

Healthcare Model for Elderly

The developed world has evolved many models for elderly care, e.g. nursing home care, health insurance, etc. No such model for older people exists in India as well as in most other societies with similar socioeconomic situation. Presently elderly people are provided health care by the general healthcare delivery system in the country. As their health problems also need specialist care from various disciplines, e.g. ophthalmology, orthopedics, psychiatry, cardiovascular, dental, urology to name a few, a model of care providing comprehensive health services to elderly at all levels of healthcare delivery is imperative to meet the growing health need of the elderly.

Ministry of Health and Family Welfare was entrusted with the agenda to attend to the healthcare needs of the elderly in the following ways:

1. Establishing geriatric ward for elderly patients at all district level hospitals.
2. Expansion of treatment facilities for chronic, terminal and degenerative diseases.
3. Providing improved medical facilities to those not able to attend medical centers; strengthening of CHCs/PHCs/mobile clinics.
4. Inclusion of geriatric care in the syllabus of medical courses including courses for nurses.
5. Reservation of beds for elderly in public hospitals.
6. Training of geriatric caregivers.
7. Setting up research institutes for chronic elderly diseases such as dementia and Alzheimer's.

Specific Objectives

1. To provide an easy access to promotional, preventive, curative and rehabilitative services to the elderly through community-based primary healthcare approach.
2. To identify health problems in the elderly and provide appropriate health interventions in the community with a strong referral backup support.

3. To build capacity of the medical and paramedical professionals as well as the caretakers within the family for providing health care to the elderly.
4. To provide referral services to the elderly patients through district hospitals, regional medical institutions.

Expected Outcomes

1. Regional geriatric centers (RGC) in eight regional medical institutions by setting up regional geriatric centers with a dedicated geriatric OPD and 30-bedded geriatric ward for management of specific diseases of the elderly, training of health personnel in geriatric health care and conducting research.
2. Postgraduates in geriatric medicine (16) from the 8 regional medical institutions.
3. Video conferencing units in the 8 regional medical institutions to be utilized for capacity building and mentoring.
4. District geriatric units with dedicated geriatric OPD and 10-bedded geriatric ward in 80–100 district hospitals.
5. Geriatric clinics/rehabilitation units set up for domiciliary visits in community/primary health centers in the selected districts.
6. Subcenters provided with equipment for community outreach services.
7. Training of human resources in the public healthcare system in geriatric care.

National Tobacco Control Program

In India, more than 2,000 persons die every day and about 8 lakh people die every year due to tobacco-related diseases. Tobacco use can cause spontaneous abortion, premature delivery and intrauterine growth retardation. Even passive smoking can cause lung cancer, respiratory illness, heart diseases, nasal sinus cancer, premature aging and intrauterine effects.

50% of all male cancers and 25% in females are tobacco related; 34% of all cancers are tobacco related. Tobacco-related cancer morbidity, during 1995–2025, is predicted to increase seven fold. The Government of India launched the National Cancer Control

Program in 1975. Its strategies were revised in 1984–85 stressing on primary prevention and early detection of cancer.

Strategies

India is in the forefront in enacting the tobacco control measures through tobacco control legislation. An Act called 'The Cigarette and other Tobacco Product (Prohibition of Advertisement and Regulation of Trade and Commerce, Production, Supply and Distribution) Act, 2003' has been enacted to curb the use of tobacco.

There is a ban on smoking in public places, ban on tobacco advertising, ban on sale of tobacco products to minors and a ban on the sale of tobacco products within a radius of 100 yards from educational institutions in India. The most recent and prominent contribution to tobacco control is the notification of the specified pictorial health warnings to be displayed on all tobacco product packs.

Rules to implement the law have been notified and revised to expand the definition of public places to include all workplaces, shopping malls, cinema halls, etc. State governments are being sensitized to accord due priority to the implementation of the law.

Government of India has launched National Tobacco Control Program (NTCP) in the 11th five year plan to implement anti-tobacco laws. School program is one of the crucial parts of the national program targeting school children as well as college going youth. The central government has instructed the states to use the National Rural Health Mission (NRHM) workforce for anti-tobacco programs.

Tobacco Free Initiatives

WHO established the tobacco free initiatives (TFI) in 1998. Long-term mission of TFI is to reduce smoking prevalence and tobacco consumption in all countries and among all groups and thereby reduces the burden of disease caused by tobacco.

The goals of the TFI are:

1. To galvanize global support for evidence-based tobacco control policies and actions.

2. To build new partnerships for action and to strengthen existing ones.
3. To heighten awareness of the need to address tobacco issues at all levels of society.
4. To accelerate the implementation of national, regional and global strategies.
5. To commission policy research to support rapid, sustained and innovative actions.
6. To mobilize resources to support required action.

WHO has developed partnership with UNICEF, World Bank, CDC, Environment Protection Agency, US National Institute of Health, international NGOs, private sector and academic centers for tobacco prevention work. In the 53rd and the 54th World Health Assembly, all member states reaffirmed for the actions required to control tobacco.

National Program for Control and Treatment of Occupational Diseases

Government of India has launched the 'National Program for Control and Treatment of Occupational Diseases' in 1998-99. The National Institute of Occupational Health, Ahmedabad (ICMR) has been identified as the nodal agency for the same.

The government has proposed to initiate the following research projects:

1. Prevention, control and treatment of silicosis and silicotuberculosis in agate industry.
2. Occupational health problems of tobacco harvesters and prevention.
3. Database generation, documentation and information dissemination on hazardous process and chemicals.
4. Capacity building to promote research, education and training (National Institute of Occupational Disease).
5. Health risk assessment and development of intervention program in cottage industries with high risk of silicosis.
6. Prevention and control of occupational health hazards among workers in the remote desert areas of Gujarat and Rajasthan.

Global Strategy for Occupational Health

The global strategy for achieving occupational health for all (WHO-SEARO 1999) includes the following 10 major areas for action:

1. Strengthening international and national policies for health at work and development of policy tools.
2. Developing healthy work environments.
3. Developing healthy work practices and promoting health at work.
4. Strengthening occupational health services.
5. Establishing support services for occupational health.
6. Developing occupational health standards based on scientific risk assessment.
7. Developing human resources for occupational health.
8. Establishing registration and data system including development of information services for experts, effective transmission of data and raising public awareness through strengthened public information system.
9. Strengthening research.
10. Developing collaboration in occupational health services and organizations.

SECTION

9

Health Care in India: Vision and Mission

CHAPTER

31

National Health Policy and Rural Health Mission

❑ NATIONAL HEALTH POLICY 2002

National Health Policy (NHP) last formulated in 1983, in a spirit of optimistic empathy for the health needs of the people, particularly the poor and underprivileged, had hoped to provide 'Health for All by the year 2000 AD', through the universal provision of comprehensive primary healthcare services. In retrospect, it is observed that the financial resources and public health administrative capacity was far short of that necessary, to achieve such an ambitious and holistic goal. The changed circumstances relating to the health sector of the country since 1983 have generated a situation in which it is now necessary to review the field and to formulate a new policy framework as the NHP-2002. The NHP-2002 will attempt to set out a new policy framework for the accelerated achievement of public health goals in the socioeconomic circumstances currently prevailing in the country.

Objectives

The main objective of this policy is to achieve an acceptable standard of good health amongst the general population of the country. The approach would be to increase access to the decentralized public health system by establishing new infrastructure in deficient areas and by upgrading the infrastructure in the existing institutions. Overriding importance would be given to ensure a more equitable access to health services across the social and geographical expanse of the country. Emphasis will be given to increasing the aggregate public health investment through a substantially increased contribution by the central government. It is expected that this initiative will strengthen the capacity of the public health administration at the state level, to render effective service delivery. The contribution of the private sector in providing health services would be much enhanced, particularly for the population group, which can afford to pay for services. Primacy will be given to preventive and first-line curative initiatives at the primary health level through increased sectoral share of allocation. Emphasis will be laid on rational use of drugs within the allopathic system. Increased access to tried and tested systems of traditional medicine will be ensured.

The existing scenario and the vision of NHP-2002 are given below.

Financial Resources

The public health investment in the country over the years has been comparatively low. As a percentage of GDP, it has declined from 1.3% in 1990 to 0.9% in 1999. The aggregate expenditure in the health sector is 5.2% of the GDP. The central budgetary allocation for health over this period, as a percentage of the total central budget, has been stagnant at 1.3%, while that in the states has declined from 7.0% to 5.5%. The current annual per capita public health expenditure in the country is no more than ₹ 200. Given these statistics, it is no surprise that the reach and quality of public health services has been below the desirable standard. Under the constitutional structure, public health is the responsibility of the states. The fiscal resources of the state governments are known to be very inelastic. This is reflected in the declining percentage of state resources allocated to the health sector out of the state budget. If the decentralized public health services in the country are to be improved significantly, there is a need for the injection of substantial resources into the health sector from the central government budget. The NHP-2002 has been formulated taking into consideration these ground realities in regard to the availability of resources.

Equity

The attainment of health indices has been very uneven across the rural–urban divide. The attainment of an equitable regional distribution was considered one of its major objectives by the central government. Given a situation in which national averages in respect of most indices are themselves at unacceptably low levels, the wide interstate disparity implies that, for vulnerable sections of society in several states, access to public health services is nominal and health standards are grossly inadequate. Applying current norms to the population projected for the year 2000, it is estimated that the shortfall in the number of SCs/PHCs/CHCs is of the order of 16%. However, this shortage is as high as 58% when disaggregated for CHCs only. The NHP-2002 will need to address itself for making good of these deficiencies so as to narrow the gap between the various states, as also the gap across the rural-urban divide.

Access to and benefits from the public health system have been very uneven between the better-endowed and the more vulnerable sections of society. This is particularly true for women, children and the socially disadvantaged sections of society.

It is a principal objective of NHP-2002 to evolve a policy structure, which reduces these inequities and allows the disadvantaged sections of society, a fairer access to public health services.

Delivery of National Public Health Programs

It is self-evident that in a country as large as India, which has a wide variety of socioeconomic settings, national health programs have to be designed with enough flexibility to permit the state public health administrations to craft their own program package according to their needs. It has been observed that the technical and managerial expertise for designing large-span public health programs exists with the central government in a considerable degree. This expertise can be gainfully utilized in designing national health programs for implementation in varying socioeconomic settings in the states. With this background, the NHP-2002 attempts to define the role of the central government and the state governments in the public health sector of the country.

Over the last decade or so, the government has relied upon a 'vertical' implementation structure for the major disease control programs. However, such an organizational structure, which requires independent manpower for each disease program, is extremely expensive and difficult to sustain. Over a long time period, 'vertical' structures may only be affordable for those diseases, which offer a reasonable possibility of elimination or eradication in a foreseeable time span.

It is a widespread perception that, over the last decade and a half, the rural health staff has become a vertical structure exclusively for the implementation of family welfare activities. As a result, for those public health programs where there is no separate vertical structure, there is no identifiable service delivery system at all. The policy will address this distortion in the public health system.

State of Public Health Infrastructure

The existing public health infrastructure is far from satisfactory. For the outdoor medical facilities in existence, funding is generally insufficient; the presence of medical and paramedical personnel is often much less than that required by prescribed norms; the availability of consumables is frequently negligible; the equipment in many public hospitals is often obsolescent and unusable; and the buildings are in a dilapidated state. In the indoor treatment facilities, again, the equipment is often obsolescent; the availability of essential drugs is minimal; the capacity of the facilities is grossly inadequate, which leads to overcrowding and consequently to a steep deterioration in the quality of the services. As a result of such inadequate public health facilities, it has been estimated that less than 20% of the population, which seek outpatient department (OPD) services and less than 45% of that, which seek indoor treatment, avail of such services in public hospitals. This is despite the fact that most of these patients do not have the means to make out-of-pocket payments for private health services except at the cost of other essential expenditure for items such as basic nutrition.

Extending Public Health Services

There is a general shortage of medical personnel in the country; this shortfall is disproportionately impacted on the less-developed and rural areas. In such a situation, the possibility needs to be examined of entrusting some limited public health functions to nurses, paramedics and other personnel from the extended health sector after imparting adequate training to them.

India has a vast reservoir of practitioners in the Indian systems of medicine and homeopathy, who have undergone formal training in their own disciplines. The possibility of using such practitioners in the implementation of state/central government public health programs, in order to increase the reach of basic health care in the country, is addressed in the NHP-2002.

Role of Local Self-government Institutions

Some states have adopted a policy of devolving programs and funds in the health sector through different levels of the Panchayati Raj institutions. Generally, the experience has been an encouraging one. The policy examines the need for a wider adoption of this mode of delivery of health services, in rural as well as urban areas, in other parts of the country.

Norms for Healthcare Personnel

It is observed that the deployment of doctors and nurses, in both public and private institutions, is ad-hoc and significantly short of the requirement for minimal standards of patient care. This policy will make a specific recommendation in regard to this deficiency.

Education of Healthcare Professionals

Medical and dental colleges are not evenly spread across various parts of the country. The quality of education is highly uneven and in several instances even substandard. It is a common perception that the syllabus is excessively theoretical, making it difficult for the fresh graduate to effectively meet even the primary healthcare needs of the population. There is a general reluctance on the part of graduate doctors to serve in areas distant from their native place. The NHP-2002 will suggest policy initiatives to rectify the resultant disparities.

The policy will make appropriate recommendations in respect of deficiencies in the area of molecular biology and gene manipulation.

Also, certain specialty disciplines, anesthesiology, radiology and forensic medicine are currently very scarce, resulting in critical deficiencies in the package of available public health services. This policy will recommend some measures to alleviate such critical shortages.

Need for Specialists in 'Public Health' and 'Family Medicine'

National Health Policy 2002 examines the possible means for ensuring adequate availability of personnel with specialization in the 'public health' and 'family medicine' disciplines to discharge the public health responsibilities in the country.

Nursing Personnel

The ratio of nursing personnel in the country vis-à-vis doctors/ beds is very low according to professionally accepted norms. There is also an acute shortage of nurses trained in superspecialty disciplines for deployment in tertiary care facilities. The NHP-2002 addresses these problems.

Use of Generic Drugs and Vaccines

India enjoys a relatively low-cost healthcare system because of the widespread availability of indigenously manufactured generic drugs and vaccines. There is an apprehension that globalization will lead to an increase in the costs of drugs, thereby leading to rising trends in overall health costs. This policy recommends measures to ensure the future health security of the country.

Urban Health

In most urban areas, public health services are very meager. Even the meager public health services, which are available, do not percolate to such unplanned habitations, forcing people to avail of private health care through out-of-pocket expenditure.

The rising vehicle density in large urban agglomerations has also led to an increased number of serious accidents requiring treatment in well-equipped trauma centers. The NHP-2002 will address itself to the need for providing this unserved urban population a minimum standard of broad-based healthcare facilities.

Mental Health

Mental health disorders are actually much more prevalent than is apparent on the surface. Sometimes, based on religious faith, mental disorders are treated as spiritual affliction. Serious conditions of mental disorder require hospitalization and treatment under trained supervision. Mental health institutions are woefully deficient in physical infrastructure and trained manpower. The NHP-2002 will address itself to these deficiencies in the public health sector.

Information, Education and Communication

A substantial component of primary health care consists of initiatives for disseminating to the citizenry, public health-related information. Information, education and communication (IEC) initiatives are adopted not only for disseminating curative guidelines (for the TB, malaria, leprosy, cataract blindness programs) but also as part of the effort to bring about a behavioral change to prevent HIV/AIDS and other lifestyle diseases. The present IEC strategy is too fragmented, relies too heavily on the mass media and does not address the needs of this segment of the population. The policy, while projecting an IEC strategy, will fully address the inherent problems encountered in any IEC program designed for improving awareness and bringing about a behavioral change in the general population.

It is widely accepted that school and college students are the most impressionable targets for imparting information relating to the basic principles of preventive health care. The policy will attempt to target this group to improve the general level of awareness in regard to 'health-promoting' behavior.

Health Research

Over the years, health research activity in the country has been very limited. The NHP-2002 will address these inadequacies and spell out a minimal quantum of expenditure for the coming decade, looking to the national needs and the capacity of the research institutions to absorb the funds.

Role of the Private Sector

Currently, the contribution of private health care is principally through independent practitioners. Also, the private sector contributes significantly to secondary-level care and some tertiary care. It is a widespread perception that private health services are very uneven in quality, sometimes even substandard. Private health services are also perceived to be financially exploitative and the observance of professional ethics is noted only as an exception. With the increasing role of private health care, the implementation of statutory regulation and the monitoring of minimum standards of diagnostic centers/medical institutions become imperative. The Policy will address the issues regarding the establishment of a comprehensive information system and based on that the establishment of a regulatory mechanism to ensure the maintaining of adequate standards by diagnostic centers/medical institutions, as well as the proper conduct of clinical practice and delivery of medical services.

Currently, non-governmental service providers are treating a large number of patients at the primary level for major diseases. However, the treatment regimens followed are diverse and not scientifically optimal, leading to an increase in the incidence of drug resistance. This policy will address itself to recommending arrangements, which will eliminate the risks arising from inappropriate treatment.

The increasing spread of information technology (IT) raises the possibility of its adoption in the health sector. The NHP-2002 will examine this possibility.

Role of Civil Society

It has become increasingly apparent that certain components of major national disease control programs cannot be efficiently implemented merely through government functionaries. A considerable change in the mode of implementation has come about in the last 2 decades with the increasing involvement of non-governmental organizations (NGOs) and other institutions of civil society. Certain disease control programs require close interaction with the beneficiaries for regular administration of drugs; periodic carrying out of pathological tests; dissemination of information regarding disease control and other general health information. The NHP-2002 will address such issues and suggest policy instruments for the implementation of public health programs through individuals and institutions of civil society.

National Disease Surveillance Network

The absence of an efficient disease surveillance network is a major handicap in providing a prompt and cost-effective healthcare system. The efficient disease surveillance network setup for polio and HIV/AIDS has demonstrated the enormous value of such a public health instrument. Real-time information on focal outbreaks of common communicable diseases such as malaria, gastroenteritis (GE), cholera and Japanese encephalitis (JE), and the seasonal trends of diseases would enable timely intervention, resulting in the containment of the thrust of epidemics. In order to be able to use integrated disease surveillance network for operational purposes, real-time information is necessary at all levels of the health administration. The policy would address itself to this major systemic shortcoming in the administration.

Health Statistics

The absence of a systematic and scientific health statistics database is a major deficiency in the current scenario. Further, the absence of proper and systematic documentation of the various financial resources used in the health sector is another lacuna in the existing health information scenario.

The NHP-2002 will address itself to the program for putting in place a modern and scientific health statistics database as well as a system of national health accounts.

Women's Health

Social, cultural and economic factors continue to inhibit women from gaining adequate access even to the existing public health facilities. This handicap does not merely affect women as individuals; it also has an adverse impact on the health, general well-being and development of the entire family, particularly children. This policy recognizes the catalytic role of empowered women in improving the overall health standards of the community.

Medical Ethics

Professional medical ethics in the health sector is an area, which has not received much attention. Professional practices are perceived to be grossly commercial and the medical profession has lost its elevated position as a provider of basic services to fellow human beings. Also, the new frontier areas of research; involving gene manipulation, organ/human cloning and stem cell research, impinge on visceral issues relating to the sanctity of human life and the moral dilemma of human intervention in the designing of life forms. Besides this, in the emerging areas of research, there is the uncharted risk of creating new life forms, which may irreversibly damage the environment as it exists today. The NHP–2002 recognizes that this moral and religious dilemma, which was not relevant even 2 years ago, now pervades mainstream health sector issues.

Enforcement of Quality Standards for Food and Drugs

There is an increasing expectation and need of the citizenry for efficient enforcement of reasonable quality standards for food and drugs. Recognizing this, the policy will make an appropriate policy recommendation on this issue.

Regulation of Standards in Paramedical Disciplines

It has been observed that a large number of training institutions have mushroomed, particularly in the private sector, for paramedical personnel with various skills such as laboratory technicians, radiodiagnosis technicians, physiotherapists, etc. Currently, there is no regulation/monitoring, either of the curricula of these institutions or of the performance of the practitioners in these disciplines. This policy will make recommendations to ensure the standardization of such training and the monitoring of actual performance.

Environmental and Occupational Health

Unsafe drinking water, unhygienic sanitation and air pollution significantly contribute to the burden of disease, particularly in urban settings. The initiatives in respect of these environmental factors are conventionally undertaken by the participants, whether private or public, in the other development sectors. In this backdrop, the policy initiatives and the efficient implementation of the linked programs in the health sector would succeed only to the extent that they are complemented by appropriate policies and programs in the other environment-related sectors.

Work conditions in several sectors of employment in the country are substandard. As a result, workers engaged in such employment become particularly vulnerable to occupation-linked ailments. The long-term risk of chronic morbidity is particularly marked in the case of child labor. The NHP-2002 will address the risk faced by this particularly vulnerable section of society.

Providing Medical Facilities to Users from Overseas

The secondary and tertiary facilities available in the country are of good quality and cost-effective compared to international medical facilities. This is true not only of facilities in the allopathic disciplines but also of those belonging to the alternative systems of medicine, particularly Ayurveda. The policy will assess the possibilities of encouraging the development of paid treatment packages for patients from overseas.

Impact of Globalization on the Health Sector

There are some apprehensions about the possible adverse impact of economic globalization on the health sector. With the adoption of Trade-related Aspects of Intellectual Property Rights (TRIPS) and the subsequent alignment of domestic patent laws consistent with the commitments under TRIPS, there will be a significant shift in the scope of the parameters regulating the manufacture of new drugs/vaccines. Global experience has shown that the introduction of a TRIPS-consistent patent regime for drugs in a developing country results in an across-the-board increase in the cost of drugs and medical services. The NHP-2002 will address itself to the future imperatives of health security in the country, in the post-TRIPS era.

Intersectoral Contribution to Health

It is well recognized that the overall well-being of the citizenry depends on the synergistic functioning of the various sectors in the socioeconomy. The health status of the citizenry would, inter alia, be dependent on adequate nutrition, safe drinking water, basic sanitation, a clean environment and primary education, especially for the girl child. The policies and the mode of functioning in these independent areas would necessarily overlap each other to contribute to the health status of the community. From the policy perspective, it is therefore imperative that the independent policies of each of these interconnected sectors be in tandem and that the interface between the policies of the two connected sectors be smooth.

Sectoral policy documents are meant to serve as a guide to action for institutions and individual participants operating in that sector. Consistent with this role, NHP-2002 limits itself to making recommendations for the participants operating within the health sector. The policy aspects relating to interconnected sectors, which, while crucial, fall outside the domain of the health sector, will not be covered by specific recommendations in this policy document. Needless to say, the future attainment of the various goals set out in this policy assumes a reasonable complementary performance in these interconnected sectors.

Population Growth and Health Standards

Efforts made over the years for improving health standards have been partially neutralized by the rapid growth of the population. It is well recognized that population stabilization measures and general health initiatives, when effectively synchronized, synergistically maximize the socioeconomic well-being of the people. Government has separately announced the `National Population Policy-2000'. The principal common features covered under the National Population Policy-2000 and NHP-2002 relate to the prevention and control of communicable diseases; giving priority to the containment of HIV/AIDS infection; the universal immunization of children against all major preventable diseases; addressing the unmet needs for basic and reproductive health services and supplementation of infrastructure. The synchronized implementation of these two policies, National Population Policy-2000 and NHP-2002, will be the very cornerstone of any national structural plan to improve the health standards in the country.

Alternative Systems of Medicine

Under the overarching umbrella of the national health framework, the alternative systems of medicine; ayurveda, unani, siddha and homeopathy, have a substantial role. Because of inherent advantages, such as diversity, modest cost, low level of technological input and the growing popularity of natural plant-based products, these systems are attractive, particularly in the underserved, remote and tribal areas. The alternative systems will draw upon the substantial untapped potential of India as one of the eight important global centers for plant diversity in medicinal and aromatic plants. The policy focuses on building up credibility for the alternative systems, by encouraging evidence-based research to determine their efficacy, safety and dosage, and also encourages certification and quality marking of products to enable a wider popular acceptance of these systems of medicine. The policy also envisages the consolidation of documentary knowledge contained in these systems to protect it against attack from foreign commercial entities by way of mala fide action under patent laws in other countries. The main components of NHP-2002 apply equally to the alternative systems of medicines. However, the policy features specific to the alternative systems of medicine will be presented as a separate document.

❑ NATIONAL RURAL HEALTH MISSION (2005–2012)

The Government of India launched a flagship program called the National Rural Health Mission (NRHM) in 2005 with the objective of expanding access to quality health care to rural populations by undertaking architectural corrections in the institutional mechanism for healthcare delivery. The mission is an articulation of the commitment of the government to raise public spending on health from 0.9% of GDP to 2%–3% of GDP.

The crucial strategies under NRHM have been the integration of family welfare and national disease control programs under an umbrella approach for optimization of resources and manpower; strengthening of outreach services by incorporation of village health worker called accredited social service activist (ASHA); efforts for communization of services through formation of health and sanitation committees at village, block and district level; registering Rogi Kalyan Samitis for improving hospital management; strengthening and upgrading the public health infrastructure to Indian Public Health Standards (IPHS) and consolidation of the district level program management unit through the induction of professionals.

State of Public Health in India

Public health expenditure in India has declined from 1.3% of GDP in 1990 to 0.9% of GDP in 1999. The union budgetary allocation for health is 1.3%; while the state's budgetary allocation is 5.5%. Union government's contribution to public health expenditure is 15%, while states' contribution is about 85%. Vertical health and family welfare programs have limited synergization at operational levels. Lack of community ownership of public health programs affects levels of efficiency, accountability and effectiveness.

There is lack of integration of sanitation, hygiene, nutrition and drinking water issues. There are striking regional inequalities.

Population stabilization is still a challenge; especially in states with weak demographic indicators. Curative services favor the non-poor. For every ₹ 1 spent on the poorest 20% population, ₹ 3 is spent on the richest quintile. Only 10% Indians have some form of health insurance, mostly inadequate. Hospitalized Indians spend on an average 58% of their total annual expenditure. Over 40% of hospitalized Indians borrow heavily or sell assets to cover expenses. Over 25% of hospitalized Indians fall below poverty line because of hospital expenses.

Goals

1. Reduction in infant mortality rate (IMR) and maternal mortality ratio (MMR).
2. Universal access to public health services such as women's health, child health, water sanitation and hygiene, immunization and nutrition.
3. Prevention and control of communicable and non-communicable diseases, including locally endemic diseases.
4. Access to integrated comprehensive primary health care.
5. Population stabilization, gender and demographic balance.
6. Revitalize local health traditions and mainstream AYUSH.
7. Promotion of healthy lifestyles.

Strategies

Core Strategies

1. Train and enhance capacity of Panchayati Raj Institutions (PRIs) to own, control and manage public health services.
2. Promote access to improved health care at household level through the ASHA.
3. Health plan for each village through village health committee of the panchayat.
4. Strengthening subcenter through an untied fund to enable local planning and action, and more multipurpose workers (MPWs).

5. Strengthening existing primary health centers (PHCs) and community health centers (CHCs), and provision of 30–50-bedded CHC per lakh population for improved curative care to a normative standard (IPHS defining personnel, equipment and management standards).
6. Preparation and implementation of an intersectoral district health plan prepared by the district health mission, including drinking water, sanitation and hygiene, and nutrition.
7. Integrating vertical health and family welfare programs at national, state, block and district levels.
8. Technical support to national, state and district health missions, for public health management.
9. Strengthening the capacities for data collection, assessment and review for evidence-based planning, monitoring and supervision.
10. Formulation of transparent policies for deployment and career development of human resources for health.
11. Developing capacities for preventive health care at all levels for promoting healthy lifestyles, reduction in consumption of tobacco, alcohol, etc.
12. Promoting non-profit sector, particularly in underserved areas.

Supplementary Strategies

1. Regulation of private sector including the informal rural practitioners to ensure availability of quality service to citizens at reasonable cost.
2. Promotion of public private partnerships (PPP) for achieving public health goals.
3. Mainstreaming AYUSH; revitalizing local health traditions.
4. Reorienting medical education to support rural health issues including regulation of medical care and medical ethics.
5. Effective and viable risk pooling and social health insurance to provide health security to the poor by ensuring accessible, affordable, accountable and good-quality hospital care.

Components

Accredited Social Health Activists

Local village woman will be trained on pedagogy of public health. She will be an honorary volunteer receiving performance-based compensation for promoting universal immunization, referral and escort services for reproductive and child health (RCH), construction of household toilets and other healthcare delivery programs. She will be given a drug kit containing generic AYUSH and allopathic formulations for common ailments.

Strengthening Subcenters

Each subcenter will have an untied fund for local action at ₹10,000 per annum in joint bank account of the auxiliary nurse midwife (ANM) and village head (Sarpanch), operated by the ANM.

Strengthening Primary Health Centers

Adequate and regular supply of essential quality drugs and equipment (including supply of auto-disabled syringes for immunization) to PHCs; 24-hour service in 50% PHCs; upgradation of 100% PHCs for 24-hours referral service and provision of second doctor at PHC level (one male, one female) would be undertaken on the basis of felt need.

Strengthening Community Health Centers for First Referral Care

Operationalizing 3,222 existing community health centers (30–50 beds) as 24-hour first referral units including posting of anesthetists.

District Health Plan

District becomes core unit of planning, budgeting and implementation. All vertical health and family welfare programs at district and state levels merge into one common 'District Health Mission' at the district level and the 'State Health Mission' at the state level. Provision of project management unit for all districts through contractual engagement of MBA, intercharter/intercost and data entry operator for improved program management.

Converging Sanitation and Hygiene Under NRHM

The district health mission would therefore, guide activities of sanitation at district level and promote joint IEC for public health, sanitation and hygiene, through Village Health and Sanitation Committee, and promote household toilets and school sanitation program. The ASHA would be incentivized for promoting household toilets by the mission.

Strengthening Disease Control Programs

Disease surveillance system at village level would be strengthened. Provision of a mobile medical unit at district level for improved outreach services.

Public-private Partnership for Public Health Goals, Including Regulation of Private Sector

District institutional mechanism for mission must have representation of private sector. Need to develop guidelines for public-private partnership (PPP) in health sector. Identifying areas of partnership, which are need-based, thematic and geographic.

Public sector plays the lead role in defining the framework and sustaining the partnership.

New Health Financing Mechanisms

Progressively the district health missions to move toward paying hospitals for services by way of reimbursement on the principle of 'money follows the patient'. Standardization of services; outpatient, inpatient, laboratory, surgical interventions and costs will be done periodically by a committee of experts in each state.

Reorienting Health/Medical Education to Support Rural Health Issues

While district and tertiary hospitals are necessarily located in urban centers, they form an integral part of the referral care chain serving the needs of the rural people. Medical and paramedical education facilities need to be created in states based on the need assessment.

Assessment

Assessments of the progress of key program interventions in 2009 (i.e. after 4 years of implementation of the program) have clearly indicated major gains, which have been made in rejuvenating the public health delivery system in India. An assessment by the sample registration system of the RGI Census of India has shown that maternal mortality ratio has declined to 254 per 100,000 births during 2004–06 compared to 301 during 2001–03. The DLHS-III survey conducted under supervision of International Institute of Population Sciences also recorded significant gains in institutional deliveries in hitherto backward states like Madhya Pradesh, Orissa, Rajasthan, Bihar, etc. The SRS data for 2007 put the infant mortality rate at 55, a two-point reduction from the previous year. The NRHM has clearly fueled accelerated progress toward provisioning of quality health care to citizens of the country and the improved indicators are testimony to the same. Faster improvements in the IMR and MMR are likely over the coming years as the NRHM interventions start yielding dividend.

SECTION

10

Epidemiology and Biostatistics

CHAPTER

32

Epidemiological Methods in Health Care

Epidemiological methods are used to study health and disease in populations in contrast to clinical medicine, which deals with the health of individuals. Data collected from frequency and distribution studies are used to formulate effective public health intervention programs in order to prevent disease and promote health. Maxcy, a pioneer epidemiologist defined epidemiology as that field of medical science, concerned with the relationship of various factors and conditions, which determine the frequency and distribution of an infectious process, a disease or a physiologic state in a community. By relating the frequencies and distribution of health parameters to the frequencies of other factors to which populations are exposed, epidemiologists are able to identify those that may be causes of a disease or promoters of good health.

❑ EPIDEMIOLOGICAL STUDIES

Epidemiological studies cannot give experimental evidence, but can provide indirect evidence of a relationship between health or disease and other factors.

Any change in relationship between the agent, environment and the host may result in loss of health. By agent, the causative agent of any disease is meant and by host, the human beings. Another triad; time, place and person is used in epidemiological studies to describe, when, where and who are affected by the disease. By describing the agent, environment and host in terms of time, place and person, it is possible to elucidate the causative agent, the natural history of a disease and the risk factors that increase the likelihood of acquiring a disease and suggest ways to intervene in the disease process and prevent disease or death.

Epidemiological studies rarely provide 'proof' of a causal relationship. However, the causal relationship will be strengthened by criteria such as the strength of association (statistical probability and risk ratio), consistency of findings across multiple studies, specificity of the relationship, temporality (outcome follows causation), biological gradient (a dose-response relationship), biological plausibility, coherence (consistency with prior knowledge), experimental evidence and analogy (relationship hypothesized similar to that known in relationships). But still, the fact remains that epidemiological studies seldom provide proof of a causal relationship in the sense of Koch's postulates, but they can be used to reveal a possible relationship and build a case that the relationship is causal.

Uses

Epidemiological studies are used to:

1. Describe the spectrum of the disease that is the varied presentation of a disease. Cohort studies have brought to light the role of high blood pressure in causing stroke, myocardial infarction and kidney disease. Measles virus infection can be manifested as a typical febrile blotchy rash disease as well as generalized hemorrhagic rash, acute encephalitis and years later, as subacute sclerosing panencephalitis (SSPE) and multiple sclerosis.
2. Describe the natural history of a disease. Natural history of AIDS was revealed by cohort studies, which assisted in the efficient use of limited treatment modalities available.
3. Identify factors that increase or decrease the risk of acquiring a disease. Smoking as risk factor for cancer, cardiovascular disease and chronic respiratory disease was identified by epidemiological studies.
4. Predict disease trends. Periodicity of infectious diseases such as measles, polio and influenza was identified by descriptive studies and the knowledge is used to control these epidemics with advance preparation.

5. Elucidate mechanisms of disease transmission. Vectors and animal reservoirs of arboviral encephalitides such as Japanese encephalitis were elucidated by epidemiological studies.
6. Test the efficiency of intervention strategies. Double blind placebo-controlled trials are the important steps in devising a behavioral intervention strategy to stop smoking.
7. Evaluate an intervention program. Serial cross-sectional studies can be used to find out whether there has been a change in the prevalence of diseases or indicators of health status over time. Cohort studies are used to compare incidence of disease in comparable populations receiving or not receiving the preventive intervention.
8. Identify health needs of a community. Cross-sectional studies are used to identify the health problem of a community or country and surveillance to identify the trends in disease, infection and/or health status over time.
9. Evaluate public health programs. Whether intervention programs are effective and cost-effective can be studied by finding out the incidence and prevalence of targeted disease in the populations.

Epidemiological Study Designs

Descriptive Studies

The first clue that a particular factor may cause a specific disease in specific locations can be obtained by correlating the prevalence or incidence of disease with the frequency of suspected causal factors. However, it has to be understood that such studies reveal only the cooccurrence, which may be purely due to chance. Therefore, descriptive studies are useful in the sense that they provide a rationale for further analytical studies.

Cross-sectional/Prevalence Surveys

The magnitude of a disease and other factors in a community are brought out by cross-sectional studies. The number of people who have the disease in a given population and the difference in frequency of the disease in different subpopulations will be known and it can be used by administrators to chalk out appropriate public health programs. Cross-sectional studies are useful in studying chronic diseases, which show a high prevalence, but low incidence, but they are not useful in studying diseases of low prevalence, e.g. SSPE.

Problems such as response bias, recall bias and undocumented confounders may be encountered. Time relationship and under-representation may be problems in cross-sectional studies.

Case-control Studies

Comparing the prevalence of suspected causal factors between cases and controls is undertaken. If the prevalence of a factor, in cases, is significantly different from that in controls, it can be presumed that the factor is associated with the disease. However, it does not measure the risk. The risk can be estimated by calculating the odds ratio.

Cases can be selected from hospitals and controls from either hospitalized patients with other diseases or by using algorithms or formulae for selecting community or other type of controls. The participants are seen only once and no follow-up is necessary. Recall bias may be a problem. For example, patients are more motivated than controls in recalling the events. These studies are particularly useful in exploring relationships noted in observational studies. A hypothesis is necessary for case-control studies, which are the methods of choice in studying rare diseases. As we conduct case-control studies after defining what constitutes the disease for the study purpose, spectrum of the disease cannot be found out.

Cohort Studies

Cohort studies establish the temporal relationship between an exposure and health outcome and then measure the risk directly. Because of the cost and complexity of cohort studies, they are usually performed only after descriptive, cross-sectional and/or case-control studies have suggested a causal relationship. These are particularly suitable for investigating health hazards associated with environmental or occupational exposures. Disease spectrum also can be studied. Cohort studies may take years or decades to yield results and therefore, time consuming and expensive. Ensuring the participation of cohorts for a prolonged period is also difficult.

The size of the cohort is dependent on the anticipated incidence of the disease resulting from exposure and so diseases with very low incidence are not suitable for cohort studies. Cohort studies can establish the risk associated with exposures, but cannot prove that the factor is causal.

Experimental Studies

In experimental studies, there is some intervention or manipulation such as deliberate application or withdrawal of suspected cause in the experimental group, while making no change in the control group. Because of the serious implications of applying an intervention that may alter the biological status of an individual, intervention studies are undertaken only after establishing a causal relationship between the suspected cause and the disease by other type of study designs. Experimental studies have ethical, cost and feasibility problems. These studies provide a strong evidence of a causal relationship, if not, proof by demonstrating a reduction in specific health outcome.

❑ RATE, RATIO AND PROPORTION

Disease magnitude is expressed as a rate, ratio or proportion.

Rate

A rate measures the occurrence of some event (disease or death) in a population during a given period. Death rate is a commonly used rate and is obtained by the formula:

$$\text{Death rate} = \frac{\text{Number of deaths in 1 year}}{\text{Midyear population}} \times 1{,}000$$

Numerator indicates the total number of events that occurred, while the denominator is the total population in which the specific events (numerator) took place. The multiplier is selected according to the incidence or prevalence of the event. Smaller the incidence bigger will be the multiplier. The usual multipliers are 1,000, 10,000 or 100,000.

The time specification is also selected as per the incidence or prevalence and it may be 1 year or 1 month or any other specified period depending upon the requirement. Rates are either crude rates or specific rates. Crude death rates measure the total deaths that have occurred without any specific identification of the cause of death. Specific death rates can be calculated for different causes of death, e.g. death due to accidents, death due to tuberculosis, etc. Death rates can also be group specific (e.g. Hindus, Muslims) or time specific (annual, monthly or weekly). Standardized rates are necessary for comparison purpose and they are calculated by making adjustments in respect of age or sex.

Mortality Rates

1. Crude death rate (CDR) =

$$\frac{\text{Total number of deaths in 1 year}}{\text{Midyear population}} \times 1{,}000$$

2. Specific death rate:

Death rate due to TB =

$$\frac{\text{Total number of deaths due to TB in 1 year}}{\text{Midyear population}} \times 1{,}000$$

3. Case fatality rate is calculated in acute infectious diseases such as cholera, food poisoning, etc. and it can be calculated by the formula:

Case fatality rate =

$$\frac{\text{Total number of deaths from a specific disease in a week}}{\text{Total number of the cases from the same disease in the same week}} \times 1{,}000$$

4. Survival rates (in cancer) =

$$\frac{\text{Total number of patients alive after 5 years of detection or specific treatment}}{\text{Total number of patients diagnosed or treated}} \times 1{,}000$$

Standardization is necessary to compare rates of events of two populations with different demographic composition. Adjustments have to be made for age, sex, parity, etc. before comparison. This is done by direct or indirect standardization.

Morbidity Rates

Sickness, illness or disability is called morbidity. Morbidity is measured in terms of frequencies, duration and severity. Incidence and prevalence rates indicate the frequency of a disease or disability.

Incidence rate

Incidence, that is how often a disease or health event occurs, is measured as a rate and it is calculated by the formula:

Incidence rate =

$$\frac{\text{Total number of new cases of a specific disease during a given period}}{\text{Population at risk in the same period}} \times 1{,}000$$

Incidence rate measures the number of new spells of a particular disease or illness per 100 or 1,000, etc. population at risk in a given period of time. The multiplier is selected according to the incidence of the event. Smaller the incidence bigger will be the multiplier.

Attack rates indicate the extent of an epidemic measured as a percentage. Secondary attack rates (SAR) indicate the infectiousness of a disease. It is the number of exposed persons who develop the disease within the range of the incubation period of that disease after exposure to a primary case. SAR is high in chickenpox, measles, etc.

Knowledge of incidence rate is used:

1. To take disease control measures.
2. To assess the efficacy of the preventive and control measures already instituted.

Prevalence rate

Prevalence refers to all the cases of specified disease existing in a given population during a specified time. It includes cases that may arise during the period and the old cases that already exist.

Point prevalence is the number of all currently seen cases of a disease in a given population at one point of time, which may be 1 day or 1 week depending upon the time taken to examine the sample population.

Point prevalence =

$$\frac{\text{Total number of all current cases at a given point of time}}{\text{Estimated population at risk at the same point of time}} \times 100$$

Period prevalence measures all cases occurring during a specified period (usually a longer period like 1 year). Prevalence can also be calculated using the incidence rate by the formula:

$$P = I \times D$$

where,

P is prevalence;

I is incidence rate;

D is duration.

Prevalence rate is used to assess the magnitude of the disease problem and to plan the various measures for the effective control of the disease.

Ratio

Ratio expresses a relation in size between two random quantities. For example, male-female ratio, doctor-population ratio, doctor-nurse ratio, etc.

Proportion

A proportion indicates the relation in magnitude of a part of the whole and it is usually expressed in percentage. For example, number of children vaccinated against a disease out of total children present in the population, is a proportion and the vaccination coverage can be calculated by the formula:

$$\frac{\text{Total number of children aged 1 year, vaccinated in an area}}{\text{Total number of children in the same age group in the area}} \times 100$$

Vaccination coverage in 1 year olds in India is about 90%.

❑ DESCRIPTIVE STUDIES

Descriptive studies identify the distribution of a disease by studying disease in respect of time, place and person distribution. The pertinent questions raised are:

1. When does the disease occur?
2. Where does it occur?
3. Whom does the disease affect?

The time may be a year, season, a month, a week or a day. The place may be climatic zones, country and region of a country, rural areas, urban towns, cities or institutions. Persons may be young or old, male or female, married or unmarried, poor or rich, educated or uneducated and so on.

Time Distribution

Time trend studies reveal three types of trends in the occurrence of diseases:

1. Short-term fluctuations.
2. Periodic fluctuations.
3. Long term or secular trends.

Short-term Fluctuations

An epidemic is a short-term fluctuation. It is defined as the occurrence, in a community or region, of cases of an illness or health-related events, clearly in excess of normally expected frequency. Three types of epidemics are described.

Common source single exposure epidemics: In these, all the affected persons are exposed to the disease agent simultaneously. The epidemic curve shows only one peak and all cases develop within one incubation period of the disease. Bhopal MIC gas tragedy is an example for this type of epidemic. Contaminated community water supply or food may also cause such an epidemic.

Common source continuous exposure epidemics: These may be caused by contaminated well water catering to a large community or by a food item distributed throughout a country over a period of time. Continuous exposure epidemics continue beyond one incubation period. However, the epidemic is not maintained by secondary cases, i.e. by person-to-person transmission. Epidemic dropsy can occur in this way.

Propagated epidemics: These are maintained by person-to-person transmission. Polio and hepatitis A occur as propagated epidemics. Continuation of the epidemic is decided by the availability of susceptibles in the community to the infectious agent.

Periodic Fluctuations

Seasonal trend is seen in diseases like measles, varicella, malaria, etc. Seasonal variation may be caused by changes in climatic conditions like rainfall, temperature, humidity, overcrowding, life cycle of vectors, etc. Upper respiratory infections show a seasonal rise in winter and gastrointestinal infections in summer months.

Cyclic trends: In the prevaccination era, measles used to occur in cycles with peaks every 2–3 years and rubella every 6–9 years. Variations in herd immunity decide this type of disease occurrence. When susceptible population increases in the community, epidemics occur. Non-communicable diseases like automobile accidents also show cyclical trend.

Long Term/Secular Trends

When there is a progressive increase or decrease in the occurrence of a disease over a long period of time, usually several years or decades, it is called a secular trend. Infectious diseases show a declining trend in developed countries. Non-communicable diseases such as diabetes mellitus, coronary heart disease (CHD), etc.

show an increasing trend due to probably changing lifestyles of populations there. Time trends indicate whether a disease is increasing or decreasing, throw light on the etiology of diseases and decide the control measures needed.

Place Distribution

In the distribution of diseases, we find there are international variations, national variations, rural-urban differences and differences in local distribution. Environment, diet and lifestyle factors may be the root cause of these differences seen and this may give a lead to the etiological hypothesis. Stomach cancer is common in Japan whereas it is rare in USA. Oral and cervical cancers are common in India. Cardiovascular diseases also show variation in their incidence between different countries.

Endemic goiter is seen more in sub-Himalayan region than the rest of the regions in India. Fluorosis is peculiar to certain regions in India.

The incidence of zoonotic diseases and helminthic infestation like hookworm disease are common in rural areas than in urban pockets. Accidents, cancer, cardiovascular diseases, drug addiction, etc. are urban problems in India.

Spot Maps

Spot maps will reveal the clustering of cases in certain areas of a city and thereby contribute to the etiological hypothesis. John Snow was able to hypothesize that water contamination was responsible for the cholera outbreak in certain areas of London by using spot maps, which showed clustering of cases even before the bacterial etiology of the disease was known.

Migration

Migration of people permanently from the country of their origin to a different country with different environment lifestyle and eating habits offer a unique opportunity to study the difference in the incidence of diseases and thereby contribute to arriving at etiological hypothesis.

Person Distribution

Variation in disease distribution is found among people of different ages, sex, occupation and subgroups. Ethnicity, marital status, social class, behavior, stress, etc. are also found to affect the disease incidence.

Epidemiological studies are often undertaken to estimate the disease load, which may be required to plan intervention programs. In cross-sectional studies single examination of a cross-section of the population at a given point of time is done and the findings are projected to the whole population. Cross-sectional studies are more useful to study chronic diseases like hypertension than acute diseases. As the prevalence rates of diseases can be found out from such studies, they are also called as prevalence studies. In longitudinal studies, observations are repeated several times, in the same population, over a prolonged period (several years or decades). Incidence rates of diseases, natural history of diseases and risk factors can be brought to light by longitudinal studies. However, longitudinal studies are time consuming, expensive and difficult to organize.

Purposes

Descriptive studies provide:

1. Data regarding disease load and the type of diseases in the community.
2. Clues to disease etiology.
3. Background data for planning, organizing and evaluating preventive and curative services.
4. Data for further research.

❑ CASE-CONTROL STUDIES

Case-control study is also known as retrospective study. Individuals with a particular disease constitute the cases and individuals without the disease act as controls. Cases and controls must be comparable in respect of age, sex, occupation, social status, etc. The definition of a case must be well defined and the diagnostic criteria for the cases should be well decided and should not be altered until the completion of the study. Only newly diagnosed cases are considered eligible for the study rather than old and advanced cases. Cases can be selected from hospitals or general population. All the cases or random samples of the cases can be used as cases for the study. Controls can be selected from hospitals, relatives, neighborhood or general population. Case-control ratio can be 1:1, if the study is large. However, if the study is small more than one control for each case should be arranged. An example of a case-control study design is given in Table 32.1.

Exposure in Case-control Study

Measurement of exposure to a suspected causal factor of both cases and controls is made by going into the history of exposure retrospectively. Exposure particulars can be obtained by interviews, questionnaires or by studying past records such as hospital records, employment records, etc. (refer Table 32.1).

Table 32.1: A case-control study design

Category	Cases (lung cancer)	Controls
Smokers	33 (a)	55 (b)
Non-smokers	2 (c)	27 (d)
Total	35 (a+c)	82 (b+d)

Exposure Rates

Controls:

$$\frac{b}{b+d} \times 100 = \frac{55}{82} \times 100 = 67.1\%$$

Cases:

$$\frac{a}{a+c} \times 100 = \frac{33}{35} \times 100 = 94.3\%$$

In the above example, the exposure rate is found to be higher among the cases than among the controls. The statistical association between exposure (cigarette smoking) and the development of disease (lung cancer) is then tested by an appropriate test of significance (Chi-square). In the present study the p value is 0.001, which is statistically significant. The association out of chance is almost ruled out when the p value is smaller.

Odds Ratio

As relative risk cannot be calculated from case-control studies because they do not provide incidence rates, hence, odds ratio can be found out. It is a measure of strength of association between the risk factor and the outcome.

$$\text{Odds ratio} = \frac{ad}{bc} = \frac{33 \times 27}{55 \times 2} = 8$$

Odds ratio of 8 means that smokers have a risk, 8 times higher than non-smokers do for developing lung cancer.

Bias in Case-control Studies

Many types of bias can occur in case-control studies. Proper matching in respect of age, sex, occupation, social class, etc. can eliminate confounding factors. Confounding factor is one, which is associated with both the cause and the effects. Age will be a confounding factor in the association between oral contraceptives and breast cancer. Old age is itself a risk for breast cancer. So if matching is not done properly with regard to age (that is both cases and controls should belong to similar age groups) it may affect the outcome and create a wrong inference due to confounding effect of age. Memory recall bias is another possibility to be borne in mind as cases are more likely to remember the past events than the controls. Interviewer's bias may be avoided by making the study a double blind one. Berksonian bias is one which arises because of different rates of admission to hospitals for people with different diseases.

Thalidomide Tragedy, as Example

A good example for case-control studies is the one that established a causal relationship between thalidomide and congenital defects in the newborn. In Britain, babies were born with congenital abnormalities when the mothers were administered thalidomide, a non-barbiturate hypnotic during pregnancy. A case-control study revealed that 41 of 46 mothers who had delivered babies with congenital defects had taken thalidomide, while none of the 300 mothers who had not taken thalidomide delivered defective babies.

❑ COHORT STUDIES

A cohort is a group of individuals who share a common characteristic or experience. All those born on a particular year may form a birth cohort. Similarly, all those doctors who graduated on a particular year will form a cohort (age, occupation, pregnancy, exposure to a drug or vaccination, etc. may be the basis for making a cohort). By following up the members of a cohort over the years, we are able to find out the occurrence of diseases in the subgroups depending upon the exposure to different axiological factors.

Cohort studies are similar to case-control studies. But the subjects for the study are selected and followed up over a period of years or decades to see how the disease under study develops in two different groups one, which is exposed to a suspected causal factor, the other not exposed. Therefore, cohort studies are also called prospective studies or forward-looking studies.

Steps

Steps in a cohort study are given below.

Selecting Study Subjects

Study subjects can be selected from general population, if the suspected exposure is fairly frequent. Special groups like doctors, nurses, lawyers, teachers, obstetric population, etc. and exposure groups like industrial workers exposed to suspected causal factors can also be selected as the study subjects. Doctors exposed to X-ray may be followed up to see whether they develop blood cancer in comparison to doctors who are not exposed. Gradation of exposure may also be made depending upon the duration of exposure.

Obtaining Data on Exposure

Data on exposure may be collected by means of interviews, mailed questionnaires, review of records, medical examination, special tests and environmental surveys. Demographic variables, which may affect the frequency of disease under study may also be needed for subsequent analysis.

Selection of Comparison Group

When degree of exposure can be collected, we can form comparison groups within the same cohort. For example, smokers can be classified into various subgroups depending upon the number of cigarettes smoked per day and compared with one another to find out how lung cancer develops in the different subgroups with different degree of exposure. This is what is called internal comparison. When degree of exposure is not available, external controls are used. For example, smokers can be compared with non-smokers and radiologists with ophthalmologists. Sometimes, comparison can be made with the rates seen in general population. For example, frequency of lung cancer among uranium miners can be compared with that in general population residing in the same area.

Follow-up

Follow-up of the study subjects can be done by mailed questionnaire, telephone enquiry, periodic home visits on an annual basis, periodic medical examination of each subject, review of physician and hospital records and routine surveillance of death records. Periodic examination of each subject is the best approach as it yields the greatest amount of information. Some percentage of loss of follow-up (attrition) may become unavoidable, due to death, change of residence, migration, etc.

Analysis

Incidence rates among the exposed and the non-exposed are found out and estimation of risk is calculated.

Study Results

Incidence Rates

The incidence rates can be calculated as follows (Table 32.2).

$$\text{Among smokers} = \frac{70}{7{,}000} \times 1{,}000 = 10 \text{ per } 1{,}000$$

$$\text{Among non–smokers} = \frac{3}{3{,}000} \times 1{,}000 = 1 \text{ per } 1{,}000$$

TABLE 32.2: Incidence of cancers in smokers and non-smokers

Group	Cancer developed	No cancer	Total
Smokers	70 (a)	6,930 (b)	7,000 (a+b)
Non-smokers	3 (c)	2,907 (d)	3,000 (c+d)

Adapted from Dr Nitin V Solanki. Department of Community Medicine, Gujarat Adani Institute of Medical Sciences, Bhuj.

Estimation of Risk

The risk of developing the disease under study (lung cancer) because of exposure to the suspected factor (smoking) is estimated from relative risk and attributable risk.

Relative risk: It is the ratio between the incidence of disease among the exposed and the same among the non-exposed.

$$\text{Relative risk} = \frac{\text{Incidence among the exposed}}{\text{Incidence among the non-exposed}}$$

That is, 10/1 = 10

Attributable risk: It indicates the extent to which the disease under study can be attributed to the exposure to cigarette smoke. It is expressed as percentage and it is calculated by the formula:

$$\text{Attributable risk} = \frac{\text{Incidence among the exposed} - \text{Incidence among the non-exposed}}{\text{Incidence among the exposed}} \times 100$$

$$\text{That is} = \frac{10-1}{10} \times 100 = \frac{9}{10} \times 100 = 90\%$$

Population attributable risk: This is the incidence of disease in the total population minus the incidence among the non-exposed.

Advantages

Incidence rates can be calculated from cohort studies, while is not possible in case-control studies. Several outcomes related to exposure to a suspected causal factor can be studied simultaneously. For example, smoking and lung cancer studies also brought to light the association between smoking and CHD, peptic ulcer, etc. Dose-response ratios can be estimated and certain forms of bias can be minimized.

Disadvantages

Cohort studies involve large number of people and so a longer duration follow-up is needed for years or decades. Attrition (loss of follow-up) may be a real problem; expensive too. Ethical problems may be encountered. Selection of representative sample and comparison group may be difficult.

❑ EXPERIMENTAL STUDIES

Experimental studies are conducted in animals or human beings. There is deliberate manipulation in the form of application or withdrawal of a suspected cause in the experimental group, while making no change in the control group. Comparison of the outcome between both the groups will reveal the difference, if any.

Purposes

Experimental studies are done:

1. To provide scientific proof of etiological factors for diseases.
2. To find out the efficacy of some specific form of therapy or vaccination or health services.

Studies in animals are conducted before the methods are applied to human beings. Ethical and time constraints may not be problems in animal studies, but the results cannot be applied to human situation in toto.

Experiments on human beings should be done only after ascertaining the benefits over the risks involved. Volunteers should be adequately briefed of all possible consequences of the study.

Randomized controlled trials and non-randomized trials are the two experimental study designs undertaken.

Randomized Controlled Trials

Randomized controlled trials are done:

1. To evaluate therapeutic agents (mainly drugs).
2. To evaluate vaccines and chemoprophylactic drugs.
3. To conduct risk factor trials for CHDs and cessation experiments (e.g. cessation of smoking to see whether lung cancer incidence gets less).
4. To conduct trial of etiological agents to confirm or refute etiological hypothesis (e.g. O_2 as a cause of retrolental fibroplasia in newborns).
5. To evaluate of health services.

Design

Design of randomized controlled trials includes the following steps:

1. Drawing up of protocol.
2. Selecting reference and experimental populations.
3. Randomization.
4. Manipulation or intervention.
5. Follow-up.
6. Assessment of outcome.

Protocol: The aims and objectives of the study are specified. Criteria for the selection of study and control groups are set. Size of the sample is decided. Procedures for allocation of subjects into study and control groups are decided. Treatments to be applied, standardization of working procedures and schedules, responsibility of the parties involved are all specified. The protocol aims at preventing bias and reducing sources of error. The protocol once evolved should be strictly adhered to throughout the study.

Preliminary test

Preliminary test runs may be necessary to see whether the protocol contains any flaw. Feasibility, operational efficiency of certain procedures or unknown effects and acceptability of certain policies are to be tested in trial runs.

Selecting the reference and experimental groups: The reference population is the one to which the study findings are to be applied. Entire population of an area or selected groups based on age, sex, occupation, social group, etc. may be taken as reference population. Experimental population is selected from the reference population. Random selection of experimental population is done to ensure that it has the same characteristics as the reference population.

Informed consent

Informed consent of the study group is a must. The participants in the study must be aware of the purpose, procedures and the possible dangers of the study.

Randomization: Once the selection of study subjects is over, randomization process begins. Randomization ensures that the groups are comparable so that like can be compared with like and the investigator has no control over the allocation of subjects to either study or control group. The entire study population is grouped into subgroups according to the variable and individuals within each subgroup are then randomly allocated into study and control groups. Random allocation is done by using a table of random numbers.

Manipulation: After randomization, administration or withdrawal of a suspected factor to study group begins. What is being administrated or withdrawn is called independent variable, while the outcome of application or withdrawal is called dependent variable.

Follow-up: Study and control groups are examined at definite intervals in a standard manner, under the same circumstances for the outcome. The duration of follow-up will depend upon the type of study undertaken. Loss of follow-up (attrition) should be minimized as it may affect generalization of the study findings.

Assessment: Blinding is adopted to reduce bias (participant bias, observer bias and evaluation bias). In single-blind designs, the participants are not aware whether they belong to study group or control groups. In double-blind trials, both the doctor and the participant are not aware of the group allocation and the treatment received by the participants. In triple-blind trials, the participants, the investigator and the persons who analyze the data are all blind. Double blinding is the most frequently used method.

The results in the study and control groups are compared and the difference, if any, is tested for statistical significance.

Types

Concurrent studies and crossover studies are the two types of study designs followed in randomized controlled trials.

Concurrent studies: In these, the study group undergoes the interventions (administration of a drug, vaccination or withdrawal of some factor) while the control group receives no intervention in the same period and the effect is compared.

Crossover studies: In these one group receives treatment and the other group receives placebo during the first phase. They are then taken off the medication or placebo for a period sufficient to wash off the effects of drugs in the study group. Now the placebo group receives the treatment and the study group receives the placebo and the effects are compared. Crossover studies may not be suitable in certain conditions.

Some Randomized Trials

Examples of some randomized trials conducted are given below.

Clinical trials: Clinical trials of Aspirin on cardiovascular diseases and folate supplementation on neural tube defects proved the beneficial effects of these medicaments. However, ethical problems may be encountered in clinical trials and blinding may not be possible sometimes.

Preventive trials: Efficacy of whooping cough vaccine in children of 6–18 months age group was tested in a preventive trial, which showed a significant reduction in the attack rates in vaccinated children (Table 32.3).

TABLE 32.3: Efficacy of whooping cough vaccine

Group	Number	Developed diseases	Attack rate per 1,000 child/months
Vaccinated	3,801	149	1.45
Unvaccinated	3,757	687	6.72

Adapted from British Medical Journal. June 30, 1951.

Risk factor trials: Trial of clofibrate on cholesterol level; a risk factor for CHD, showed a significant reduction in the incidence of non-fatal cardiac infarction. But unfortunately, 25% more deaths were observed in the study group probably due to the toxic effect of clofibrate.

Cessation experiments: Stopping of smoking can be tested to see whether the incidence of lung cancer gets less.

Trial of etiological agents: The relationship between the incidence of retrolental fibroplasia in the newborn and the use of 50% oxygen was tested in a trial conducted in premature babies weighing 1,500 g or less for 28 days. The result proved the role of oxygen in causing retrolental fibroplasia.

Evaluation of health services: A study conducted by Tuberculosis Research Center at Egmore, Chennai found that the domiciliary treatment of tuberculosis cases was equally effective as hospital or sanatorium treatments, which led to the adoption of domiciliary treatment as a standard procedure that reduced the cost of treatment.

Non-randomized Trials

When randomized controlled trials are not possible because of ethical, administrative and other reasons, non-randomized trials are the methods of choice. When it is known that smoking is associated with lung cancer, it is unethical to allow smokers to continue smoking and look for the development of lung cancer in them. When the incidence of disease is low, controlled trial may be time consuming and costly.

Some Non-randomized Trials

Uncontrolled trials: Here, there is no control group, but still historical control is being compared. Usefulness of PAP test in reducing mortality from cervical cancer was found out by uncontrolled trials.

Natural experiments: John Snow, in 1853, was able to find out that people who drank water collected from the polluted area of Thames river in London suffered from cholera, while those who used water from unpolluted area of the river did not suffer. This he was able to do even before the bacterial etiology of cholera was known by making use of the natural difference observed between the two areas.

Before and after comparison studies without control: John Lind in 1750 demonstrated that fresh fruits prevented scurvy in his sailors.

Before and after comparison studies with control: The usefulness of seat belts in reducing the incidence of deaths in car accidents was demonstrated in a study conducted in the state of Victoria in Australia. The other states of Australia were used as the control for comparison.

❑ ASSOCIATION AND CAUSATION

When two variables occur together more often than by chance, association is said to be present between the two. Association does not necessarily mean it is a causal relationship between the two variables. If correlation coefficient is one, a perfect linear relationship between the two variables is said to occur.

Spurious Association

Sometimes the association is spurious and not real. In a study in UK on perinatal mortality, it was found that perinatal mortality was higher in hospital deliveries than in home deliveries. However, it can be inferred that the higher prenatal mortality in the hospital was not due to any deficiency in the service in hospitals, but because it attracted serious and complicated cases for delivery. The association between the two variables was due to the fact that like was not compared with like. In this comparison, factors like age, parity, prenatal care, disease state of the women, etc. were not matched.

Indirect Association

Sometimes the association is indirect and it is due to the presence of confounding variables that influence both the suspected causal factor and the disease. For example, high prevalence of goiter in hilly areas is not due to high altitudes, but due to iodine deficiency in the soil of the hilly terrain.

Direct Association

When one-to-one causal relationship between two variables is observed it is direct association. In communicable diseases (e.g. tuberculosis), one-to-one relationship is seen. However, sometimes a single cause may produce many manifestations. Hemolytic streptococcal infection can manifest as tonsillitis, scarlet fever and erysipelas. In humans, multiple factors may operate to cause a single disease. The individual factors either independently or synergistically can contribute to the development of the disease. In the same tuberculosis example, it is possible that there are other factors like the cell-mediated immunity and nutritional status, which decide an individual's susceptibility to tuberculosis. It is now well known that not all people who have been exposed to tubercle bacilli develop tuberculosis. This phenomenon is seen in diseases like poliomyelitis. Acute flaccid paralysis develops only in less than 1% of children exposed to poliovirus.

Additional Criteria for Uncontrolled Trials

In uncontrolled trials, some additional criteria are looked for to incriminate a causal relationship.

Temporal Association

In acute diseases like food poisoning, the temporal relationship-causal factor preceding the disease is quite evident. However, in chronic diseases, because the diseases have insidious onset, it is difficult to establish the temporal sequence between the cause and the disease.

Strength of Association

When the relative risk is high and there is dose-response or duration-response relationship between a suspected causal factor and a disease, the association is likely to be causal in nature. Cigarette smoking causing lung cancer satisfies both high relative risk (RR) and dose-response relationship.

Specificity of Association

When one-to-one relationship is seen between a cause and a disease, there is specificity. But it is difficult to establish such a specific relationship as development of a disease may require other factors as well in addition to the one known to be associated. Therefore, while specific association strengthens the causal relationship lack of it cannot negate it.

Consistency of Association

Evidence from a single study is not sufficient to infer a causal relationship. Repeated studies should show consistent results to strengthen the causal association.

Biological Plausibility

The hypothesis that cigarette smoking causes lung cancer is biologically plausible. Cigarette smoke is known to contain carcinogens. Experimental tracheobronchial implantation of tobacco extracts in animal studies has produced cancer. Therefore, it is quite possible that carcinogens from cigarette smoke deposited on the epithelial tissues of respiratory passage over long periods can induce neoplastic changes.

Coherence of Association

There is an increase in the habit of smoking the world over. There is also an increase in the incidence of lung cancer the world over. Both the findings are coherent. As more and more females take to smoking, the incidence of lung cancer among them is seen rising.

CHAPTER

33

Basic Statistics in Health Care

Statistical methods are applied in the dispensation of medical and health care to the community. Some elementary statistics useful in the practice of public health are discussed here.

Statistics is the study of methods and procedures for collecting, classifying, summarizing and analyzing data and for making scientific inferences from such data. It has two distinct categories, viz. descriptive statistics and inferential statistics. Biostatistics concerns with the application of statistics to problems of biology including human biology, medicine and public health. Statistics dealing with vital events like birth, death, stillbirth, marriage and divorce is known by the name vital statistics.

Health statistics deals with three aspects concerning health and they are:

1. Health status of populations (e.g. morbidity rate, mortality rate, etc.).
2. Factors affecting health (e.g. housing, nutrition, social, economic and environmental factors).
3. Health services provided in the community (e.g. number of hospitals, dispensaries, doctors, nurses, etc. in a given population).

❑ COLLECTION OF STATISTICS

Data can be collected by means of interview, observation or focus group discussion and it is done by using tools such as schedules or questionnaires.

1. Schedule: This is the most widely used method. Enumerators or field workers fill in the questionnaire or schedules. Questions in the schedule should be simple, unambiguous, easily understood, relevant, brief, arranged in logical order and capable of eliciting a precise answer.
2. Questionnaires also are used to collect data. They are sent by post to the respondents who will fill in and send back to the investigator.

Sampling

Covering each and every member of a given population (the universe) in the course of an enquiry is called complete enumeration. But when a large population is to be studied, it is impossible to cover all members in the population. Only samples from the population concerned are selected for the enquiry. Data obtained from the samples is extrapolated to the whole population (the universe). In sampling, representativeness of the sample to the universe must be ensured to make the data useful.

Many types of sampling techniques are employed to collect data. Some of them are described below.

Simple Random Sampling

In simple random sampling, a number is assigned to each unit of the universe to be studied. By using the table of random numbers, samples are selected for the study.

Systematic Random Sampling

In systematic random sampling, every 5th or 10th unit of the universe at regular interval is selected as samples for the study. The units of the universe are numbered first and then a number is selected at random between 1 and 10. For taking a 10%, sample every 10th unit is selected as samples for the study.

Stratified Random Sampling

In stratified random sampling, the population (the universe) is categorized into different strata and samples are drawn from each stratum. For example, separate samples may be drawn from each religious denomination like Christians, Muslims, Hindus, etc. to be representative of the whole population in a given area for a common enquiry.

Standard Error

If random samples are taken repeatedly from the same universe every sample will have a different mean. The mean of the sample means will be the same as the population mean. The standard deviation of the sample means from the mean of the sample means is a measure of the sample error, which is called the standard error or the standard error of the mean and it is given by the formula:

$$\sigma/\sqrt{n}$$

Standard error enables us to judge, whether the mean of a given sample is within the set confidence limits or not.

❑ PRESENTATION OF STATISTICS

Data collected should be arranged purposively. Many methods are used to present data and they are the following:

- Tables
- Charts
- Diagrams
- Graphs.

Tabular Presentation of Data

Tabulation is the first step before the data is used for analysis and interpretation. A table can be simple or complex depending upon the number or measurement of a single set or multiple sets of items. Whether simple or complex there are certain simple principles, which should be followed, while designing tables:

1. Table should be numbered, e.g. Table 1, Table 2, etc.
2. A title must be given to each table. The title must be brief and self-explanatory.
3. Headings of columns or rows should be clear and concise.

4. Data must be presented according to size or importance—chronologically, alphabetically or geographically.
5. If percentages or averages are to be compared, they should be placed as close as possible.
6. No table should be too large.
7. Footnotes may be given wherever necessary providing explanatory notes or additional informations.

Some examples of tabulation are simple table and frequency distribution table.

Simple Table

The most populous countries in the world are detailed in Table 33.1.

Frequency Distribution Table

When the data to be presented is large, simple tables will not be useful. So, we go for frequency distribution tables. To construct a frequency distribution table, the huge data is first arranged into convenient groups (class intervals) and then the number of items (frequency) occurring in each group is shown in the adjacent column. As a rule a maximum of 20 and a minimum of 5 groups are chosen depending upon the amount of data. Tally marks are used to count the frequency of the items.

The following are the ages of patients admitted to a hospital with poliomyelitis: 8, 24, 18, 5, 6, 12, 4, 3, 3, 2, 3, 23, 9, 18, 16, 1, 2, 3, 5, 11, 13, 15, 9, 11, 11, 7, 10, 6, 9, 5, 16, 20, 4, 3, 3, 3, 10, 3, 2, 1, 6, 9, 3, 7, 14, 8, 1, 4, 6, 4, 15, 22, 2, 1, 4, 7, 1, 12, 3, 23, 4, 19, 6, 2, 2, 4, 14, 2, 2, 21, 3, 2, 9, 3, 2, 1, 7, 19.

TABLE 33.1: Most populous countries in the world—2012

Country	Population (million)
China	1,350
India	1,260
United States	314
Indonesia	241
Brazil	194
Pakistan	180
Nigeria	170
Bangladesh	153
Russia	143
Japan	128

Adapted from 2012 World Population Data Sheet (PRB)

Frequency distribution table prepared from the above numerals is given in Table 33.2. In the example, the age distribution is arranged into groups of five (class interval).

TABLE 33.2: Age distribution of polio patients

Age group (class interval)	Number of patients (frequency)
0–4	35
5–9	19
10–14	10
15–19	8
20–24	6

Diagrammatic Representation of Data

Charts and diagrams are also used in presenting simple numerical data. Diagrams are better retained in memory than the statistical tables. Therefore, they are a popular method of presenting statistical data, especially in newspapers and magazines.

Bar Charts

Bar chart is a way of presenting a set of data by means of bars.

Simple Bar Charts

In simple bar charts, each item of a series is represented by a bar, the length being proportional to the magnitude of the corresponding item. For data varying over time, vertical bars are used and for data varying over space, horizontal bars are used. The bars are usually separated by appropriate spaces for clear presentation. A suitable scale must be chosen to present the length of the bar and this scale must, at all times, start from zero; otherwise the relative lengths of the bar would give a wrong impression.

The horizontal bar chart (Fig. 33.1) shows the mean age at marriage in different states of India.

In the vertical bar diagram (Fig. 33.2), each bar represents the population in a census year from 2004 to 2011.

Multiple Bar Charts

In multiple bar charts, two or more bars each representing a certain item are grouped together. In the chart given (Fig. 33.3), births

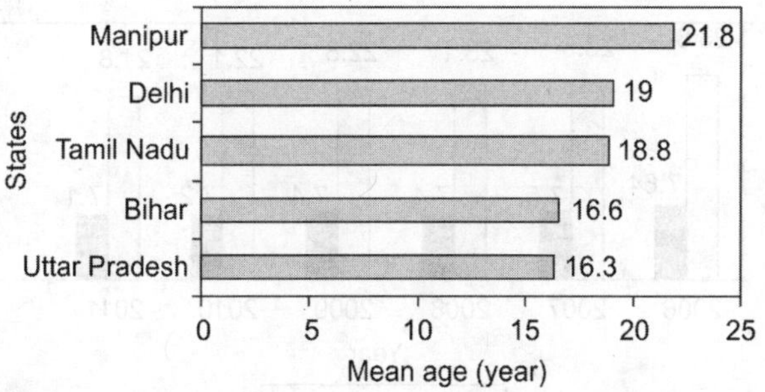

Figure 33.1: Mean age at marriage in different state of India [*Source:* National Family Health Survey (NFHS) (1998–1999)]

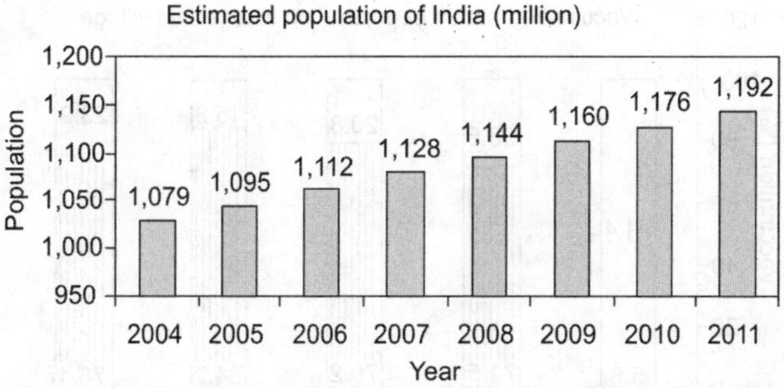

Figure 33.2: Estimated population of India in a census year from 2004 to 2011 (*Source:* Census of India—Office of the Registrar General and Census Commissioner, India)

and deaths have been grouped for comparison between one year and another, and also over the years.

Component Bar Charts

Here, each bar is divided into two or more parts; each part representing a certain item, proportional to the magnitude of that particular item. In the component bar chart (Fig. 33.4), the percentages of the vaccinated and the unvaccinated children of a particular age group are shown in the same bar.

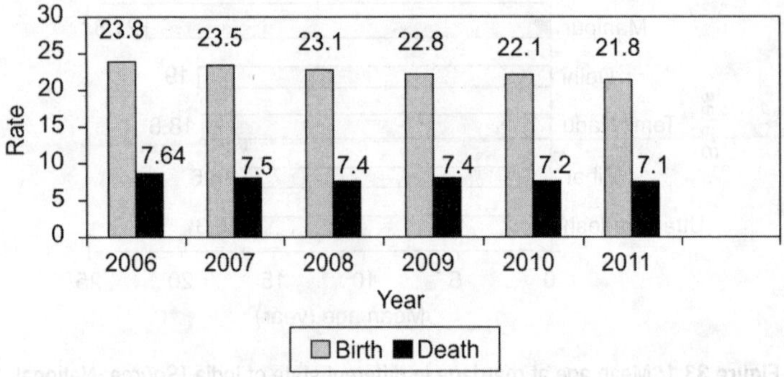

Figure 33.3: Birth and death rates in India (2006–2011) [*Source:* Sample Registration System (SRS) Bulletin (2006–2012)]

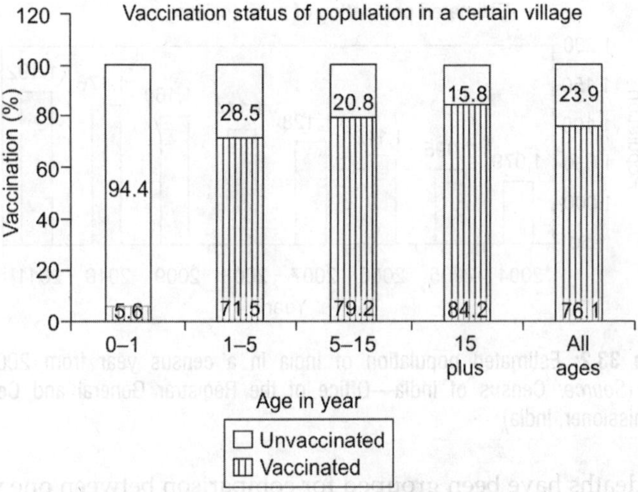

Figure 33.4: Vaccination percentage in different age groups

Frequency Graphs

Histogram

In histogram, a frequency distribution is presented as a series of blocks leaving no gaps between consecutive blocks. The class intervals are given along the horizontal axis and the frequencies along the vertical axis. The Figure 33.5 is the histogram of the frequency distribution of houses according to the number of occupants.

Frequency Polygon

A frequency polygon also can be drawn to present a frequency distribution. It is obtained by joining the midpoints of the histogram blocks. The Figure 33.6 is the frequency polygon of the above histogram showing the frequency distribution of houses according to the number of occupants.

If a smooth curve connecting all the midpoints of the histogram, replacing straight lines, is drawn, it is called frequency curve.

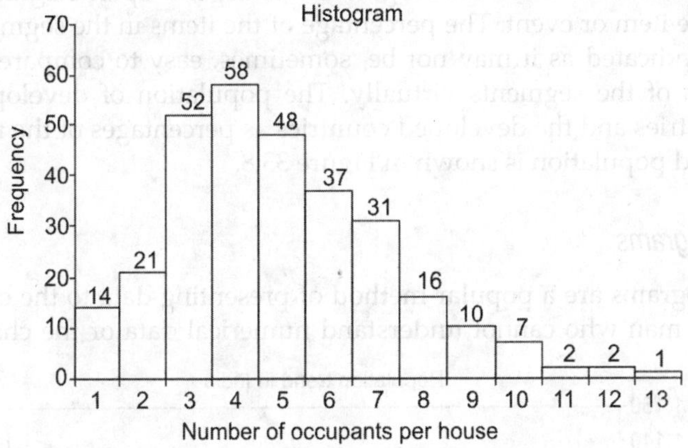

Figure 33.5: Frequency distribution of occupants in houses

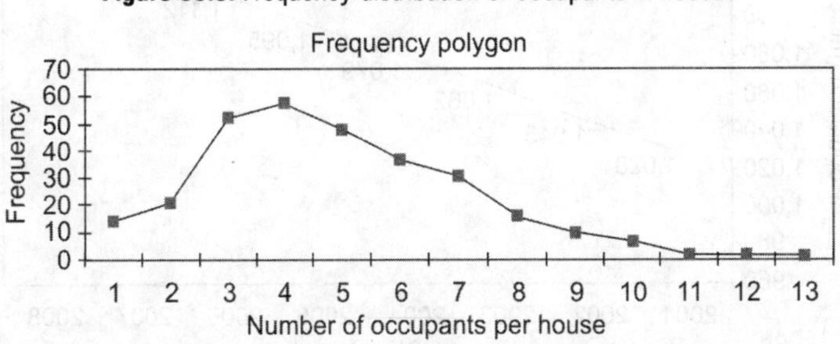

Figure 33.6: Frequency distribution of occupants in houses

Graph

The commonest method to depict the trend of events in time is a graph or line drawn with time points plotted on the horizontal axis and the frequency or magnitude of the event in question on the vertical axis. The population growth of India over the years is shown in Figure 33.7.

Diagrams

Pie Diagram

Pie charts are a method of presenting a set of data, each item being shown as a percentage of the whole, in a circle. In pie charts, segments of a circle are used to represent different items of a series of data. The area of the each segment will depend upon magnitude of the item or event. The percentage of the items in the segments are indicated as it may not be, sometimes, easy to compare the areas of the segments virtually. The population of developing countries and the developed countries as percentages of the total world population is shown in Figure 33.8.

Pictograms

Pictograms are a popular method of presenting data to the common man who cannot understand numerical data or the charts.

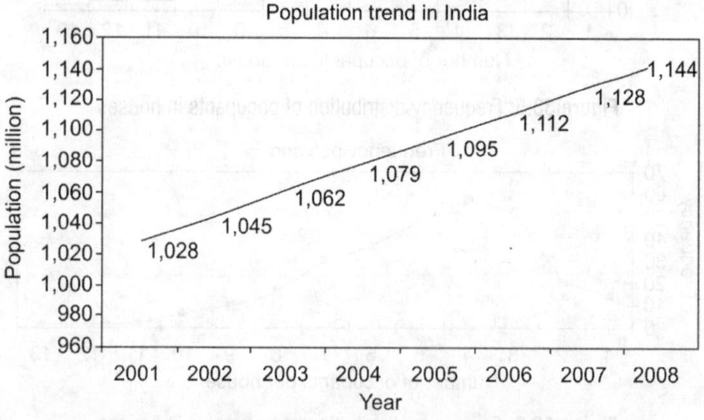

Figure 33.7: Annual population growth in India between 2001 and 2008

Small pictures or symbols are used to present the data. For example, tiny pictures of infants can be used to present infant mortality.

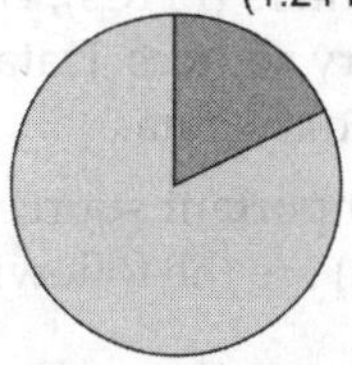

Figure 33.8: Population of developing and developed countries [*Source:* Population Reference Bureau (PRB), 2012]

Statistical Maps

Maps can be drawn to show the geographic distribution of certain events or things diagrammatically. These maps are mainly of two types namely:

1. Dot map.
2. Shaded or colored map.

Dot map: In dot map, the locality of occurrence of an event is shown by a properly placed dot on the map. This type of map is frequently used in epidemiological work wherein individual cases or deaths due to a disease are indicated by dots on the map. By using different sorts of dots a number of facts and relations (e.g. cases and deaths due to various diseases) can be indicated on the same dot map.

Shaded map: In this, different sorts of shading, cross batching or coloring of areas are done to indicate different absolute magnitudes. For example, mortality rates or case rates of a certain disease, population density, etc. can be shown in this type of maps.

❑ SOURCES OF HEALTH INFORMATION

The sources of data are of two major types. They are the primary and secondary sources.

The primary sources provide first hand raw data, which is further processed to give useful information. Data from primary sources called primary data are collected by methods such as interview, mailed questionnaire, etc. The secondary sources give ready-made information. But, the quality of information collected will not be known. All matters published in newspapers, magazines, research bulletins, etc. and unpublished matters available in registers and records maintained by the institutions like primary health centers (PHCs), community nutrition centers will form the secondary sources. Data collected from secondary sources are called secondary data.

Some important sources of health and population data (secondary data) are the following:

1. Census.
2. Civil registration system (CRS).
3. Sample registration system (SRS).
4. Survey of specific diseases.
5. National sample survey (NSS).
6. Registration of causes of death (RCD).
7. National family health survey (NFHS).
8. Rapid household survey on RCH (RHS-RCH).
9. Notification of infectious diseases.

Census

Census of population is defined as the total process of collection, compilation and publication of demographic, economic and social data pertaining to all persons in a country or delimited area, at specified time or times. In India, the first synchronous census was undertaken in 1881 and it is being carried out once in every 10 years thereafter. The census is carried out by the office of the Registrar General and Census Commissioner of India, Delhi, an office in the Ministry of Home Affairs, Government of India, under the 1948 Census of India Act. The act gives Central Government many powers like to notify a date for census, power to ask for the services of any citizen for census work. The law makes it compulsory for every citizen to answer the census questions truthfully. The Act provides penalties for giving false answers or not giving answers at all to the census questionnaire. One of the most important provisions of law is the guarantee for the maintenance of secrecy of the information collected at the census of each individual. The census records are not open to inspection and also not admissible in evidence.

The census provides information on size, distribution and socioeconomic, demographic and other characteristics of the country's population. The data collected are used for administration, planning and policy making as well as management and evaluation of various programs by the government, non-governmental organizations (NGOs), researchers, commercial and private enterprises, etc. Researchers and demographers use census data to analyze growth and trends of population and make projections. The census data is also important for business houses and industries for strengthening and planning their business for penetration into areas, which had hitherto remained uncovered.

The census is conducted in two phases: first, house listing and house numbering phase and second, the actual population enumeration phase. The census is carried out by the canvassing method. In this method, each and every household is visited and the information is collected by specially trained enumerator. They collect data related to households, e.g. number of members, water and electricity supply, ownership of land, vehicles, computers and other assets, and services. In the second phase, total population is counted and statistics related to individuals are collected.

The latest census in the series was carried out in the year 2011, which was the 15th census in the continuous series as reckoned from 1872 and the 7th since independence. The Government of India has permitted to conduct caste-based enumeration in 2011 census.

In 2003, the Census Commissioner's office has been assigned the work of a pilot project on Multipurpose National Identity Card (MNIC). This pilot project is under implementation in 12 states and one union territory covering a population of 3.1 million.

Civil Registration System

Births and deaths in India are compulsorily registered under the Registration of Births and Deaths (RBD) Act, 1969. The civil registration system is in operation since 1st April, 1970 throughout the country. The Registrar General of India, appointed by the Central Government under the Act, coordinates and unifies the activities of the state governments in respect of registration of births and deaths and prepares national report annually based on states reports.

Each state has a chief registrar of births and deaths who executes the various provisions of the Act. The actual registration is carried by the local registrars of births and deaths; births and deaths in villages should be reported to the village administration officer (VAO) and in urban areas, health inspectors act as registrars for registration.

Domiciliary events are to be reported by the head of the household and the institutional events by the in charge of the institution within the prescribed period of 21 days. The event has to be registered at the place of occurrence. Events occurring in moving vehicles such as bus, train, ship, flight, etc. have to be registered at the next authorized stop.

Delayed Registration

Births and deaths not reported within the prescribed period, but within 30 days of occurrence, can be registered after payment of a late fee. After 30 days, but within 1 year of occurrence, the event can be registered only on written permission from the prescribed officer (usually Tahsildars/Commissioners/Chief Officers), on production of an affidavit and payment of late fee. After 1 year of occurrence, the event can be registered only on an order of First Class Magistrate and on payment of late fee.

Penalties on persons/establishments not reporting the events and the registration functionary who neglects or refuses without reasonable cause to register are levied.

Issue of Certificates

As soon as the registration is completed a certificate is to be issued free of cost to the informant. The Section 17 of the Act provides for giving certified extracts from the birth and death register on payment of prescribed fee. Such extracts are admissible under the Indian Evidence Act as evidence of the birth or death the entry relates to. Such extracts will not include the cause of death entered in the register.

Entry of the name of the child later on: If the birth was registered without name of the child, the name can be got entered without any fee within 12 months of registration of a birth. After 12 months, but within 15 years of registration, it can be entered only after payment of a prescribed fee.

Correction or cancellation of entries made: Erroneous, fraudulent or improper entry in the birth and death registers, if proved to the satisfaction of the registrar, he may correct the error or cancel the entry, subject to the rules.

Sample Registration System

Sample Registration System (SRS) is a large-scale demographic survey for providing reliable annual estimates of birth rate, death rate, and other fertility and mortality indicators at the national and subnational levels. Initiated on a pilot basis in a few selected states by the Office of the Registrar General, India in 1964–1965; it became fully operational during 1969–1970 with about 3,700 sample units. The field investigation consists of continuous enumeration of births and deaths in selected sample units by resident part-time enumerators, generally Anganwadi workers and teachers, and an independent survey every 6 months by SRS supervisors. On completion of the half-yearly survey, the forms 9 and 10 filled in by the supervisors are compared with those in the forms 4 and 5 filled in by the enumerators and matched. The unmatched and partially matched events are reverified in the field and thereafter an unduplicated count of births and deaths is obtained. The sample unit in rural areas is a village or a segment of it, if the village population is 2,000 or more. In urban areas, the sampling unit is a census enumeration block with population ranging from 750 to 1,000. The SRS sample is replaced every 10 years based on the latest census frame. It had been a practice to stagger the replacement process over 2–3 years. However, the latest replacement has been carried out in one go effective from January 2004; this sample is based on the 2001 Census frame. At present, SRS is operational in 7,597 sample units (4,433 rural and 3,164 urban) spread across all states and union territories, and covers about 1.5 million households and 7.18 million population.

Health and Population Surveys/ Survey of Specific Diseases

Routine statistics collected do not provide complete information about health and disease, and therefore population surveys become necessary. For example, information on abortion, contraception, etc. essential for the study of fertility, can never be obtained from a census, but only through a special sample survey.

The Government of India has established some special statistical bodies to conduct population surveys. They are:

1. Office of the Registrar General of India.
2. Bureau of the health statistics; unit of the Central Ministry of Health.
3. Central Statistical Organization.
4. National Sample Survey Organization.

National Sample Survey

National Sample Survey Organization (NSSO) conducts nationwide sample surveys on various socioeconomic issues in successive rounds, each round covering subjects of current interest in a specific survey period by using the technique of sample survey.

The organization has four divisions namely:

1. Survey Design and Research Division (SDRD).
2. Field Operations Division (FOD).
3. Data Processing Division (DPD).
4. Coordination and Publication Division (CPD).

The main objective of the National Sample Survey (NSS) has been to collect data on some important socioeconomic aspects on a comprehensive basis for the whole country through its various rounds of survey. The first survey was conducted in 1950. Since then, data on different aspects of the population have been collected through various rounds; each round concentrating on one aspect. Information on fertility, mortality, population growth, economically active population, family planning (FP), employment and unemployment, consumers' expenditure patterns, housing conditions and many other aspects have been collected so far by NSS survey unit.

Registration of Causes of Death—Rural

Registration of causes of death (RCD) was started on a limited scale in 1965 and is now in operation in about 1,400 PHC head quarter villages. One of the paramedical personnels known as the field agent, contacts households and enquires about symptoms and conditions observed in individuals before their death. He uses a non-medical list on causes of death supplied by United Nations to arrive at the cause of death. Another member of PHC, known as recorder, conducts baseline survey and half-yearly surveys to have a complete count of vital events. Recorder checks the register of field agent every month. Medical officer of the PHC scrutinizes the death register; the symptoms recorded for every death and investigates up to 2 or 1/10th of deaths reported to him/her in a month. Copies of entries of registration every month are sent to the chief registrar of birth and death, the state level official. The state official in turn consolidates and sends it to the Registrar General of India.

National Family Health Survey

National Family Health Survey (NFHS) is a large-scale, multi-round survey conducted in a representative sample of households throughout India.

The NFHS has had two specific goals:

1. To provide essential data on health and family welfare needed by the Ministry of Health and Family Welfare, and other agencies for policy and program purposes.
2. To provide information on important emerging health and family welfare issues.

Three rounds of the survey have been conducted: first survey in 1992–93 (NFHS-1), second in 1998–99 (NFHS-2) and the third in 2005–06 (NFHS-3). The survey provides state and national information for India on fertility, infant and child mortality, the practice of family planning, maternal and child health, reproductive health, nutrition, anemia, utilization and quality of health, and family planning services.

In NFHS-3, information was collected about households and individual interviews were conducted with women aged 15–49 years and men aged 15–54 years. The NFHS-3 also included height and weight measurement, and blood tests for HIV and anemia.

Rapid Household Survey on RCH

Decentralized district based planning need district level data as district is the basic nucleus of administration. Hence, Ministry of Health and Family Welfare (MOHFW), Government of India decided to undertake district level household survey in all the districts in the country. The first round of the RCH survey (RHS-RCH) in India was conducted during the year 1998–1999 in two phases (each phase covered half of the districts from all states/union territories). International Institute for Population Sciences (IIPS), Mumbai was designated as the nodal agency. Particulars on RCH issues, such as fertility, knowledge of FP, current use of FP methods, unmet need for FP, antenatal checkups, tetanus toxoid (TT) immunization, supply of iron and folic acid, institutional delivery, home delivery, child care, immunization, reproductive morbidity, home visit by health worker, utilization of government health services are being collected in this survey. In Round II, the survey was completed during 2002–04 in 593 districts. In addition to the information in various RCH issues, Round II had a significant nutritional component also. Measuring weight of children to assess the nutritional status, testing of blood of children (aged below 72 months), adolescents and pregnant women to assess the level of anemia and testing of cooking salt for iodine levels were undertaken.

Notification of Infectious Diseases

Notification is a valuable source of data on the incidence and distribution of certain notifiable diseases. Though notifiable diseases vary from country to country, usually diseases, which are considered to be serious menace to the society are listed as notifiable diseases.

Notification is implemented through legal acts such as Madras Public Health Act, 1939 in the states. On 23 May 2005, the World

Health Assembly adopted the new International Health Regulations, IHR (2005), which came into force on 15 June 2007 in 193 member countries of the World Health Organization (WHO). The IHR (2005) are an update of the IHR (1969), which were limited to the reporting of just three infectious diseases—cholera, plague and yellow fever. The IHR (2005) are broader in scope and require each country to report to the WHO any public health emergency of international concern, whether nuclear, biological or chemical in nature, irrespective of the origin.

The infectious diseases reportable under the IHR (2005) include unusual diseases such as smallpox, wild poliovirus infection, human influenza (new subtype), SARS; epidemic-prone diseases such as cholera, pneumonic plague, yellow fever, viral hemorrhagic fevers, West Nile fever and diseases of special regional concern such as dengue fever.

Notification, though useful, has limitations also. Reporting of only a small part of the total sickness, under reporting due to non-recognition and lack of diagnostic facilities especially in rural areas may affect the usefulness of the notification system.

Besides the above, hospital records, disease registers and other health service records also may provide useful information.

❑ INTERNATIONAL POPULATION STATISTICS

1. Popline CD-ROM.
2. MEDLARS CD-ROM.
3. Demographic year book.
4. Statistical year book.
5. Monthly bulletin of statistics.
6. Epidemiological and vital statistics (VS) report, WHO.

Adapted from Population Index by Population Association of America and the Office of Population Research, Princeton University, USA.

Uses of Vital Statistics

Registration system provides statistical data on birth, death, marriages, divorces, etc.

Apart from being an important source of fertility and mortality statistics to the nation, it is also useful to the individuals in many ways.

The birth certificate is useful to an individual as a legal document having evidential value to establish his/her identity, rights of citizenship and nationality, school admission, employment, establishing legal dependency, maternity and paternity, proof of age for obtaining passport, voting rights, for settling inheritance or insurance claims and claiming old age pension.

Death certificate is used for settling questions of inheritance or insurance claims.

The statistical data on birth, death, marriages, divorces, etc. can be utilized for research in demography, medicine and public health. They are used for:

1. For population estimation and projection.
2. For studying the changes in the proportion of higher order births and for evaluating the impact of family planning program.
3. For planning and implementing various disease control and eradication programs. Death certificate usually contains a column on cause of death. Based on the analysis of death statistics various public health control programs on diseases such as malaria, TB and leprosy, and immunization can be planned.

❑ MEASURES OF CENTRAL TENDENCY

Measurements obtained in a study cannot be meaningfully and adequately described by the values of all the individual measurements. Appropriate summary indices are therefore necessary. The arithmetic mean, the median, the mode and the geometric mean are the measures of the central tendency, which indicate the central point or the most characteristic value around which all the values of the measurements scatter. To compare say the height and weight of people of one country or region with another, the mean height and weight of the respective countries or regions are used for getting a meaningful inference.

Mean

Individual values of observations are added together and then divided by the number of observations to get the mean. If n observations are denoted as $x_1, x_2, x_3, \ldots, x_n$, their sum $x_1 + x_2 + x_3 + \ldots + x_n$ is denoted by the symbol $\sum x$. The mean is denoted by $\bar{X}$ and it is calculated by the formula:

$$\bar{X} = \sum x / n$$

For example, hemoglobin (Hb) values of 10 persons (in g) were 11, 12, 15, 12, 9, 10, 10, 12, 13 and 16. Total of these values is 120. The mean hemoglobin value is obtained by dividing the total 120 by 10, i.e.

$$\bar{X} = \sum x / n = 120/10 = 12 \text{ g}$$

Median

Median is the middle value of observations. Data is first arranged in an ascending or descending order of magnitude. Then the value of the middle observation is found out, which is called the median. If there is no single middle observation, average of the two middle observations is found out to get the median, i.e. if n is the size of the sample, the median value will be:

- $(n + 1)/2$th item, if n is an odd number
- The average of $n/2$th and ($n/2$th + 1) items, if n is even.

For example, Hb values of nine persons (in g) are as follows: 11, 12, 15, 13, 9, 10, 12, 13 and 16.

Data arranged in ascending order:

9

10

11

12

12 → Median

13

13

15

16

Since the number of observations (n = 9), is found to be odd we get a single median, which lies in the (9 + 1)/2th position, i.e. the 5th item in the table namely 12.

If there are 10 values instead of 9, the middle two values should be added and the average taken to get the median.

Mode

Most commonly occurring value in a distribution of data is called the mode.

For example, Hb values of 15 persons (in g) are as follows: 12, 11, 10, 9, 13, 14, 16, 12, 8, 9, 12, 11, 10, 13, 15.

Here, 12 is the mode as it is the most frequently occurring value.

❑ MEASURES OF VARIABILITY (DISPERSION)

Variability is the essential feature of biological systems. For example, not all people are of the same height and weight. The range, the mean or the average deviation and the standard deviation are the measures used to measure the dispersion or variations seen.

Range

Range is the difference between the highest and the lowest values in a distribution of observations. For example, if the heights of a sample population ranged between 4 and 6.5, the range lies 2.5 apart.

Mean Deviation

Mean deviation explains how the values of the observations deviate on an average from the mean (arithmetic mean) of the distribution. First the deviations of each value of observations from arithmetic mean are computed. Then all the absolute deviations (that is ignoring the plus or minus) are added and the average is taken. This average is called 'mean deviation'.

For example, the absolute deviation of heights is shown in Table 33.3.

TABLE 33.3: Absolute deviation of heights

Sl No	Height (X)	Mean ($\bar{X}$)	Deviation ($X-\bar{X}$)	Absolute deviation $\lvert X-\bar{X} \rvert$
1.	150	160	–10	10
2.	145	160	–15	15
3.	135	160	–25	25
4.	135	160	–25	25
5.	180	160	20	20
6.	185	160	25	25
7.	160	160	0	0
8.	170	160	10	10
9.	175	160	15	15
10.	165	160	5	5
Total	1,600			150

From the above Table,

Mean = $\bar{X}$ = 1,600/10 = 160

$$\text{Mean deviation} = \frac{\Sigma \lvert X-\bar{X} \rvert}{n} = \frac{150}{10} = 15$$

Standard deviation (SD) is the roots means square deviation (Table 33.4) and the formula for calculation of SD is:

$$SD = \sqrt{\frac{\Sigma(\bar{X}-X)^2}{n}}$$

For example, the standard deviation (from the earlier example) is calculated as follows:

$$\text{Mean } (\bar{X}) = \frac{\Sigma X}{n} = 1{,}600/10 = 160$$

$$SD = \sqrt{\frac{\Sigma(\bar{X}-X)^2}{n}} = \sqrt{\frac{2{,}950}{10}} = 17.17$$

TABLE 33.4: Squared deviation of heights

Sl No	Height (X)	Mean ($\bar{X}$)	Deviation ($\bar{X} - X$)	Squared deviation $(\bar{X} - X)^2$
1.	150	160	–10	100
2.	145	160	–15	225
3.	135	160	–25	625
4.	135	160	–25	625
5.	180	160	20	400
6.	185	160	25	625
7.	160	160	0	0
8.	170	160	10	100
9.	175	160	15	225
10.	165	160	5	25
Total	1,600			2,950

Regression and Correlation

Correlation

Correlation analysis is concerned with measuring the strength of relationship between different variables, e.g. literacy and family size. The relationship between only two variables is called simple correlation and that between more than two variables is called multiple correlation. These relationships may be further categorized either as linear or non-linear. The variable (factor), which causes a change in another variable is called independent (or the predictor) variable, while the variable, which gets changed is called dependent variable, e.g. good food (predictor) and growth (dependent).

The relationship between two variables can be vaguely shown in a table or a scatter diagram.

The relationship between per capita income and the monthly weight gain of babies is shown in Table 33.5.

The relationship of the above same variables is shown in Figure 33.9.

TABLE 33.5: Family income and weight gain of babies

Per capita income of family (₹)	1,000	2,000	3,000	4,000	5,000
Monthly weight gain of babies (g)	40	40	80	100	120

Here, the variable per capita income is taken on the X-axis and gain in weight is taken on the Y-axis. An inspection of this scatter plot shows that small values of X are associated with small values of Y and vice versa. The scatter is found to occur in a straight line indicating a positive correlation between the income and the monthly weight gain of babies.

Some of the possible scatters of data are given Figure 33.10.

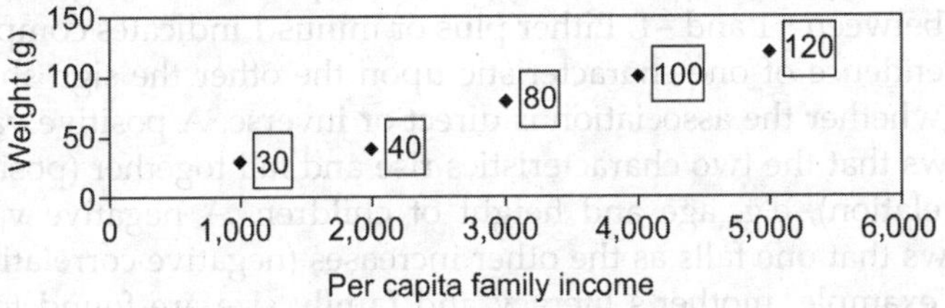

Figure 33.9: Family income and weight gain of babies

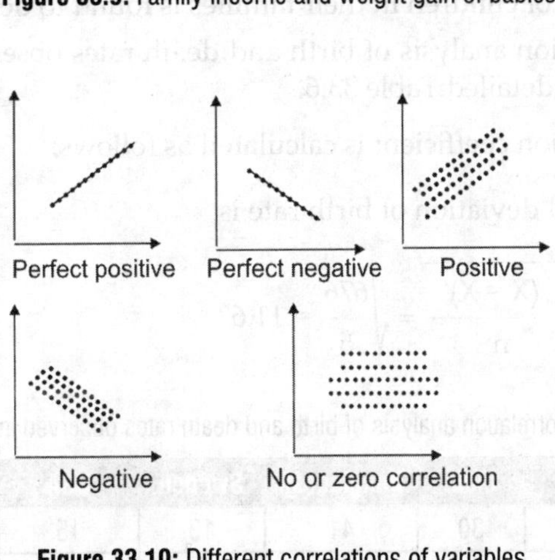

Figure 33.10: Different correlations of variables

The degree of relationship between two variables can also be measured by what is called coefficient of correlation denoted as 'r'. It is calculated by the formula:

$$r = \frac{\Sigma (X - \overline{X})(Y - \overline{Y})}{n \sigma_x \sigma_y}$$

where, σ_x and σ_y are the standard deviations of the variables x and y respectively.

If no association at all exists between two variables r equals 0. If there is a complete dependence r equals 1. For any other degree of association r must lie between 0 and 1, being low as its value approaches 0 and high as it approaches 1. The r is calculated in such a way that its value may be either positive or negative lying between +1 and –1. Either plus or minus 1 indicates complete dependence of one characteristic upon the other the sign showing whether the association is direct or inverse. A positive value shows that the two characteristics rise and fall together (positive correlation), e.g. age and height of children. A negative value shows that one falls as the other increases (negative correlation). For example, mother's literacy and family size are found to be negatively correlated. As the mothers' education level increases, the number of children in their families is found to decrease.

Correlation analysis of birth and death rates observed in five countries is detailed Table 33.6.

Correlation coefficient is calculated as follows:

Standard deviation of birth rate is:

$$\sigma_X = \sqrt{\frac{\Sigma (X - \overline{X})^2}{n}} = \sqrt{\frac{676}{5}} = 11.63$$

TABLE 33.6: Correlation analysis of birth and death rates observed in five countries

	India	Bangladesh	Sweden	USA	Japan
Birth rate (BR)	30	41	13	15	11
Death rate (DR)	11	15	10	9	7

Standard deviation of death rate is:

$$\sigma_Y = \sqrt{\frac{\Sigma (Y - \bar{Y})^2}{n}} = \sqrt{\frac{35.2}{5}} = 2.65$$

Correlation coefficient is given by the formula:

$$r = \frac{\Sigma (X - \bar{X})(Y - \bar{Y})}{n\, \sigma_X\, \sigma_Y}$$

$$r = \frac{143}{5 \times 11.63 \times 2.65} = 0.927$$

As r = 0.927 is nearer to the value 1, the inference is that the birth and death rates are positively correlated (Table 33.7).

Rank correlation analysis is also done in some situations where the observations cannot be exactly measured, but only can be ranked. For example, different states can be ranked according to say infant mortality rate (IMR) and immunization coverage.

Regression

Regression analysis is done to assess the relationship among the variables. Simple or linear regression studies the relationship between one dependent variable and one independent (predictor)

TABLE 33.7: Calculation of correlation coefficient

Sl No	BR (X)	DR (Y)	$X - \bar{X}$ (X – 22)	$Y - \bar{Y}$ (Y–10.4)	$(X - \bar{X})^2$	$(Y - \bar{Y})^2$	$(X - \bar{X})(Y - \bar{Y})$
1.	30	11	8	0.6	64	0.36	4.8
2.	41	15	19	4.6	361	21.16	87.4
3.	13	10	–9	–0.4	81	0.16	3.6
4.	15	9	–7	–1.4	49	1.96	9.8
5.	11	7	–11	–3.4	121	11.56	37.4
Total (Σ)	110	52	0	0	676	35.2	143.0
Mean	$\bar{X}$= 22	$\bar{Y}$= 10.4					

variable. Multiple Regression studies deal with the relationship between more than two variables. Association between the prevalence of disease or mortality and environmental factors is well known, e.g. prevalence of typhoid and insanitary nature of water supply. However, in most real life situations a simple one- to-one cause and effect mechanism is unlikely to prevail. The effect is more likely brought about by a number of causes, some interrelated, some independent of each other. The other factors that may decide the prevalence of typhoid are the immune status of the given population, poor standard of life and unhealthy lifestyle practices.

Correlation coefficient is a useful measure of the degree of association between two characteristics, but only when their relationship is adequately described by a straight line. The regression equation allows the value of one characteristic to be estimated when the value of the other characteristic is known. But the error of this estimation may be very large even when the correlation is very high. Evidence of association is not necessarily evidence of causation and the possible influence of other common factors must be remembered in interpreting correlation coefficients.

Normal Distribution

Variables may be distributed in many ways, but the distribution occupying central position in statistical theory and practice is the normal distribution. It has been shown that many natural phenomena such as the heights and weights of the people conform to the normal distribution. Statisticians have also been able to demonstrate that several important sample statistics tend towards the normal distribution as the sample size increases (Fig. 33.11).

When a frequency curve is drawn using the frequency distribution with narrow class interval, obtained from a very large sample of the universe, the curve will appear as a smooth and symmetrical curve. The shape of the curve will depend upon the mean and the standard deviation. Statisticians, to estimate the area under the normal distribution curve, have devised a standard normal curve. Any frequency distribution with mean and standard deviation can be converted into a standard normal curve. It is a smooth, bell-shaped, perfectly symmetrical curve based on an infinitely large number of observations. The total area of the curve

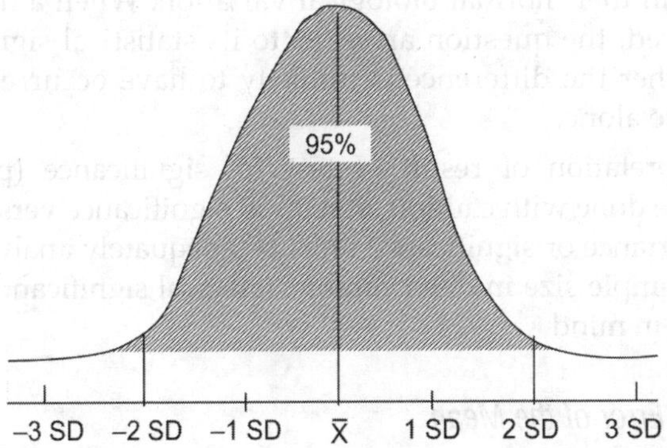

Figure 33.11: Normal distribution curve (SD, standard deviation)

is taken as 1; it is mean 0 and the standard deviation 1. The mean, median and mode all coincide in a normal distribution.

The area of one SD on either side of the mean will include approximately 68%, two SDs almost 95% and three SDs 99.7% of the values in the distribution. These estimates are called confidence limits. Normal distribution curve is used for estimation of population parameters from the sample statistics and for hypothesis testing.

If the mean and the variance of a normal distribution are known the probability of various events can be determined. The range of values within which the unknown parameter lies can be found out and it is called estimation.

In hypothesis testing, we make some statements about the population about its form or about the numerical value of one or more of its parameters. Then inspecting a random sample from the population, we can infer whether the sample is consistent or inconsistent with the stated hypothesis.

Tests of Significance

Tests of significance are standard statistical procedures for drawing inferences from sample estimates about unknown population parameters. Sample estimates are never exact, being subject to sampling errors. Tests of significance allow us to decide whether sample estimates or the difference between estimates are within their normal biological variation. When a difference is observed, the question arises as to its statistical significance, i.e. whether the difference is unlikely to have occurred purely by chance alone.

Interpretation of result of tests of significance (p values) should be done with caution. Statistical significance versus medical importance or significance must be adequately analyzed. The role of sample size in determining statistical significance should be borne in mind.

Standard Error of the Mean

When the result of a study is expressed in averages, the standard error (SE) of the mean is used to assess the result of the study. The SE concept is used to find out, whether a sample mean obtained in a study is significantly different from the population mean or the difference has occurred merely by chance.

For example, in a study of systolic blood pressure of 566 males in a region of a district, the mean systolic pressure was 128.8 mm Hg. The question here is whether this observed mean systolic pressure is the true mean of the males of the entire district. Let us see how this question can be answered.

Suppose that the true mean systolic pressure of males is M. Then using the principle of normal distribution, we can say that the mean of the sample may well, differ from the true mean by as much as twice the standard error $\sigma/\sqrt{n}$, where σ is the standard deviation of the blood pressure of the individuals in the universe from which the sample was taken and n is the number of individuals in the sample. It is not likely to differ by more than that amount, i.e. the observed mean is likely to lie within the range $M \pm 2\,(\sigma/\sqrt{n})$. Here, we do not know the value of the σ of population mean and as an estimate of it we must use the standard deviation of the values in the sample. In this study of 566 males, the SD of the values of systolic blood pressure (BP) was 13.05 mm. We therefore, estimate that the SD of means in samples of 566 would be $13.05/\sqrt{566} = 0.55$ mm.

Therefore, we can conclude that the observed mean (128.8 mm) may differ from the true mean by as much as ± 2 (0.55) and the true mean is likely to lie within the limits of 128.8 ± 2 (0.55), i.e. between 127.7 mm and 129.9 mm.

So, if we conclude that the true mean is two SE away (plus or minus) from the sample mean we can expect to be wrong in that conclusion once in 20 times. To be more confident we can estimate that the true mean of the universe is not more than 2½ times the SE and we are likely to go wrong in that conclusion once in 80 times. This estimation is not applicable to small sized samples (say less than 20 observations).

Standard Error of Proportion

In studies like drug trials, the results are expressed in percentages (proportions) and not in averages as in the earlier example. In such situations the SE of the proportions is found out to arrive at an inference of the study. When a study is conducted with no control group for comparison, the result of a past similar study is utilized to find out the expected result. Standard error of the proportion is given by the formula:

$$\sqrt{pq/n}$$

where, p is the percentage of individuals belonging to one category and q is the percentage of in the other category, and n is the number of individuals in the sample.

For example, past experience has shown that in a particular line of treatment in 100 patients, 20 (20%) persons died and 80 (80%) survived. Then SE of proportions (i.e. between the percentage survived and the percentage died) is given by the formula $\sqrt{pq/n}$ where, p is the percentage of individuals who died; q is the percentage of individuals who survived; n is the number of individuals in the sample.

In the study quoted above, the SE will be $\sqrt{20 \times 80/100} = 4.0$. In other words on the basis of past experience, we should expect 20 of the 100 patients on a similar line of treatment to die. But in different samples of the same size we may not observe the same proportion dying and the percentage of deaths will be scattered around 20 with a SD of 4, i.e. percentage of deaths will lie between 28[20 + 2(4)] and 12[20 – 2(4)]. Suppose we observe a value of 10 deaths in a study much lower than the expected lowest value (i.e. 12), we can deduce that the new treatment has actually lowered the fatality. But it is always better to interpret such inferences with caution taking other factors into consideration besides the one we have presently considered in the study.

Standard Error of Difference Between Two Means

In a study, the mean height of 6,194 English men was 171 cm with a standard error of 6.51 and the mean height of 1,304 Scottish men was 174 cm with a standard deviation of 6.34. Whether this difference in the height between the two countrymen was just by chance or real can be worked out as given in Table 33.8.

Standard error of difference (SEd) between means is calculated by the formula:

$$SE = \sqrt{\frac{\sigma_1^2}{n_1}} + \sqrt{\frac{\sigma_2^2}{n_2}}$$

where, σ_1 is the SD of the heights of English men; σ_2 is the SD of the heights of Scottish men; n_1 is the sample size of the former and n_2 is the sample size of the latter, i.e.

$$SE = \sqrt{\frac{(6.5)^2}{6,194} + \frac{(6.34)^2}{1,304}} = 0.083 + 0.176 = 0.20 \text{ cm}$$

The actual difference between the two mean heights was 3 cm, which is 15 times more than the SEd between the two means. Therefore, it is inferred that Scottish men are, on the average, taller than English men.

TABLE 33.8: Standard error in height deviation

	Sample size	Mean height	Standard deviation
English men	6,194	171	6.51
Scottish men	1,304	174	6.34

Standard Error of Difference Between Two Proportions

Result of a study to test the effect of vitamin C supplementation on the incidence of common cold is given in Table 33.9.

TABLE 33.9: Effect of vitamin C in common cold

	Sample size	Cold affected	Not affected
Control group	50	48 (96%)	2 (4%)
Supplemented group	50	43 (86%)	7 (14%)

From the results, it is observed that in the supplemented group the incidence of common cold is less. Whether this effect is real or by chance can be decided by finding out the SEd between the two proportions, i.e. between the percentage affected and the percentage unaffected in both the groups.

Standard error of difference between two proportions is given by the formula:

$$\text{SEd} = \sqrt{\frac{p_1q_1}{n_1} + \frac{p_2q_2}{n_2}}$$

where, p_1, q_1 represent the percentages of the effect in the control group, while p_2, q_2 represent the same in the supplemented group; n_1 and n_2 are the sample sizes respectively of both the groups, i.e.

$$\text{SEd} = \sqrt{\frac{4 \times 96}{50} + \frac{14 \times 86}{50}} = \sqrt{7.68 + 24.08} = 5.64$$

The SEd is 5.64. The observed difference is (96 – 86) 10. The observed difference between the two groups is less than twice the SEd, i.e. 5.64 × 2. Therefore, it can be easily inferred that the observed difference may be due to chance.

Chi-square (χ^2) Test

Difference between two proportions can also be tested by chi-square test. To study the association between two discrete variables like say religion and family planning adoption the results of which are expressed in percentages, χ^2 test is applied. The χ^2 test measures the discrepancy between the observed frequency (O) and the expected frequency (E). If the value of χ^2 is zero, the observed and expected frequencies completely coincide. Greater the value of χ^2, bigger is the difference between the proportions.

The result of a study to find out the association between religion and adoption of family planning (FPA) is detailed in a Table 33.10.

First we make a tentative null hypothesis (H_0), i.e. there is no difference in the adoption process of family planning between different religious groups and an alternate hypothesis (H_1), i.e. there is difference between different religious groups in the adoption of family planning. And then proceed to prove or disprove the Null hypothesis. When null hypothesis is rejected based on the chi-square value, alternate hypothesis is automatically accepted.

Next, we calculate the expected frequencies (E) from the observed frequencies (O). For example, out of 470 total eligible couples belonging to all religions studied, 250 couples have undergone sterilization (permanent family planning method). Then the expected frequency of sterilizations among 300 Hindus is calculated as follows, i.e.

$$\frac{250}{470} \times 300 = 160$$

Similarly, the expected frequency can be calculated for each religious category. The expected frequencies in respect of sterilization and intrauterine device (IUD) are shown in brackets alongside the observed frequencies in the Table 33.11.

The difference between the observed and the expected frequencies is found out and squared for each category. These values are given in the Table 33.12.

TABLE 33.10: Family planning adoption status of a community by religion

Religion	FP adopters		Non-adopters	Total
	Sterilization	IUD*		
Hindu	200	50	50	300
Muslim	40	20	40	100
Christian	10	20	40	70
Total	250	90	130	470

*IUD, intrauterine device

TABLE 33.11: Sterilization and IUD frequencies

Religion	FP adopters		Non-adopters	Total
	Sterilization	IUD		
Hindu	200 (160)	50 (57)	50 (83)	300
Muslim	40 (53)	20 (19)	40 (28)	100
Christian	10 (37)	20 (13)	40 (19)	70
Total	250	90	130	470

TABLE 33.12: Observed and expected frequencies (for Table 33.11)

Observed (O)	200	50	50	40	20	40	10	20	40
Expected (E)	160	57	83	53	19	28	37	13	19
O – E	40	–7	–33	–13	1	12	–27	7	21
$(O - E)^2$	1,600	49	1,089	169	1	144	729	49	441

The χ^2 value is found out by the formula:

$$\chi^2 = \frac{\Sigma (O - E)^2}{E}$$

$$\chi^2 = \frac{1,600}{160} + \frac{49}{57} + \frac{1,089}{83} + \frac{169}{53} + \frac{1}{19} + \frac{144}{28} + \frac{729}{37} + \frac{49}{13} + \frac{441}{19}$$

$$= 10 + 0.86 + 13.12 + 3.19 + 0.05 + 5.14 + 19.70 + 3.77 + 23.21 = 79.04$$

The calculated value of χ^2 is 79.04.

Degrees of freedom = (number of rows – 1) (number of columns – 1) = 2 × 2 = 4

The table value at 5% level ($x^2 0.05$) for 4 degrees of freedom is 9.49 (obtained from ready made tables)

Since the calculated value 79.04 is greater than the table value, i.e. 9.49, the null hypothesis (H_0) is rejected and the alternative hypothesis (H_1) is accepted. Therefore, the inference is that adoption of family planning varies with religion significantly.

Student's 't'-test

When the sample size is small (less than 30) t-test is applied instead of normal test criterion Z for testing the difference between any two sample statistics, such as means and proportions. The calculated value of 't' denoted by t_c is given by the formula:

$$t_c = \frac{\bar{X}_1 - \bar{X}_2}{SE \text{ of } (\bar{X}_1 - \bar{X}_2)}$$

The calculated value t_c is compared with the theoretical t-value from the t-table obtained for an appropriate degrees of freedom given by $df = n_1 + n_2 - 2$.

If $t_c < t_\alpha$, for a given degrees of freedom, the null hypothesis H_0 is taken as significant.

That is:

If $t_c < t_{0.05}$, for the given degrees of freedom, the H_0 is significant at 5% level.

If $t_c < t_{0.01}$, for the given degrees of freedom, the H_0 is significant at 1% level.

If $t_c < t_{0.001}$, for the given degrees of freedom, the H_0 is significant at 0.1% level.

Index

Page numbers followed by *f* refer to figure and *t* refer to table

T